TARGET JIPMER

(Model Questions with Solved Explanatory Answers)

"Get the inside edge! Authored by Jipmerites"

December 2019 (Supplement)

Dr. T. ARUN BABU
MD Pediatrics (JIPMER), DAA (CMC, Vellore), MBA (HM)
Fellow in Neonatal Perinatal Medicine (Canada)
Associate Professor and Head, Department of Pediatrics
All India Institute of Medical Sciences (AIIMS)
Mangalagiri, Andhra Pradesh
Puducherry – 605009
Website: www.drarunbabu.in

Peepee Publishers and Distributors (P) Ltd.®

TARGET JIPMER DECEMBER 2019 (Supplement)

Published by
Pawaninder P. Vij and Anupam Vij

Peepee Publishers and Distributors (P) Ltd.
Head Office: 160, Shakti Vihar, Pitam Pura, Delhi-110 034 (India)

Correspondence Address:

7/31, First Floor, Ansari Road, Daryaganj
New Delhi-110 002 (India)

Ph: 41512412, 23246245, 9811156083

e-mail: peepee160@yahoo.co.in

e-mail: peepee160@gmail.com

www.peepeepub.com

join us on facebook.com/pp.publishers

First Edition: 2020

ISBN: 978-81-8445-278-5

Dedication

***To my Parents, Teachers,
my wife Dr. Sharmila,
my kids Akshaya and Akash***

Disclaimer:

This book fully complies with the non-disclosure agreement (NDA) levied by JIPMER. This book contains Model questions with solved explanatory answers. No questions included in this book have been obtained from any candidates registered for JIPMER exam. Any resemblance to the original JIPMER questions, if present, is purely coincidental. The author, contributors, publisher or sellers cannot be held responsible for any damage or loss caused to anyone, directly or indirectly.

PREFACE

We are very happy in bringing out yet another supplement of TARGET JIPMER Book. Big thanks for making TARGET JIPMER series the best book for JIPMER PGMEE preparation. This book series was started with the sole purpose of making model JIPMER questions accessible to PG aspirants. The questions have been solved by a team of subject experts from reputed academic backgrounds. This book is tailor made for JIPMER PG entrance exam preparation. Most of our contributors are JIPMER alumni and have personally written JIPMER PG exams in the last few years and are well experienced and aware of the examination pattern. JIPMER questions are mostly taken from standard textbooks and articles. Though the pattern of JIPMER questions have changed in the last few years, the high yield area remains the same.

We have incorporated a systematic approach in solving each and every question which can be appreciated while reading this book. The schematic diagrams, tables, illustrations, bulleted key points and references are the highlights of this book and will make reading and understanding of the material easier and effective. Every solved question will have a valid reference citing a standard textbook or article in order to increase the credibility of the answers. The focused explanations should help you solve questions from same topics in the future easily.

I would like to thank all the contributors for their commitment and hard work that has led to the tremendous success of this book series. I wish to thank our publishers, Mr. Pawaninder Paul Vij and Mr. Anupam Vij, the Directors of Peepee Publishers and Distributors (P) Ltd, who have always been a pillar of support to our team. I would also like to thank our publishing team for their relentless efforts in releasing this book in a short notice. I am deeply indebted to students for their overwhelming support, feedback and critical appraisal. We are looking forward to hear your feedback and are fully committed in bringing out better editions in the future. For JIPMER students, a JIPMERITE tag is a matter of pride which they carry as a badge of honour throughout their professional life. For most others it is a dream. I believe and hope that this book will make your dream come true.

All the best!

T. Arun Babu

Website: www.drarunbabu.in

Email: babuarun.t@gmail.com

"Books are infinite in number and time is short. The secret of knowledge is to take what is essential."

–Swami Vivekananda

CONTRIBUTORS

Dr. Arun Babu T, MD Pediatrics (JIPMER), DAA (CMC)
Fellow NPM (Canada)
Associate Professor, Department of Pediatrics
All India Institute of Medical Sciences (AIIMS)
Mangalagiri
Andhra Pradesh
(Chief Editor)

Dr. Arundhathi S, MD Pathology
Associate Professor, Department of Pathology
All India Institute of Medical Sciences (AIIMS)
Mangalagiri – 522 503
(Pathology)

Dr. Arul Varman, MD Psychiatry (JIPMER)
Assistant Professor, Department of Psychiatry
Indira Gandhi Medical College and Research Institute (IGMC&RI)
Puducherry – 605009
(Psychiatry)

Dr. Dinesh Kumar, MD Pediatrics
Assistant Professor, Department of Pediatrics
All India Institute of Medical Sciences (AIIMS)
Mangalagiri
Andhra Pradesh
(Pediatrics)

Dr. Jean Fredrick, MD Physiology
Assistant Professor
Department of Physiology
Mahatma Gandhi Medical College and Research Institute (MGMC&RI), Pillaiyarkuppam, Puducherry
(Physiology)

Dr. Madhav Rao, MD Pharm (JIPMER)
Associate Professor, Department of Pharmacology
All India Institute of Medical Sciences (AIIMS)
Mangalagiri– 522 503
(Pharmacology)

Dr. Mugunthan N, MS Anatomy, DNB, PhD, MBA
Professor of Anatomy
Sree Mookambika Institute of Medical Sciences
Kulasekaram, Kanyakumari District,Tamil Nadu–629161
(Anatomy)

Dr. Mukul Mohindra, MS (Ortho), DNB, MNAMS, Dip.SICOT (Belgium)
Fellow National Board (Arthroscopy and Sports Medicine)
Sports Injury Center, Safdarjung Hospital and VMM College
New Delhi
(Orthopedics)

Dr. Prasanna S, MD Microbiology (AFMC, Pune)
Associate Professor, Department of Microbiology
Shri Sathya Sai Medical College and Research Institute
Kancheepuram, Tamil Nadu – 603108
(Microbiology)

Dr. Priyanka Choudhary, MD Community Medicine
Senior Resident, Department of Community Medicine
PGIMS, Rohtak, Haryana
(Preventive and Social Medicine)

Dr. R. Rajamahendran, MS, MRCS (UK), FMAS, MCh (SGE)
Assistant Professor in Surgical Gastroenterology
GVMCH, Villupuram, Tamil Nadu
Consultant Surgical Gastroenterologist and Advanced Lap GI Surgeon
RRM Gastro Surgical and Research Centre, Villupuram
Director, "KONCPT NEET" Medical Coaching Centre
(Surgery)

Dr. Sangeeta Dhanger, DA, DNB, MNAMS
Assistant Professor, Department of Anesthesiology
Indira Gandhi Medical College and Research Institute (IGMC&RI)
Puducherry – 605009
(Anesthesiology)

Dr. Satvinder Singh Bakshi, MS ENT (JIPMER), DNB
Associate Professor, Department of Otorhinolaryngology
All India Institute of Medical Sciences (AIIMS)
Mangalagiri, Andhra Pradesh
(ENT)

Dr. Sharmila Arun Babu, MS OBG (JIPMER)
Additional Professor and Head, Department of OBG
All India Institute of Medical Sciences (AIIMS)
Mangalagiri
Andhra Pradesh
(OBG)

Dr. Sindhujha Sekar G, JIPMER, DGO, DNB OG
Assistant Professor, Department of OBG
Sri Venkateswara Medical College Hospital and Research Centre
Puducherry
(OBG)

Dr. Soumya Sathyan, MD General Medicine
Senior Resident
MES Medical College
Perintalmanna
(Medicine)

Dr. Usha S Adiga, MBBS MD PhD
Professor, Department of Biochemistry
KS Hegde Medical Academy
Mangalore, Karnataka
(Biochemistry)

Dr. Venipriya, MS Ophthalmology
Senior Resident, Department of Ophthalmology
Indira Gandhi Medical College and Research Institute
(IGMC&RI)
Puducherry – 605 009
(Ophthalmology)

Dr. Yatiraj Singi, MD Forensic Medicine
Professor, Department of Forensic Medicine
Sree Mookambika Institute of Medical Sciences
Kulasekharam, District Kanya Kumari, TN
(Forensic Medicine)

Editorial Assistance

Gaurang Narayan, CRRI
Indira Gandhi Medical College and Research Institute
(IGMC&RI)
Puducherry – 605009

Dr. Padmapriya, MD Pathology
Resident, Department of Pathology
Andhra Medical College
Visakhapatnam – 605009

Balakrishnan Ramanan, CRRI
Indira Gandhi Medical College and Research Institute
(IGMC&RI)
Puducherry – 605009

ACKNOWLEDGEMENTS

Target JIPMER – Previous Edition Contributors

Dr. Udayashankar C, Professor and Head of Dermatology, IGMC&RI, Puducherry
Dr. Prudhvinath Reddy A, Assistant Professor of Radiodiagnosis, AIIMS, Mangalagiri
Dr. Ranjith AR, Molecular Pathologist, Bangalore
Dr. Vinoth Kumar S, Assistant Professor of General Medicine, IGMC&RI, Puducherry
Dr. Bharath Kumar VD, MD Assistant Professor of Pharmacology, BGSGIMS, Bangalore, Karnataka
Dr. Abhishek Bhaumik, MS Senior Resident, Department of Surgery, West Bengal HS
Dr. Kantamani Bala Teja, MS (ENT) MCh, Head and Neck Surgery, Senior Resident, Mumbai
Dr. Nishanth Sampath, MD Clinical Neurophysiologist, SIMS, Chennai, Tamil Nadu
Dr. Suthanthira Kannan, MD Assistant Professor of Community Medicine, ESI Medical College, Hyderabad
Dr. Pratheep, MS General Surgery MCh Oncosurgery Resident
Dr. Balamurugan N, DCH, DNB, MRCPCH, Assistant Professor, Department of Pediatrics, SLIMS, Puducherry
Dr.Tejswita Rajpal Hande, MBBS, DGO, MUHS, Nashik
Dr. Saranya K, MD Physio (JIPMER), Assistant Professor of Physiology, JIPMER, Puducherry
Dr. Abarna Devi S, DDVL (JIPMER), MD Medicine, Assistant Professor of Medicine, ESIMC, Chennai
Dr. Anshu Bahl, MD Anatomy (AIIMS), New Delhi
Dr. Ankit Agarwal, MD RT (JIPMER), Senior Resident, GMCH, Chandigarh, Sector 32
Dr. Naga Dharshan Devendra, MD (JIPMER), Associate Professor and Course Director, Department of Biochemistry and Genetics, Trinity School of Medicine, Saint Vincent and Grenadines
Dr. Saseendar S, MS (Ortho), DNB, Dip SICOT (Belgium), MNAMS, Care Sports Injury, Chennai
Dr. Srirangaraj S, MD, Professor, Department of Microbiology, MGMCRI, Puducherry
Dr. Sri Vengadesh Gopal, MS (JIPMER), Assistant Professor, Department of Surgery, IGMC&RI, Puducherry
Dr. Sumanth MM, MD (JIPMER), DNB, Associate Professor of PSM, MMCRI, Mysore, Karnataka
Dr. Sentitoshi, JIPMER, MD Forensic Medicine, Former Assistant Professor, MGMCRI, Puducherry
Dr. Asayas Bosco Chandrakumar, MS, Associate Professor of Surgery, SLIMS, Puducherry
Dr. Mahesh Nagappa, MD Anesthesia (JIPMER), DNB, MNAMS, Assistant Professor, SLIMS, Puducherry
Dr. Sinhasan SP, MD, Associate Professor of Pathology, IGMC&RI, Puducherry
Dr. Amiya Kumar Nath, MD (JIPMER), Associate Professor of Dermatology, IGMC&RI, Puducherry
Dr. Venkateswaran R, MD, Associate Professor of Medicine, JIPMER, Puducherry
Dr. Niranjan G, MD Biochem (JIPMER), Associate Professor of Biochemistry, AIIMS Nagpur
Dr. VishnuKanth, MD (JIPMER), Associate Professor, Department of Respiratory Medicine, JIPMER, Puducherry
Dr. Dilli Kumar, MD (JIPMER), Associate Professor of Pediatrics, JIPMER, Puducherry
Dr. Dilip Kumar R, MD (JIPMER), MRCP (UK), Dr. Mehta's Hospitals, Chetpet, Chennai - 31
Dr. Sachidananda Adiga, MD, Professor of Pharmacology, KS Hegde Medical Academy, Mangalore
Dr. Giriyanna Gowda, MD, Associate Professor of Community Medicine, KIMS, Bangalore, Karnataka
Dr. Gomathi Shankar V, MS (JIPMER), DNB, MNAMS, Associate Professor of Surgery, JIPMER, Puducherry
Dr. Karthik, MD Physiology (JIPMER), Associate Professor of Physiology, JIPMER, Puducherry
Dr. Lourdu Jafrin, MD, Associate Professor of Pharmacology, IGMC&RI, Puducherry
Dr. Mahalakshmy T, MD PSM (JIPMER), Associate Professor of PSM, JIPMER, Puducherry
Dr Melvin George, MD, DM Clin Pharm (JIPMER), Assistant Professor, Cardiac Clinical Trials and Research, Department of Cardiology, SRM Medical College and Hospital, Potheri, Tamil Nadu
Dr. Naveen Nair, MS Orthopedics (JIPMER), Associate Professor of Orthopedics, IGMC&RI, Puducherry
Dr. Noyal Mariya Joseph, MD (JIPMER) Associate Professor of Microbiology, JIPMER, Puducherry
Dr. Raveendranath, MS Anatomy (St. Johns), Associate Professor of Anatomy, JIPMER, Puducherry
Dr. Rupa Vani, DNB, Assistant Professor of Obstetrics and Gynecology, IGMC&RI, Puducherry

Sincere Thanks to:

Dr. Nivedhan, MBBS, Stanley Medical College, Chennai
Dr. Anoop Singh, MBBS, HIMS, Hassan
Dr. Nadim Anjum, MBBS, North Bengal Medical College, Siliguri, West Bengal
Dr. Mimi Janet, MBBS, Velammal Medical College, Madurai
Dr. Abdul Hazan, MD (Physician) Russia, Rostov State Medical University
Dr. Allan Deepak, Chennai
Dr. Arunima Das, MBBS, Midnapore Medical College, Paschim Medinipur, West Bengal
Dr. Brijesh Chandra Yadav, Anesthesia Resident, Motilal Nehru Medical College, Allahabad
Dr. Sumi Maniraju, MBBS, Vinayaka Mission's Medical College and Hospital, Karaikal
Dr. Vennila Krishnan, MBBS, Sri Muthukumaran Medical College and Hospital, Chennai
Dr. Zubaida Begum A, MBBS (MGMCRI), Junior Resident in Department of PSM, IGMCRI, Puducherry
Dr. Priyadharshini A, MBBS (SVMCHRC), MRB, Tamil Nadu
Dr. Maheswaran, MBBS, Government Stanley Medical College, Chennai
Dr. Vishnu Venkatesan, MBBS, SVMCHRC, Puducherry
Dr. Supriya Jeevanthanam, MBBS, Government Vellore Medical College, Vellore
Dr. Rachit Singhania, MBBS, North Bengal Medical College and Hospital, Darjeeling, West Bengal
Dr. Renuga Devi, MBBS, Junior Resident in Pediatrics, MAPIMS, Melmaruvathur, Tamil Nadu
Dr. Shahul Hamid, MBBS Intern, IGMCRI, Puducherry
Dr. Ashwin Reddy, MBBS, IGMCRI, Puducherry
Dr. Jayaram Saibaba, MBBS, Medicine Resident, JIPMER, Puducherry
Dr. Immaneul Joshua, MBBS, IGMCRI, Puducherry
Dr. GK Raman, MBBS, IGMCRI, Puducherry
Dr. Ashok E, MBBS, DCH, Salem, Tamil Nadu
Dr. Anandhasayanan Sriramalu, MBBS, Tirukkoyilur, Tamil Nadu

and

Mr. Thirunavukkarasu D, Government School English Lecturer (Retd), Puducherry
Mrs. Sampurnam, Principal (Retd), SSVHSS, Puducherry
Mr. Vijayan D, Cash Officer (Retd), SBI, Puducherry
Mrs. Sagoundala, Under Secretary (Retd), Government of Puducherry
Mr. Srinivasan@Babu, PWD, Puducherry
Mr. Dhinesh Shankar, EC Software, Chennai
Mr. Rajkumar, System Engineer, Apple, CA, USA

Write to Us

Any observations, suggestions, criticisms are welcome. Write to the author at babuarun.t@gmail.com

Errata

Please visit: www.drarunbabu.in & www.peepeepub.com

Follow Author in Facebook: www.facebook.com/targetjipmer/& Dr. Arun Babu's Pediatrics Discussion group (TARGET Pediatrics by Dr. Arun Babu)

CONTENTS

JIPMER–DECEMBER 2019

ANATOMY

1. A female patient visited ortho OPD with history of trauma left leg. On examination, foot drop is present, muscle power in tibialis anterior, extensor digitorum longus and extensor hallucis longus is 0/5. Muscle power in tibialis posterior and gastrocnemius is 4/5. Most likely injury is:

(a) Supracondylar fracture of left femur
(b) Fracture neck of left fibula
(c) Left hip posterior dislocation
(d) Left ankle fracture

Explanation:

- Most likely injury in this case is ***fracture neck of left fibula*** and ***injury to common peroneal (fibular) nerve***
- The ***common fibular nerve*** crosses posterolateral to the ***neck of fibula*** and can be ***rolled against*** the underlying bone at this location
- Presence of ***foot drop*** indicates injury to ***common peroneal nerve***
- ***Loss of muscle power*** in ***anterior compartment of leg*** (***dorsiflexors of foot***) muscle indicates injury to ***deep peroneal nerve*** – a division of common peroneal nerve
- ***Common peroneal nerve*** is one of the terminal branches of ***sciatic nerve*** with root value of ***L4,L5,S1 and S2***
- ***Common peroneal nerve*** is divided into deep peroneal nerve and superficial peroneal nerve
- Deep peroneal nerve/anterior tibial nerve/ **nervi hesitans** supplies the **dorsiflexors of foot** (**anterior** compartment of leg)
- **Superficial peroneal nerve/musculocutaneous nerve of leg** supplies **evertors of foot** (**lateral** compartment of leg)

Dorsiflexors and evertors of foot and their nerve supply

Name of muscle	Nerve supply	Action(s)
Tibialis anterior	Deep peroneal nerve	Dorsiflexion and inversion of foot
Extensor hallucis longus	Deep peroneal nerve	Dorsiflexion of foot and extends the hallux
Extensor digitorum longus	Deep peroneal nerve	Dorsiflexion of foot and extends lateral four toes
Peroneus tertius	Deep peroneal nerve	Dorsiflexion and eversion of foot
*Peronius longus (Fibularis longus)	Superficial peroneal nerve	Eversion of foot
*Peroneus brevis (Fibularis brevis)	Superficial peroneal nerve	Eversion of foot

(* lateral compartment of leg others are belongs to anterior compartment of leg)

Ans: (b) Fracture neck of left fibula

Ref: *Gray's Anatomy, The Anatomical Basis of Clinical Practice, 41st Edition, 2015, page 1405-1409*

2. In a patient with head injury, fracture involves the floor of middle cranial fossa and structures passing through foramen ovale are damaged. Which of the following will be lost?

(a) Sensory supply to forehead
(b) Sensory supply over zygomatic arch
(c) Chewing movement
(d) Ability to blow up the cheeks

Explanation:

Foramen ovale transmits: (MALE structures)

- **M**andibular nerve
- **A**ccessory meningeal artery
- **L**esser petrosal nerve
- **E**missary vein

Mandibular Nerve

- ***Mandibular nerve*** is a branch from **trigeminal** nerve and it is a ***mixed nerve***
- ***Motor branches*** supply the ***muscles of mastication, tensor velipalatini, tensor tympani, mylohyoid and anterior belly of digastric.***
- ***Sensory branches*** supply the ***lower 1/3 of face (V3) and an area in front of auricle***

High Yield

- ***Lesser petrosal nerve*** carries ***preganglionic parasympathetic secretomotor fibers*** from inferior salivatory nucleus to ***otic ganglion (for parotid gland secretion)***
- ***Sensory supply to forehead*** by ***ophthalmic division*** of **trigeminal** nerve ***(V1)***
- ***Sensory supply over zygomatic arch*** by zygomatico facial and zygomatico temporal branches from ***maxillary division of*** *trigeminal nerve* ***(V2)***
- Ability to ***blow up the cheeks*** by actions of buccinators, which is supplied by ***facial nerve***.

Extra Edge:

Mandibular nerve: is the ***largest*** trigeminal division and is a ***mixed nerve***.

- Trunk of the mandibular nerve passes from floor of middle cranial fossa through ***foramen ovale*** to reach infratemporal fossa.
- **Branches of mandibular nerve**

Trunk of mandibular nerve	Anterior division of mandibular nerve	Posterior division of mandibular nerve
• ***Meningeal branch*** (nervus spinosus) – (sensory) • Nerve to ***medial pterygoid, tensor tympani and tensor veli palatine***- (motor)	• ***Buccal nerve*** (sensory) • ***Nerve to masseter*** (motor) • ***Deep temporal nerves*** (motor) • ***Nerve to lateral pterygoid*** (motor)	• ***Auriculotemporal nerve*** (sensory) [carries postganglionic parasympathetic secretomotor fibers from otic ganglion to parotid gland] • ***Lingual nerve*** (sensory) • ***Inferior alveolar nerve /dental nerve*** (mixed) [myelohyoid branch carries motor fibersand alveolar and mental branches sensory]

Ans: (c) Chewing movement

Ref: *Gray's Anatomy, The Anatomical Basis of Clinical Practice, 41st Edition, 2015, page 430, 550 and 551*

3. False regarding Ligamentum teres of femur:

(a) Stabilize the hip joint

(b) Carries blood vessel to supply femur head

(c) Relaxed on abduction

(d) Become stretched on adducting with semiflexed hip

Explanation:

Ligamentum teres femoris

- The degree to which the ligament of the head of the femur offers functional stability to the adult hip is uncertain
- The ligament of the head of the femur is known primarily for lending structural support to the blood vessels that travel to and from the femoral head
- The ligament of the head of the femur is taut when the hip joint is semi-flexed, laterally rotated, and adducted.

Extra Edge:

- The **ligament of the head ofthe femur (Ligamentum teres femoris**) is a triangular, flattened band of connective tissue
- Its apex is attached to fovea for the ligament of the head of the femur and base is attached to edges of the acetabular notch, between which it blends with the transverse acetabular ligament
- It is ensheathed by synovial membrane
- Free nerve endings within this ligament may be a source of pain when it is injured or degenerating
- The afferent innervation may serve as a source of proprioception or protection of the joint

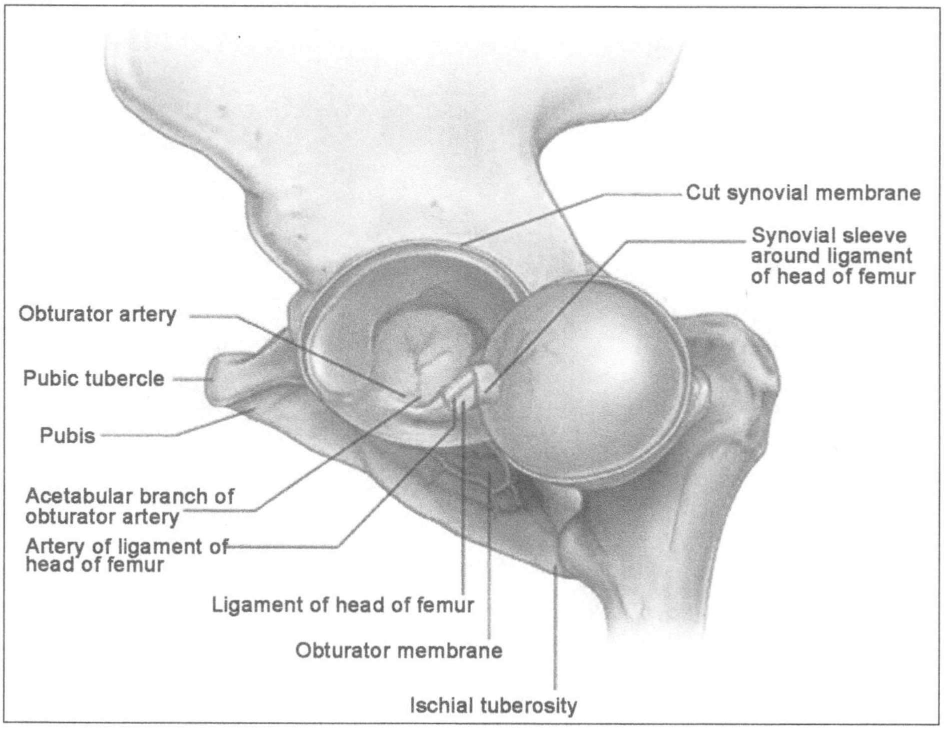

Ans: (a) Stabilize the hip joint

Ref: *Gray's Anatomy, The Anatomical Basis of Clinical Practice, 41st Edition, 2015, page 1378 and 1379*

4. Hyperextension of knee is prevented by:

(a) PCL
(b) ACL
(c) Arcuate ligament
(d) Oblique popliteal ligament

Explanation:

Anterior cruciate ligament (ACL):

- It ***prevents*** posterior displacement of the femur on the tibia and ***hyperextension of the knee joint***
- Attached from the ***anterior intercondylar area of the tibia*** (just posterior to the attachment of the medial meniscus) to the posterior part of the medial side of the ***lateral condyle of the femur***
- It limits posterior rolling (turning and traveling) of the femoral condyles on the tibial plateau during flexion, converting it to spin (turning in place)
- When the knee joint is flexed at a right angle, the tibia cannot be pulled anteriorly (like pulling out a drawer) because it is held by the ACL

Posterior cruciate ligament (PCL):

- It prevents anterior displacement of the femur on the tibia or posterior displacement of the tibia on the femur and helps ***prevent hyperflexion of the knee joint***
- Attached from the ***posterior intercondylar area of the tibia*** to the anterior part of the lateral surface of the ***medial condyle of the femur***
- PCL limits anterior rolling of the femur on the tibial plateau during extension, converting it to spin
- In the weight-bearing flexed knee, the PCL is the main stabilizing factor for the femur (e.g., when walking downhill)

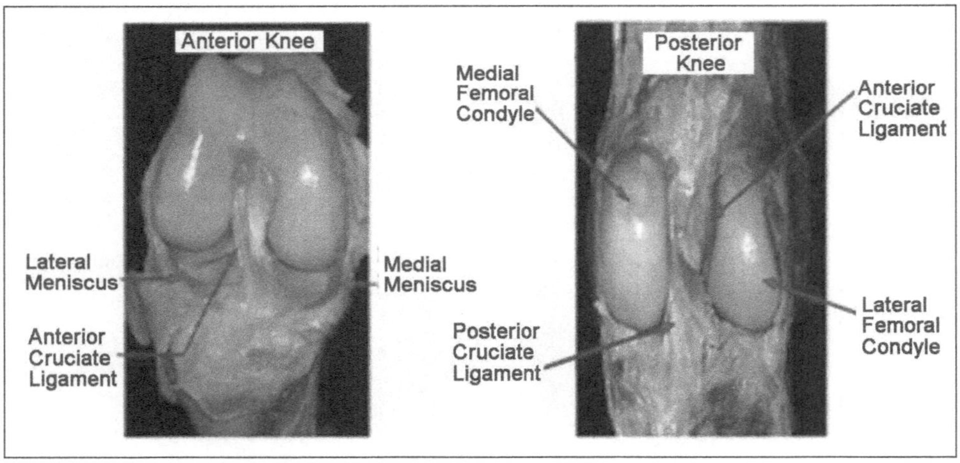

Figure: Cruciate ligaments of knee and its attachments

Oblique popliteal ligament:

- Is an expansion of the tendon of the semimembranosus that ***reinforces the joint capsule posteriorly***
- Arises posterior to the ***medial tibial condyle*** and passes superolaterally toward the ***lateral femoral condyle***, blending with the ***central part of the posterior aspect of the joint capsule***

Arcuate popliteal ligament:

- Also ***strengthens the joint capsule posterolaterally***
- It arises from the posterior aspect of the ***fibular head***, passes superomedially ***over the tendon of the popliteus***, and spreads over the ***posterior surface of the knee joint***

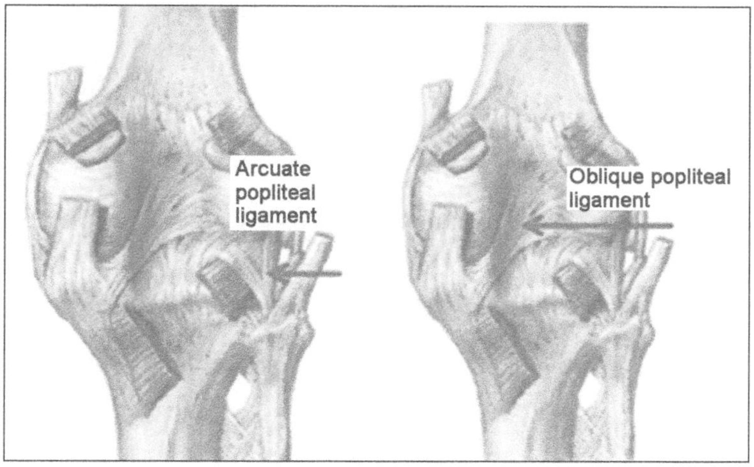

Figure: Attachments of arcuate and oblique popliteal ligaments

Ans: (b) ACL

Ref: *Clinically Oriented Anatomy, Moore, Keith L, Dalley, Arthur F., 5th Edition, 2006, page 690*

5. Which muscle spasm can give rise to symptom similar to cervical rib?

(a) Scalenus anterior
(b) Scalenus medius
(c) Scalenus minimus
(d) Scalenus posterior

Explanation:

Scalenus Anticus Syndrome: (symptoms similar to cervical rib)

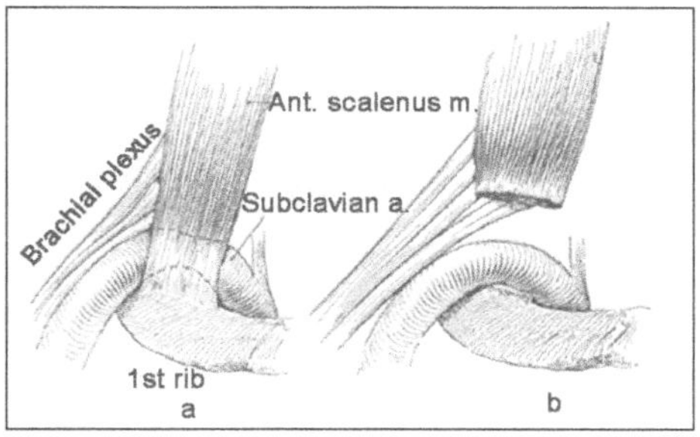

- Development of symptoms is attributable to two factors:
  - The muscular development of the young adult, whose bulging scalenus anticus muscle produces the symptoms, and
  - The sagging of the shoulder girdle of older persons, when there is an additional pull of the scalenus anticus muscle.
- Either one or both of these abnormalities will result in ***compression of the subclavian structures because of stretching of the brachial plexus and the subclavian vessels over a fixed cervical or first thoracic rib***
- Elevation of the shoulder girdle cause produces the same symptoms as do cervical ribs, and the condition has been designated as "the scalenus anticus syndrome"
- Cervical ribs have been classified according to size into 'four groups. Their size, however, is no index to the severity of symptoms, as the determining factor is their relation to the adjacent structures, the ***most important of which is the scalenus anticus muscle***
- This muscle ***arises from*** the ***anterior tubercles of the transverse processes*** of the ***third to sixth cervical vertebrae*** and it is ***inserted*** into the ***scalene tubercle of the first rib***
- It is this muscle that compresses the subclavian artery and the brachial plexus against the cervical rib; it may also elevate the first rib, producing an abnormal lift to that rib, compressing the subclavian artery, and elevating and irritating the brachial plexus
- This in turn causes ***spasm of the scalenus anticus muscle***, which is innervated by the irritated brachial plexus

Ans: (a) Scalenus anterior

Ref: *Textbook of Anatomy, Inderbir Singh, 5th Edition, 2011, Volume-1, page 61 and Winchell McK, Craig and Paul A and Knepper, Cervical Rib and The Scalenus Anticus Syndrome, Annals of Surgery, 1937 April, 105(4) 556–563*

6. Which of the following helps to differentiate between high and low radial nerve injuries?

(a) Extensor digitorum (b) Extensor pollicis longus

(c) Extensor carpi radialis brevis (d) Brachioradialis

Explanation:

- ***High radial nerve injury*** (injury to radial nerve in the arm) involves loss of function of
  - Triceps
  - Lateral part of brachialis
  - Brachioradialis
  - Anconeus
  - Extensor carpi radialis longus
- ***Low radial nerve injury*** (injury to deep branch of radial nerve [***posterior interossous nerve***]) involves loss of function of
  - Extensor carpi radialis brevis
  - Extensor digitorum
  - Extensor digitiminimi
  - Extensor carpi ulnaris
  - Supinator
  - Abductor pollicis longus
  - Extensor pollicis brevis
  - Extensor pollicis longus
  - Extensor indicis

Muscles supplied by Motor branches of radial nerve:

In the Arm			In the Forearm
Above the spiral groove	**In the spiral groove**	**Below the spiral groove**	**Posterior interosseous nerve**
• Long head of triceps • Medial head of triceps	• Lateral head of triceps • Medial head of triceps • Anconeus	• Brachialis (lateral part) • Brachioradialis • Extensor carpi radialis longus	• Extensor carpi radialis brevis • Extensor digitorum • Extensor digitiminimi • Extensor carpi ulnaris • Supinator • Abductor pollicis longus • Extensor pollicis brevis • Extensor pollicis longus • Extensor indicis

Ans: (d) Brachioradialis

Ref: *BD Chaurasia's Human Anatomy, Volume 1, 4th Edition, 2004, page 94-96,131-137*

7. Which of the following is the site of anastomosis between internal and external carotid artery?

(a) Angle of mandible (b) Angle of mouth

(c) Medial canthus of eye (d) Condyle of mandible

Explanation:

Anastomosis exist between the external and the internal carotid arteries around the eye

Four groups of anastomotic vessels have been described:

a. Branches of the ***superficial temporal artery*** anastomose with the ***lacrimal and palpebral branches of the ophthalmic artery***
b. The ***angular artery*** (terminal branch of the facial artery) anastomoses with the ***inferior palpebral and the dorsonasal branch of the ophthalmic artery***
c. ***Orbital branches of the middle meningeal artery*** (from maxillary artery) pass through the lateral part of superior orbital fissure and anastomose with the ***lacrimal branch of the ophthalmic artery***
d. The ***infra-orbital branch of the maxillary artery anastomoses with the dorsonasal branch of the ophthalmic artery***

Ans: (c) Medial canthus of eye

Ref: *Gray's Anatomy, The Anatomical Basis of Clinical Practice, 41 Edition, 2015, page 499*

8. Which of the following cranial nerves have parasympathetic component?

(a) 3, 5, 6, 10
(b) 3, 7, 9, 10
(c) 3, 7, 10, 11
(d) 1, 2, 3, 4

Explanation:

- **Preganglionic parasympathetic** neuronal cell bodies are located in certain cranial nerve nuclei of the brainstem:
  - Oculomotor nerve
  - Facial nerve
  - Glossopharyngeal nerve
  - Vagus nerve
  - Second to fourth sacral spinal nerves.

Extra Edge:

- Parasympathetic nerves system (**craniosacral** outflow) has two component
- ***(a) Cranial component:*** Arises from
  - **Edinger Westphal nucleus** (3rd)
  - **Lacrimal** and**superior salivatory nucleus** (7th)
  - **Inferior salivatory nucleus** (9th) and
  - **Dorsal nucleus** of **vagus** (10th)
- ***(b) Sacral component:***
  - S2, S3 and S4 segments of spinal cord (**Nervi Erigentes-pelvic splanchnic nerves)**

Cranial Nerves	Preganglionic neuron location [within CNS]	Postganglionic neuron location [outside the CNS]	Effector organ
Oculomotor Nerve [3rd CN]	EdingerWestpaul Nucleus [midbrain]	Ciliary ganglion [orbit]	Sphincter pupillae and Ciliary body
Facial Nerve [7th CN]	Superior Salivatory Nucleus and Lacrimatory Nucleus [lower pons]	Pterygopalatine ganglion, [pterygopalatine fossa] Submandibular ganglia/Langlay's ganglia [submandibular region]	Lacrimal, submandibular, sublingual, nasal, palatine and pharyngeal glands.

Contd.

Contd.

Glossopharyngeal Nerve [9th CN]	Inferior Salivatory Nucleus [medulla oblongata]	Otic ganglion [infratemporal fossa]	Parotid gland
Vagus Nerve [10th CN]	Dorsal nucleus of vagus [medulla oblongata]	Visceral ganglia located close or on the surface of organs	Heart, lungs and intestine

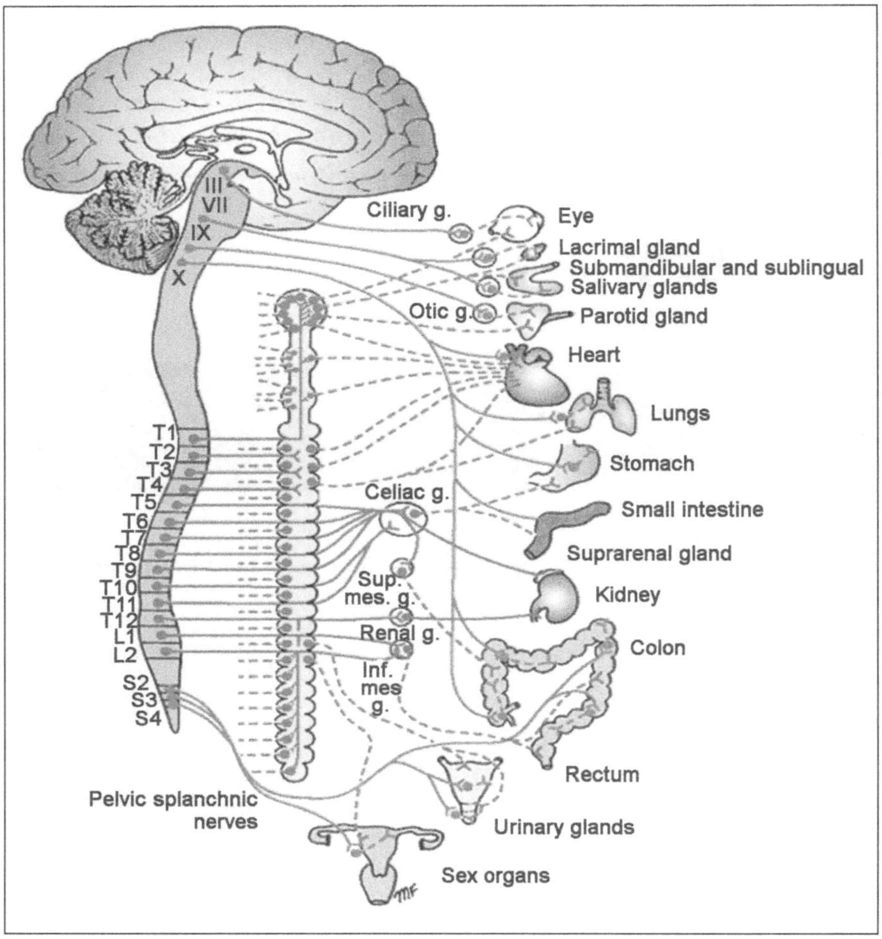

Figure: Efferent part of the autonomic nervous system

Ans: (b) 3, 7, 9, 10

Ref: *Gray's Anatomy, The Anatomical Basis of Clinical Practice, 41st Edition, 2015, page 235*
Richard S Snell Clinical Neuroanatomy, 7th Edition, 2010, page 399

9. Patient with long standing use of axillary crutches presents with restricted abduction of shoulder and extension of elbow. Which part of brachial plexus is affected?

(a) Upper trunk
(b) Lateral cord
(c) Medial cord
(d) Posterior cord

Explanation:

- ***Crutch palsy*** occurs when improper use or fitting of crutches causes ***prolonged compression of branches of posterior cord of brachial plexus at the axilla***

- Branches of **posterior cord** of **brachial plexus** are:
  - Upper subscapular nerve
  - Lower subscapular nerve
  - Thoracodorsal nerve
  - Axillary nerve
  - Radial nerve
- ***Abduction of the shoulder*** is mainly produced by middle fibers of ***deltoid muscle*** which is supplied by ***axillary nerve (C5 and C6)***
- ***Extension of elbow*** is produced by ***triceps***, which is supplied by ***radial nerve (C5, C6, C7, C8 and T1)***.

Ans: (d) Posterior cord

Ref: *Gray's Anatomy, The Anatomical Basis of Clinical Practice, 41 Edition, 2015, page 831-833*

10. Patient when standing on right side leg alone, opposite side hip drops/sags. Which nerve is affected?

(a) Left superior gluteal nerve
(b) Right superior gluteal nerve
(c) Right inferior gluteal nerve
(d) Left inferior gluteal nerve

Explanation:

- The ***gluteus medius and minimus*** are supplied by ***superior gluteal nerve***
- The gluteus medius and minimus are the ***principal abductors of hip*** when ***acting from above (pelvis)***
- The gluteus medius and minimus are ***preventing sagging down of unsupported side hip*** when ***acting from below (femur)***
- ***Acting from the femur***, they play an essential part in ***maintaining the trunk upright*** when the ***foot of the opposite side is raised from the ground*** in walking and running. In this phase, the body weight tends to make the pelvis sag downwards on the unsupported side. This is counteracted by the ***gluteus medius and minimus of the supporting side, which, acting from below,*** exert such ***powerful traction on the hip bone that the pelvis is actually raised a little on the unsupported side***
- The ***supportive effect of*** the gluteus medius and minimus or ***superior gluteal nerve*** on the pelvis when the contralateral foot is raised ***depends on the following conditions***

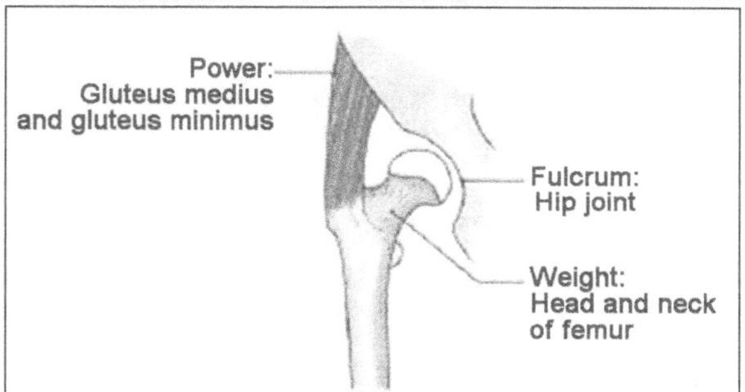

Figure: Abductor mechanism at the hip joint

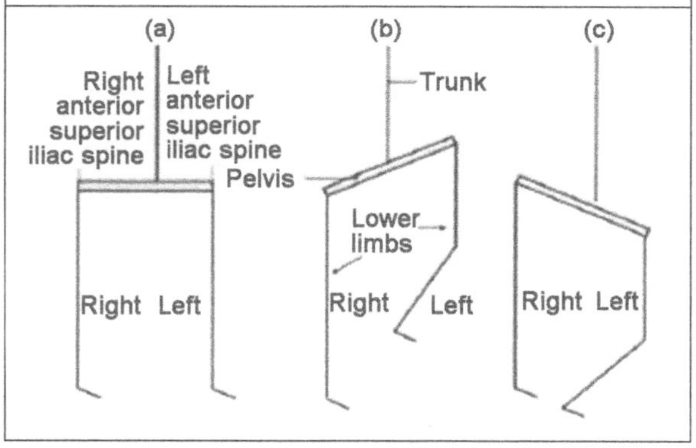

Figure: Trendelenburg sign

  - The gluteus medius and minimus muscles and its nerve supply (superior gluteal nerve) must be functioning normally
  - The components of the hip joint, which forms the fulcrum, must be in their usual relation
  - The neck of the femur must be intact, with its normal angulation to the shaft.
- When any one of these conditions is not fulfilled, e.g. in paralysis of the gluteus medius and minimus or superior gluteal nerve, developmental dysplasia of the hip or coxa vara, the supporting mechanism is upset and the ***pelvis sinks on the unsupported side when the patient tries to stand on the affected limb***. This is known clinically as ***positive Trendelenburg's sign***
- Individuals with ***paralysis of superior gluteal nerve*** have a characteristic ***lurching gait***

- ***Superior gluteal nerve*** or gluteus medius and minimus may be ***tested together by medial rotation of the thigh*** against resistance, in the supine position with hip and knee flexed

Ans: (b) Right superior gluteal nerve

Ref: *Gray's Anatomy, The Anatomical Basis of Clinical Practice, 41st Edition, 2015, page 1358, BD Chaurasia's Human Anatomy, Volume 2, 6th Edition, 2004, page 71*

11. Which cartilage of larynx doesn't ossify?

(a) Thryoid
(b) Cricoid
(c) Cuneiform and corniculate cartilage
(d) Arytenoid lower part

Explanation:

- The ***thyroid, cricoid and the greater part of the arytenoid cartilages*** consist of ***hyaline cartilage*** and may undergo ***mottled calcification*** as age advances.
- Calcification ***starting*** about the ***25th year in the thyroid*** **cartilage** and somewhat ***later in the cricoid and arytenoids***.
- By the ***65th year*** these cartilages commonly ***appear patchily dense in radiographs***.
- The ***epiglottic, corniculate, cuneiform, tritiate*** (tiny cartilage in the lateral thyrohyoid ligament) and the ***apices of the arytenoid cartilages*** are composed of ***elastic fibrocartilage***, with ***little tendency*** to calcify.

Ans: (c) Cuneiform and corniculate cartilage

Ref: *Gray's Anatomy, The Anatomical Basis of Clinical Practice, 41st Edition, 2015, page 586*

12. Tympanic membrane is supplied by all *except:*

(a) Vagus nerve
(b) Glossopharyngeal nerve
(c) Trigeminal nerve
(d) Vestibulocochlear nerve

Explanation:

- **Vestibulocochlear nerve is concerned with balance and hearing.**
- The ***tympanic membrane*** is ***mainly innervated by the auriculo temporal nerve*** (branch from posterior division of mandibular nerve [***V3***], which is a branch from trigeminal nerve) and appears to perceive only pain
- There is a ***minor, inconstant and overlapping*** sensory supply from the ***facial, glossopharyngeal and vagus nerves***
  - ***Anterior half of the lateral surface*** of tympanic membrane is supplied by the ***auriculotemporal nerve (V3)***
  - ***Posterior half of the lateral surface*** of tympanic membrane is supplied by the ***auricular branch of vagus (Alderman's nerve)***
  - ***Medial surface*** of tympanic membrane by tympanic branch of the ***glossopharyngeal nerve*** through tympanic plexus
- During myringotomy incision is usually given in the posteroinferior quadrant of tympanic membrane to avoid injury to the chorda tympani nerve, which crosses the inner aspect of the membrane in the upper part
- Fibres of the nervus intermedius (sensory root of facial nerve) may pass to the auricular branch of the vagus (Alderman's nerve) here, which may explain the cutaneous vesiculation that sometimes accompanies geniculate herpes

Ans: (d) Vestibulocochlear nerve

Ref: *Gray's Anatomy, The Anatomical Basis of Clinical Practice, 41st Edition, 2015, page 633*

13. Most dependent pleural recess is?

(a) Anterior costophrenic recess

(b) Posterior costophrenic recess

(c) Anterior costomediastinal recess

(d) Lateral costophrenic recess

Explanation:

- Normally a few milliliters of fluid in the pleural space
- About ***75 ml are required to blunt the posterior costophrenic sulcus*** (seen on the ***lateral view***) and about ***200-300 ml to blunt the lateral costophrenic sulcus*** (seen on the ***frontal view***)

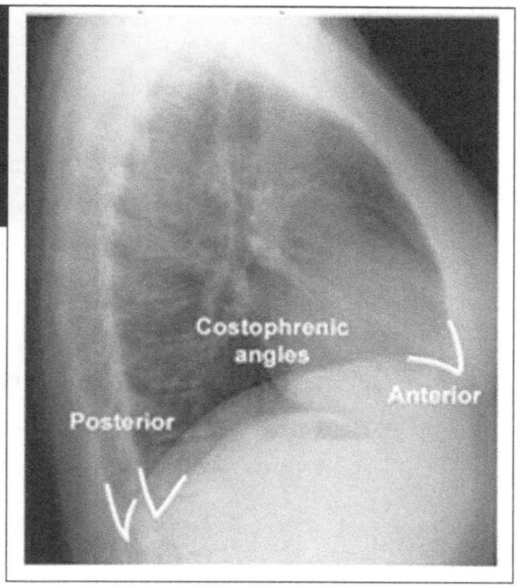

Figure: Anterior and posterior costophrenic angle in lateral chest radiograph (https://www.radiologymasterclass.co.uk)

Extra Edge:

- Pleural recesses serve as ***reserve spaces*** of pleural cavity for the lungs to ***expand during deep inspiration***.
  1. Right and left costodiaphragmatic recesses
  2. Right and left costomediastinal recesses

Costodiaphragmatic recess:

- It is located inferiorly between the ***reflections of costal and diaphragmatic pleurae***
- Vertically it measures about 5 cm and lies opposite the ***8th to 10th ribs along the midaxillary line***
- The costodiaphragmatic recesses are the ***most dependent parts of the pleural cavities***, hence the ***fluid of pleural effusion first collect*** at these sites

Costomediastinal recess:

- It is located anteriorly between the ***reflections of costal and mediastinal pleurae*** and lies between sternum and costal cartilages
- The ***right costomediastinal recess*** is possibly ***occupied*** by the anterior margin of the right lung even ***during quiet breathing***
- The ***left costomediastinal recess is large*** due to the ***presence of cardiac notch*** in the left lung. Its location can be confirmed clinically by percussion (tapping) of the chest wall (***superficial cardiac dullness***).

Ans: (b) Posterior costophrenic recess

Ref: *Text Book of Anatomy, Vishram Singh, Vol.1, 2nd Edition 2014, page 231 and www.learningradiology.com*

14. Cranial nerve is devoid of:

(a) Nodes of Ranvier (b) Neurilemma

(c) Myelin sheath (d) Oligodendrocytes

Explanation:

Neurolemma

- Also known as **neurilemma**, **sheath of Schwann**, or **Schwann's sheath**
- Outermost nucleated cytoplasmic layer of Schwann cells (also called neurolemmocytes) that surrounds the axon of the neuron. It forms the outermost layer of the nerve fiber in the **peripheral nervous system**

- The neurolemma is underlain by the **myelin sheath** (referred to as the medullary sheath in the included illustrations)
- In the **central nervous system**, axons are myelinated by **oligodendrocytes**, thus **lack neurolemma***
- The myelin sheaths of Oligodendrocytes **do not have neurolemma** because excess cytoplasm is directed centrally toward the oligodendrocyte cell body
- Neurolemma serves a protective function for **peripheral nerve fibers**

Myelin Sheath

- The axons of many neurons are insulated by a myelin sheath, which increases the rate at which an axon can conduct an action potential.
- **Myelin** is formed by **oligodendrocytes** in the **central nervous system**
- Myelin is formed by **Schwann** cells in the **peripheral nervous system**
- Oligodendrocytes myelinate several axons from different nerves (up to around 50).

Myelin in the Peripheral and Central Nervous Systems

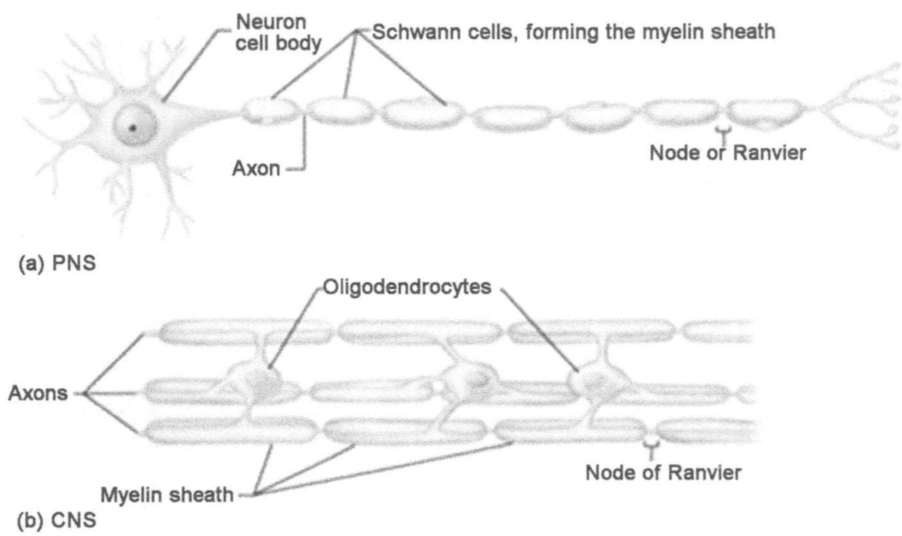

Ans: (b) Neurilemma

Ref: *www.histology.leeds.ac.uk*

15. Superior part of IVC directly develops from:

(a) Right Vitelline vein (b) Left Vitelline vein
(c) Right umbilical vein (d) Left umbilical vein

Explanation:

Superior part of IVC (terminal part) develops from the ***supra-hepatic part of the right vitelline vein.***

Development of IVC

IVC developed from the following sources from below upwards

- Persistent caudal part of the ***right posterior cardinal vein***
- ***Right supra-cardinal vein*** [this part receives 3rd and 4th pairs of lumbar veins]
- ***Anastomosis*** between ***right supra-cardinal and right sub-cardinal veins*** [this part receives the right gonadal vein]

- Upper part of the ***right sub-cardinal vein*** [this part receives both renal veins and right supra-renal vein].
- A ***new vessel*** grows dorsal to the liver and ***communicates the right sub-cardinal vein with the common hepatic vein*** [intrahepatic part of IVC]
- ***Common hepatic vein*** –which is developed from the ***supra-hepatic part of the right vitelline vein*** [terminal part of IVC]

Ans: (a) Right Vitelline vein

Ref: *Essentials of Human Embryology, A.K. Datta, 5th Edition, 2005, page 205-208*

16. Which of the following artery gives rise to posterior gastric artery?

(a) Left gastric artery (b) Right gastric artery
(c) Splenic artery (d) Left gastroepiploic artery

Explanation:

- Posterior gastric artery arises from the **splenic artery** in its middle section posterior to the body of the stomach
- It ascends behind the peritoneum of the lesser sac towards the fundus
- It reaches the posterior surface of the stomach in the gastrophrenic fold

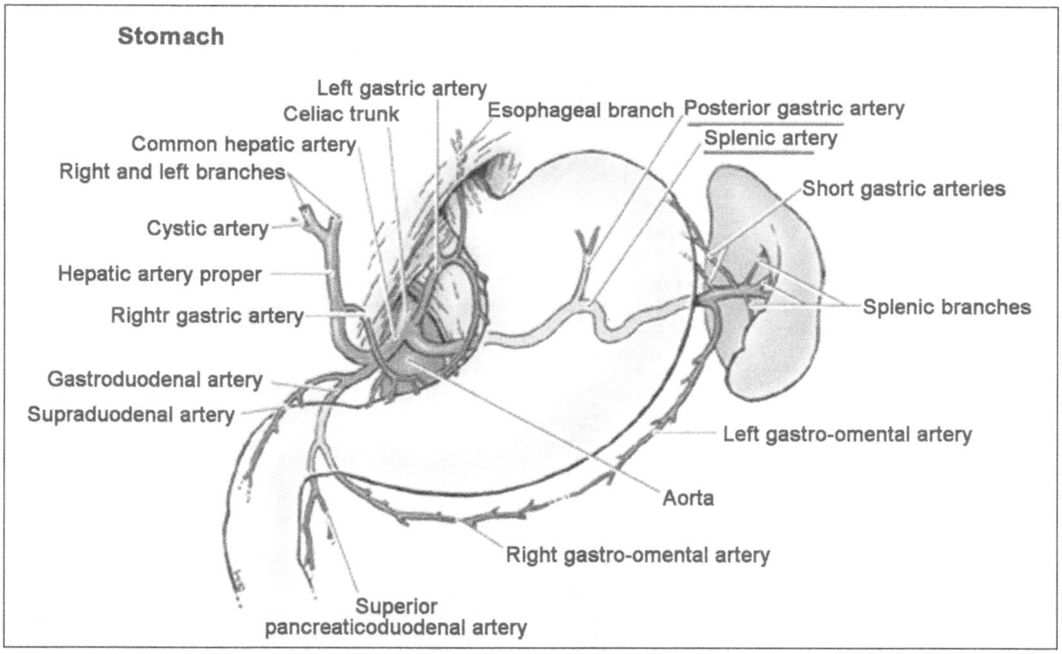

Ans: (c) Splenic artery

Ref: *Gray's Anatomy, 39th Edition, 2008, page 1147*

PHYSIOLOGY

1. A 35-year-old male patient was admitted to casualty with history of Road traffic accident. He was conscious, HR – 140/min, blood pressure was normal in supine position however there was postural hypotension. His urine output was decreased. What grade of shock is the patient is likely in:

(a) Very mild hypovolemic shock
(b) Mild hypovolemic Shock
(c) Moderate hypovolemic Shock
(d) Severe hypovolemic Shock

Explanation:

Hypovolemic shock

- Most common form of shock
- Results from decrease in blood volume due to hemorrhage or loss of extravascular fluid volume resulting in reduced venous return and inadequate cardiac output
- To maintain the perfusion to brain and heart certain homeostatic responses are seen such as increase in sympathetic activity, hyperventilation, collapse of venous capacitance vessels and release of stress hormones
- To replace the loss of intravascular fluid volume there may be decrease in urine output

Grades of hypovolemic shock and their features

Grades of hypovolemic shock	Features
Mild	< 20% loss of blood volume, mild tachycardia, cool extremities, increased capillary refill time, Diaphoresis, Collapsed veins, Anxiety
Moderate	20-40% loss in blood volume, Tachycardia, Tachypnea, Oliguria, Postural hypotension along with features of mild hypovolemic shock.
Severe	>40% loss of blood volume, hemodynamic instability, marked tachycardia, hypotension, mental status deterioration (agitation, confusion and then may lead to coma)

Ans: (c) Moderate hypovolemic Shock

Ref: *Harrison's Principles of Internal Medicine,19th Edition, page 1748*

2. At high altitudes, how work capacity is increased?

(a) Decrease the intensity of exercise and decrease the duration of exercise
(b) Decrease the intensity of exercise and increase the duration of exercise
(c) Increase the intensity of exercise and decrease the duration of exercise
(d) Increase the intensity of exercise and increase the duration of exercise

Explanation:

- At high altitudes, due to reduced barometric pressure there is **decrease in alveolar PO_2** and thereby **decrease in arterial PO_2**. There is decrease in muscle work capacity due to decreased availability of oxygen at the mitochondrial level
- **Maximal oxygen uptake (VO_2 max)** is the product of **cardiac output** and **arteriovenous difference** in **oxygen content**

- At high altitude both cardiac output and arterial oxygen content are reduced and hence decrease in **work output**
- On ascending upwards, there is a **decrease in VO_2 max** approximately from 1,500 m and thereafter by a ≈1% reduction for every 100 m
- Due to hypoxia, decreased in work capacity is seen at high altitude
- Decrease in work capacity is proportionate to the decrease in maximum oxygen uptake that a body can achieve
- At an altitude of 17000 feet, an **unacclimatized** person will have less than **50%** of normal work capacity but **after 2 months** of **acclimatization** he will have **68%** of normal work capacity
- Work capacity is directly proportional to the workload and duration of exercise. Since the oxygen uptake is limited at high altitudes, increase in duration of work may increase the work capacity of an individual

Adaptation to High altitude

- **Decrease in alveolar PO_2** due to decrease in barometric pressure
- **Decrease in arterial PO_2** (Hypoxemia)
- Stimulation of **peripheral chemoreceptors** leads to **hyperventilation** and hence resulting in **respiratory alkalosis** (due to increase in arterial pH)
- Due to **hypoxemia** there is increase in erythropoietin production resulting in polycythaemia (increase in haemoglobin concentration)
- Shift of oxygen haemoglobin dissociation curve to the **right** (Increase in 2,3 DPG concentrations)
- **Pulmonary vasoconstriction** due to hypoxemia.

Ans: (b) Decrease the intensity of exercise and increase the duration of exercise

Ref: *Guyton and Hall, Textbook of Medical Physiology, Thirteenth International Edition, page 564*

3. Tetanizing frequency is calculated by:

(a) 1 / Contraction Period
(b) 1 /Relaxation Period
(c) 1/ Contraction period + Relaxation period
(d) 1/ Contraction period - Relaxation period

Explanation:

Simple Muscle Twitch

- Contraction of a muscle in response to electrical stimulation is called as **simple muscle twitch**. The contraction recorded is called as **simple muscle curve**
- **Latent Period** – Point of stimulus to the point of onset of contraction
- **Contraction period** – Point of onset of contraction to the point of peak of contraction

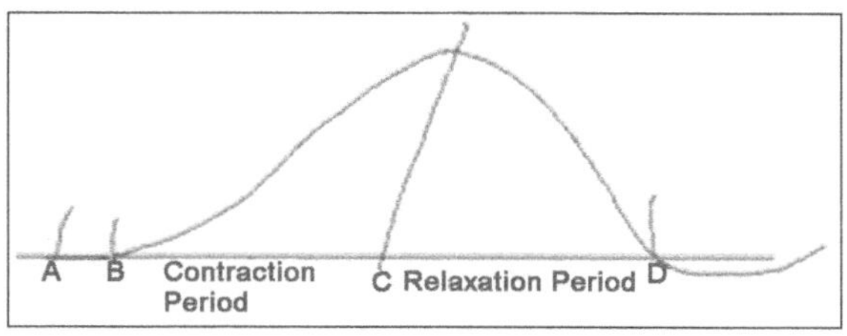

- **Relaxation Period** – Peak of contraction to the end of relaxation

Tetanus

- When muscle is repeatedly stimulated at higher frequency, it reaches a state of sustained contraction without relaxation known as tetanus
- The minimum frequency of stimulation above which tetanus occurs is called as "**minimum tetanizable frequency" or "tetanizing frequency" or "fusion** frequency"

From a simple muscle curve,

Tetanizing frequency can be calculated by formula

$$\textit{Tetanizing frequency} = \frac{1}{\textit{Contraction Period}}$$

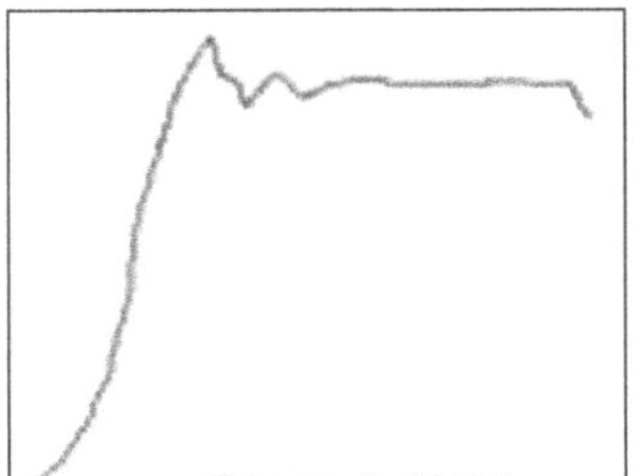
Tetanus (> 40 Hz)

Example If the contraction period is 0.06 seconds, the tetanizable frequency will be 17 Hz

TF in slow muscle fibers are less due to longer contraction period. TF in fast muscle fibers are higher due to less contraction period

Cardiac muscle cannot be tetanized because of its longer refractory period.

Treppe

- On repeatedly stimulating the muscle (15 – 20Hz), there is progressive increase in force of contraction for the first two or three contractions. This is called as **treppe or staircase effect**
- This occurs due to accumulation of calcium in the sarcoplasm due to application of repeated stimuli

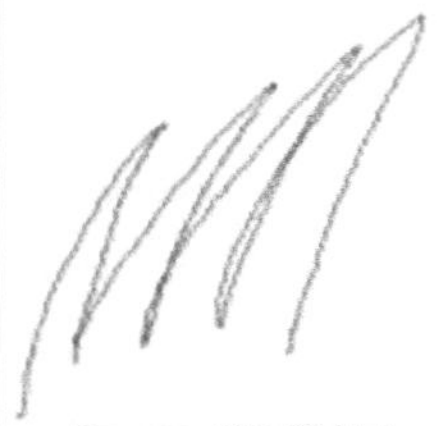
Treppe (15-20 Hz)

Ans: (a) 1 / Contraction Period

Ref: *Guyton and Hall, Textbook of Medical Physiology, Thirteenth International Edition, page 85 and GK Pal, Textbook of Practical Physiology, 4th Edition, page 395*

4. A motor cyclist suffered head injury 6 months back and presents with persistent memory deficits following injury. Choose the most appropriately matched option relating to memory:

(a) Hippocampus and implicit memory
(b) Neocortex and Associative learning
(c) Medial temporal lobe and declarative memory
(d) Angular gyrus and Procedural memory

Explanation:

- **Learning** is acquisition of the information that alters the behaviour based on previous experience and **memory** is the retention and storage of that information

Physiologically memory can be classified into explicit and implicit memory.

Type of memory	Function	Area of brain involved
Explicit memory (Declarative memory): Memory of facts such as people, place and things. Explicit memory is further classified as semantic memory and episodic memory		
• **Semantic memory**	Memory of facts (word, rules and languages)	Lateral and anterior **temporal** cortex, **prefrontal** cortex
• **Episodic memory**	Memory of events	**Hippocampus**, **medial temporal lobe**, **neocortex**
Implicit memory (Non declarative memory): Important for training reflexive motor or perceptual skills. This is further classified into Priming, procedural memory, associative learning and non-associative learning.		
• **Priming**	Facilitation of the recognition of words or objects by prior exposure to them	**Neocortex**
• **Procedural memory**	Skills and habits, which, once acquired, become unconscious and automatic	**Striatum, cerebellum and motor cortex**
• **Associative learning**	Classical conditioning and Operant conditioning– Human or animal learn the association between one stimulus and another stimulus	**Amygdala – emotional responses** **Cerebellum – Motor responses**

Contd.

Contd.

• **Non-Associative learning**	**Habituation:** Decrease in response to a benign (neutral type) stimulus, when the stimulus is presented repeatedly. **Sensitization:** Repeated application of a distinctly pleasant or unpleasant (strong) stimulus produces greater and greater response.	**Various reflex pathways**

Ans: (c) Medial temporal lobe and declarative memory

Ref: *Ganong's Review of Medical Physiology, 25th Edition, page 284-285*

5. Water absorption is maximum in :

(a) Duodenum (b) Ileum

(c) Jejunum (d) Large intestine

Explanation:

- Water moves passively into and out of the gastrointestinal lumen, driven by electrochemical gradients established by the active transport of ions and other solutes
- **2000 mL** of ingested fluid reach the intestines along with **7000 mL** of endogenous secretions from the mucosa of gastrointestinal tract and associated glands. These endogenous secretions are from stomach, salivary glands, bile, pancreas and intestine
- Majority of the water is reabsorbed by **jejunum (5500 mL**) followed by ileum and colon
- Of these **98%** of the fluid is reabsorbed and only **200 mL** of the fluid is **excreted** in **stools**
- In between meals, Sodium and chloride are absorbed together from the lumen by Sodium hydrogen exchanger and chloride bicarbonate exchanger
- Sodium enters across the apical membrane of the large intestine via ENaC (epithelial sodium) channels.
- **Iron** is mainly absorbed in **duodenum***
- **Vitamin B12** is absorbed in **ileum***. Intrinsic factor secreted from oxyntic cells of stomach is necessary for the absorption of vitamin B12
- **Large intestines*** absorb **water and electrolytes**

Ans: (c) Jejunum

Ref: *Ganong's Review of Medical Physiology, 25th Edition, page 464-465*

6. Electromyographic finding in denervation is:

(a) Myotonic discharges (b) Positive sharp waves

(c) Short polyphasic waves (d) Multiple motor neuron firing (or spikes)

Explanation:

Electromyography:

- Technique of recording the electrical activity of a **muscle** and its **motor nerve**
- EMG can be recorded at rest or activity using a needle electrode inserted into the muscle
- At rest, Spontaneous activity such as insertion activity (insertion of needle evokes discharge of action potentials) and end plate noise (non-propagated miniature end plate potentials generated by acetylcholine release) is seen

- Normal activity of the muscle is observed by recruitment of motor units on voluntary contraction of muscle. As the intensity of contraction increases, more recruitment occurs

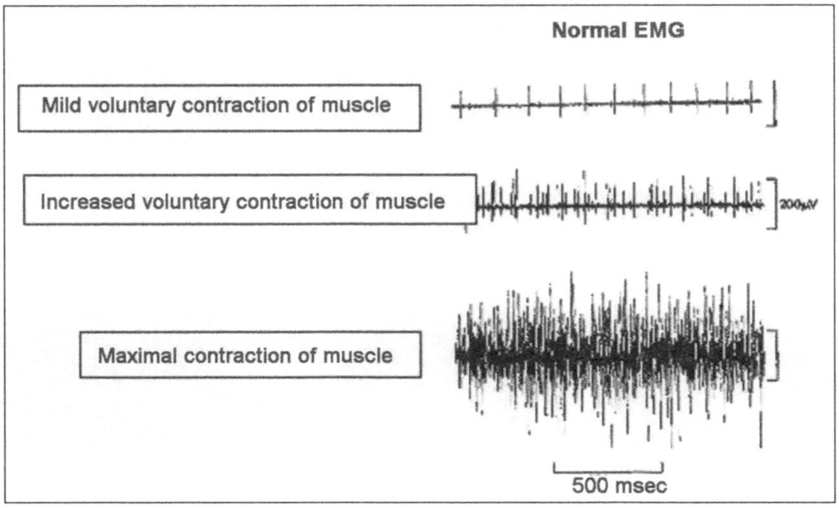

- Abnormal spontaneous activity occurs in various neuromuscular disorders, especially those associated with denervation or inflammatory changes in affected muscle
- Features of **EMG in Denervated muscle**
  - Spontaneous activity such as **fibrillation potentials**
  - **Positive sharp waves**
  - **Complex repetitive discharges**

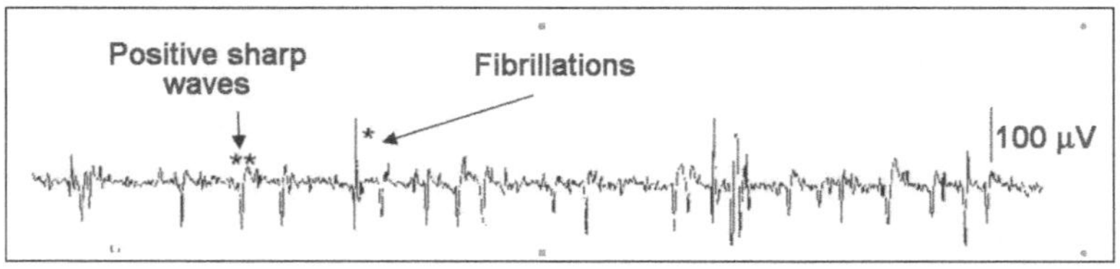

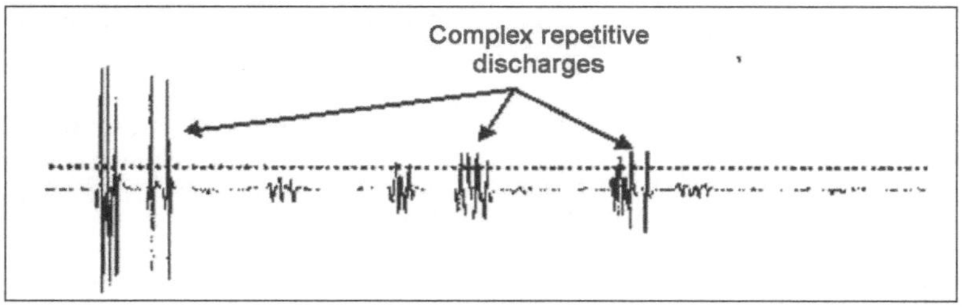

- **Fibrillation potentials** are characteristic of slowly progressive **neuropathic disorders (Amyotrophic lateral sclerosis)**
- **Myotonic discharges** are found in myotonic disorders such as **myotonic dystrophy** or **myotonia congenita**

Ans: (b) Positive sharp waves

Ref: *Neurologic Disorders, Harrison's Principles of Medicine, 19th Edition, page 442, Edition, e-4*

7. Cardiovascular effect of negative G is:

(a) Decrease in cardiac output (b) Increase in cardiac output
(c) Decrease in venous return (d) Decrease in cerebral arterial pressure

Explanation:

Positive gravity (centrifugal acceleratory force on the body)

- The force due to acceleration acting on the long axis of the body from head to foot when the body moves upwards in an aircraft is called as *positive G* (G represents the unit of gravity force). refers to the force of gravity on earth's surface. E.g., take off of flight, Pilots in fighter aircrafts

- Since the 'positive G and negative g' effects are experienced when there is a acceleration or deceleration along the long axis of the body, the astronauts avoid these effects by positioning themselves perpendicular to the direction of G, i.e. in a ***chest-to-back direction***

Effects of positive G

- Blood volume is pulled towards the lower part of the body when a person is in positive G. Depending on the speed of acceleration the movement of blood volume towards the lower part of the body will occur
- At an acceleration below 5G, the compensatory mechanisms maintain the cardiac output and cerebral circulation. Cardiac output is maintained from the blood drawn from the pulmonary reservoir. Cerebral circulation is maintained by the associated fall in JVP and intracranial pressure
- At an acceleration more than 5G, **Venous return** and **cardiac output** is markedly reduced
- There may be **"black out"**of vision (temporary loss of vision) for 5 seconds between 4 and 6 G and further increase may lead to unconsciousness and death

Negative G

- When the body moves downwards from height towards the earth, the force due to deceleration acting in the long axis of the body from footto head is called *negative G*
- *Negative G effects* are experienced during landing of space rockets, landing of airplanes and parachute jumping

Effects of negative G

- Cardiac output is increased due to general increase in venous return. Most of the cardiac output, however, moves towards upper parts of the body and hence there is accumulation of blood in head and neck
- Cerebral arterial pressure is increased markedly. There is also increase in intracranial pressure which prevents the rupture of the vessels inspite of rise in cerebral arterial pressure
- Blood vessels of head and neck show intense congestion
- Ecchymosis appears around the eyes
- Severe throbbing headache, pain, and eventually
- Mental confusion (red out)

Ans: B. Increase in cardiac output

Ref: *Indu Khurana, Textbook of Medical Physiology, page 1078 and Guyton and Hall, Textbook of Medical Physiology, Thirteenth International Edition, page 565*

8. Cardiac vascular effect of Ghrelin is:

(a) Decrease in blood pressure
(b) Decrease in myocardial contractility
(c) Constriction of peripheral vessels
(d) Decrease in coronary blood flow

Explanation:

Ghrelin

- **Ghrelin** is secreted primarily by endocrine cells in the **oxyntic gland** area of the stomach
- Some amount of ghrelin is also produced in the **hypothalamus**, **small and large intestines**, **pancreas**, and the **kidney**
- Ghrelin binds to the **growth hormone secretagogue receptor** and stimulates the release of **growth hormone** from the **pituitary**
- **Actions of Ghrelin**
  - ↑ Appetite

- ↑ Gastric motility
- ↑ Secretion of gastric acid
- ↑ Adipogenesis
- ↑ Insulin secretion

- **Leptin** and **ghrelin** are peripheral factors that act reciprocally on food intake
- **Ghrelin**, is predominantly fast-acting **orexin** that stimulates food intake. It increases synthesis and/or release of **central orexins**, including **neuropeptide Y and cannabinoids**, and suppresses the ability of leptin to stimulate the anorexigenic factors such as pro-opiomelanocortin (POMC), cocaine- and amphetamine-regulated transcript (CART), neurotensin and corticotropin-releasing hormone (CRH)

Cardiovascular effects of Ghrelin

- Ghrelin has **cardioprotective effects**
- **CVS effects of Ghrelin**
  - Reduction of mean arterial blood pressure
  - Increase in myocardial contractility
  - Protection of endothelial cells
  - Improvement of energy metabolism of myocardial cells
- Exogenous administration of ghrelin also results in
  - Improvement in coronary flow
  - ↑ heart rate
  - Dilatation of peripheral blood vessels
  - Constriction of coronary arteries
  - Improvement in ventricular and endothelial function.
- Ghrelin **promotesnitric oxide synthesis** which **cause vasodilatation**. In patients with Congestive heart failure it was found to decrease peripheral vascular resistance resulting in an increase in stroke volume and cardiac index.

Actions of Ghrelin:

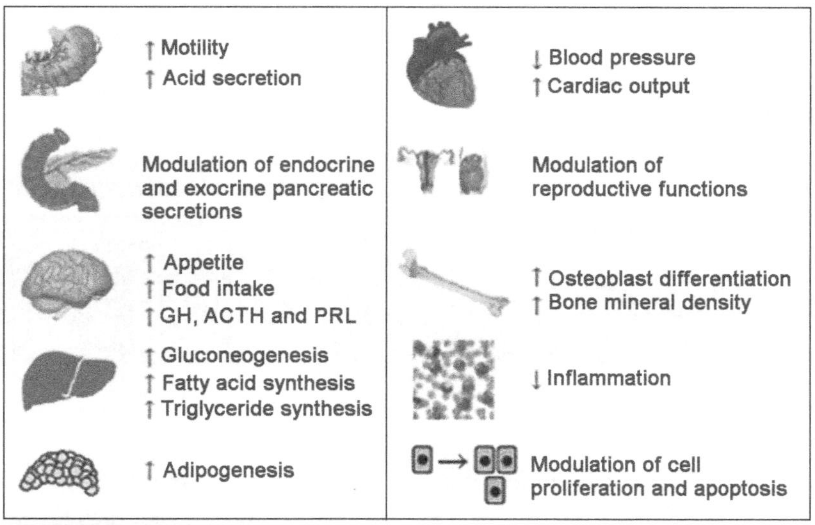

Ans: (a) Decrease in blood pressure

Ref: *Zhang G, Yin X, Qi Y, Pendyala L, Chen J, Hou D, Tang C, Ghrelin and Cardiovascular Diseases, Curr Cardiol Rev., 2010 February 6(1):62-70, Leonard R Johnson Gastrointestinal physiology, 8th Edition, page 142 and Ganong's Review of Medical Physiology, 25th Edition, page 486*

9. Which of the following parts of brain contains dopaminergic neurons?

(a) Locus coeruleus system (b) Cerebellum
(c) Nigro striatal system (d) Midline raphe nucleus

Explanation:

Dopaminergic system

- Meso-cortical system
- Tubero-infundibular system
- Nigro-striatal system
- Incerto-hypothalamic system

Noradrenergic system

- Locus coeruleus system
- Tegmental system

Adrenergic system

- From Medulla to spinalcord, hypothalamus, thalamus, periaqueductal gray

Serotonergic system

- Midline raphe nucleus of hypothalamus

Histaminergic system

- Tubero-mamillary nucleus of posterior hypothalamus

Cholinergic system

- Nucleus basalis of Meynert to amygdala and neocortex

Ans: (c) Nigro striatal system

Ref: *Pal GK, Limbic System, In: Textbook of Medical Physiology, Ahuja Publishing House, 2007, 120: 910-13*

10. Secretory phase of endometrium is due to which hormone?

(a) Estrogen (b) Progesterone
(c) Prolactin (d) Pregnanediol

Explanation:

Phases of endometrial cycle

- The endometrial cycle of 28 days can be divided into three phases
  - **Menstrual phase** (1–5 days)
  - **Proliferative Phase** (6–14 days)
  - **Secretory Phase** (15–28 days)

	Proliferative Phase	Secretory Phase	Menstrual Phase
Extent	• **6 – 14 days** • Follows Phase of menstruation, following which only a **thin basal layer** of original endometrium is left	• **15 – 28 days** • Aka **Postovulatory phase**	• **First five** days • Average duration 3 – 5 days • Aka **Bleeding phase**

Contd.

Contd.

Hormones	• **Estrogen** secreted from developing graafian follicle in the ovary • This phase **coincides** with **follicular phase** of **ovarian cycle**	• **Progesterone** secreted by corpus luteum formed after ovulation • **Estrogen**	• About 24 hours before this phase, there is **sharp decline in plasma levels of estrogen and progesterone** which causes **bleeding**
Changes in Endometrium	• Thickness of **endometrium** is **increased** (From <1 mm to 3-4 mm) • **Angiogenesis in Stratum functionalis** leads to proliferation of vessels and spiral arterioles formation • Growth of **endometrial glands** • They contain **glycogen** but are **non-secretory**	• **Elongation** and **coiling** of endometrial **mucous glands**. • The glands become secretory, secrete thick **viscous fluid containing glycogen** • Further increase in blood supply and **spiraling of blood vessels** due to progesterone effect • **Prominent corkscrew shaped glands** • **Thickness of endometrium** increases to **5 – 6 mm** • If fertilization does not occur and there is no pregnancy, the corpus luteum in the ovary involute to form **corpus albicans on Day 26** of cycle • The levels of **estrogen and progesterone fall suddenly**	• Endometrial debris contains necrosed sloughed off tissue, blood, serous fluid containing prostaglandins and fibrolysins • Average blood loss is **30 ml** • **Menstrual blood clots immediately** in uterine cavity but gets **liquefied by fibrolysins** present in endometrial debris • Around **2/3rd of the superficial endometrium is sloughed** off and only a thin basal layer is left behind (1 – 2 mm)
Cervix	• The **secretions** of mucosal cells of endocervix **become thin**, **watery** and **alkaline** • During **ovulation**, cervical mucous is **thinnest** and has **maximum elasticity** • Mucous can be **stretched** like a long, thin elastic thread up to 8 – 12 cm (**Spinnbarkeit effect**) • Produces characteristic **Fern-like pattern** on drying on glass slide (**Fern Test**) • Cervical mucous makes conditions favourable for transport of sperms and fertilization	• Cervical secretions decrease in quantity and becomes **thick, tenacious and cellular** • **Fern pattern NOT** seen • These changes make a plug and prevent entry of sperms through cervical canal • **Persistence of Fern pattern** throughout the cycle indicates '**Anovulatory cycle'**	• Does **NOT** undergo desquamation like endometrial mucosa
Vagina	• Epithelium becomes **thickened** and **cornified** (estrogen effect)	• Epithelium **proliferates** and gets **infiltrated with leucocytes** • Vaginal secretions become **thick and viscid**	

Ans: (b) Progesterone

Ref: *Guyton, 12th Edition, page 995 and Essentials of Medical Physiology by Khurana, page 509*

BIOCHEMISTRY

1. Which of the following statements is NOT true about Bence jones protein?

(a) It is associated with poor prognosis

(b) Precipitates at 20-30 degree celsius

(c) Due to Monoclonal light chains in urine

(d) This paraprotein can be demonstrated by serum electrophoresis

Explanation:

Bence Jones' protein

- Can be detected in **blood** and **urine** of patients suffering from **multiple myeloma (**Plasma cell tumor), a group of diseases characterized by proliferation of a single plasma cell clone
- This protein is a **dimer of kappa** and **lambda chains of paraprotein**
- This condition can be diagnosed by demonstration of a spike and an extra band called, **'M'band** in between beta and gamma region on serum electrophoresis

Classical heat test:

- When slightly **acidified urine is heated to 40°–50°C**, Bence Jones proteins get precipitated. On further heating urine to boiling point, crystals dissolve. Upon cooling urine to 70°, crystals reappear
- Molecular weight of this protein is **45000** and sedimentation coefficient is **3.5S**

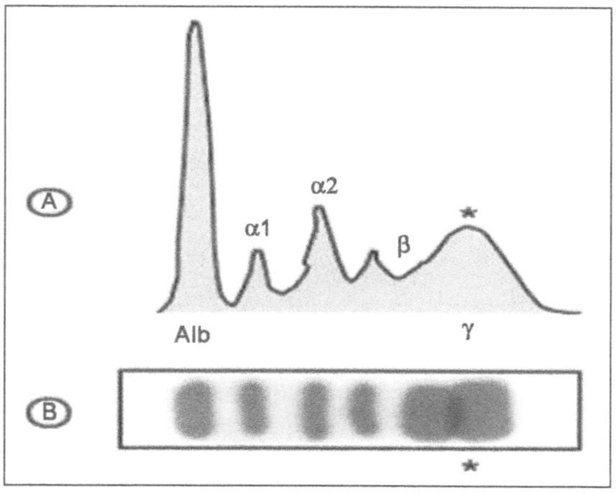

The diagram shows the electrophoretic pattern in multiple myeloma

*M spike and M band seen in gamma region, hypergammaglobulinemia

Ans: (b) Precipitates at 20-30 degree celsius

Ref: *Textbook of Medical Biochemistry by Dinesh Puri, 3rd Edition, Chapter 5, page 91*

2. A child present with depigmented iris, hypopigmented skin and photosensitivity. Which of the following enzymes is deficient in this child?

(a) Tyrosinase

(b) Tryptophan hydroxylase

(c) Tyrosine hydroxylase

(d) Tyrosine Carboxylase

(e) Tyrosine transaminase

Explanation:

Albinism

- Albinism includes a spectrum of clinical syndromes characterized by **hypomelanosis**, arising from inherited defects in the **pigment cells** (melanocytes) of **eye** and **skin**. There are various forms of the disease
- The classical form of albinism is due to the deficiency of the enzyme tyrosinase

Types:

- **Tyrosinase negative** individuals lack detectable pigment in the skin, hair, or eyes. For this reason, this disorder is sometimes called complete perfect albinism
- Other forms of albinism called complete imperfect albinism occur in tyrosinase-positive individuals. These individuals have some detectable tyrosinase activity, but fail to synthesize melanin in adequate amounts. This may be because of a transport defect, a decreased ability to transport tyrosine to a site where it has to form melanin
- Various clinical forms of albinism have been recognized

These are: **Ocular, oculocutaneous and cutaneous**, depending on the tissue involved

- A. **Oculocutaneous**: Decreased pigmentation of skin and eyes
- B. **Ocular albinism**: Affects only eye and not the skin. Occurs both as autosomal recessive and as an X-linked trait

The albinos are abnormally sensitive to light; even a slight exposure to light causes burns and can lead to skin cancer

Pathway for the conversion of tyrosine to melanin in brief:

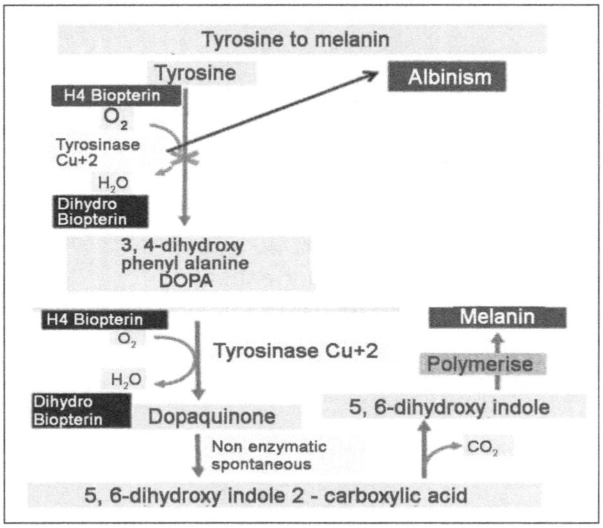

Ans: (a) Tyrosinase

Ref: *Textbook of Medical Biochemistry by Dinesh Puri, 3rd Edition,Chapter 13, Page 295-296 and Textbook of Medical Biochemistry by MN Chatterjee, 8th Edition, Chapter 27, page 503*

3. Abnormal glycogen stored in liver in all the following conditions *except:*

(a) Gaucher's disease (b) Cori's disease
(c) Mcardle's disease (d) Pompe's disease

Explanation:

Gaucher's disease

- Genetic disorder in which a **glucocerebroside** accumulates in the organs. It is due to the defect in **beta glucosidase**
- Glycogen storage diseases (GSDs): These are a group of inherited disorders associated with **glycogen metabolism**, familial in incidence and characterized by deposition of normal or abnormal type and quantity of glycogen in the tissues

Type I: Von Gierke's Disease

- Enzyme deficiency: **Glucose-6-phosphatase**
- Inheritance: **Autosomal recessive**
- Liver cells, intestinal mucosa and cells of renal tubular epithelial cells are loaded with glycogen which is normal in structure but metabolically not available
- **Features**
  - Since very little glucose is derived from the Liver, children with this disease tend to develop hypoglycaemia. **Glucose-1-P** cannot be converted to **glucose-6-P** due to deficiency of the enzyme and it is "**locked**" in the cells
  - **Fat** is utilised as energy source, which leads to **Lipaemia, Academia and Ketosis**
  - Excess acetyl-CoA is diverted for cholesterol synthesis resulting to **increase in cholesterol level**, which may produce **xanthomas**
  - Increased FA synthesis can produce **fatty infiltration of liver**
  - **Persistent hypoglycaemia** can have two effects:
    - Hypoglycaemia **inhibits insulin** secretion which in turn **inhibits protein synthesis** which causes **stunted growth (dwarfism)**
    - Hypoglycaemia stimulates secretion of **catecholamines**, which cause **muscle glycogen** to breakdown producing **Lactic acid** and **lactic acidosis**
  - **Increased blood Lactic acid** competes with **urate excretion** by kidneys leading to **increased** blood **uric acid level**. There is also evidence that there is increase in uric acid synthesis in those children who develop symptoms of gout

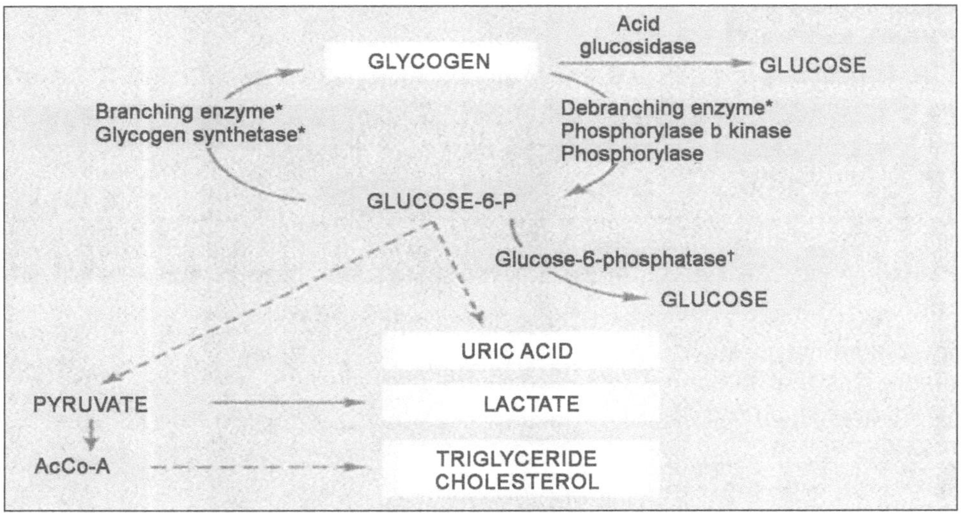

Prognosis: Although many of these children die young, a number of them have survived for adolescence, when for some unknown reason much improvement can occur

Other types of glycogen storage disorders as given in the table:

Table for Glycogen Storage Diseases			
Type: Name	**Enzyme Affected**	**Primary Organ**	**Manifestations**
Type 0	Glycogen synthase	Liver	Hypoglycemia, early death, hyperketonemia
Type Ia: von Gierke's	Glucose-6-phosphatase	Liver	Hepatomegaly, kidney failure, thrombocyte dysfunction
Type Ib	Microsomal glucose-6-phosphate translocase	Liver	Like Ia, also neutropenia, bacterial infections

Contd.

Contd.

Type Ic	Microsomal P_i transporter	Liver	Like Ia
Type II: Pompe's	Lysosomal α-1,4-glucosidase, lysosomal acid α glucosidase acid maltase	Skeletal and cardiac muscle	Infantile form = death by 2; juvenile form = myopathy; adult form = muscular dystrophy-like
Type IIIa: Cori's or Forbe's	Liver and muscle debranching enzyme	Liver, skeletal and cardiac muscle	Infant hepatomegaly, myopathy
Type IIIb	Liver debranching enzyme normal muscle enzyme	Liver, skeletal and cardiac muscle	Liver symptoms same as type IIIa
Type IV: Anderson's	Branching enzyme	Liver, muscle	Hepatosplenomegaly, cirrhosis
Type V: McArdle's	Muscle phosphorylase	Skeletal muscle	Excercise-induced cramps and pain, myoglobinuria
Type VI: Her's	Liver phosphorylase	Liver	hepatomegaly
Type VII: Tarui's	Muscle PFK-1	Muscle, RBC's	Like V, also hemolytic anemia
Type VIb, VIII or Type IX	Phosphorylase kinase	Liver, leukocytes, muscle	Like VI
Type XI: Fanconi-Bickel	Glucose transporter-2 (GLUT-2)	Liver	Failure to thrive, hepatomegaly, rickets, proximal renal tubular dysfunction

Ans: (a) Gaucher's disease

Ref: *Textbook of Medical Biochemistry by MN Chatterjee, 8th Edition, Chapter 23, page 353-355*

4. Which of the following will be raised in an overnight fasting patient compared with a patient who took meal?

(a) Glucose
(b) Insulin
(c) Triacylglycerol
(d) Non-esterified Free fatty acid

Explanation:

Following flow diagram explains various metabolisms that take place in different organs, both in well fed and fasting states:

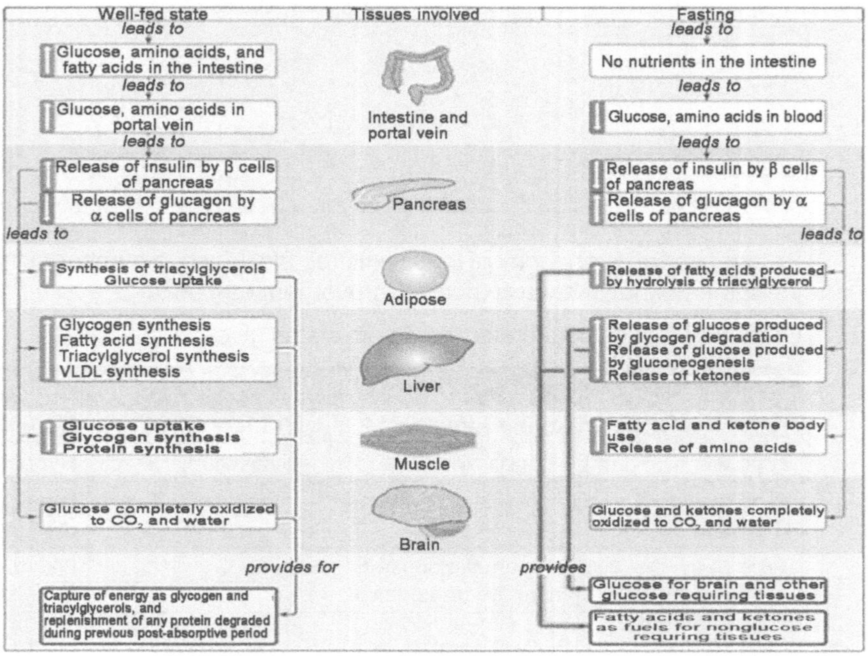

The graph below shows that glycogen is the source of energy for the first 24 hours of fasting. After depletion of glycogen stores, gluconeogenesis has a major role

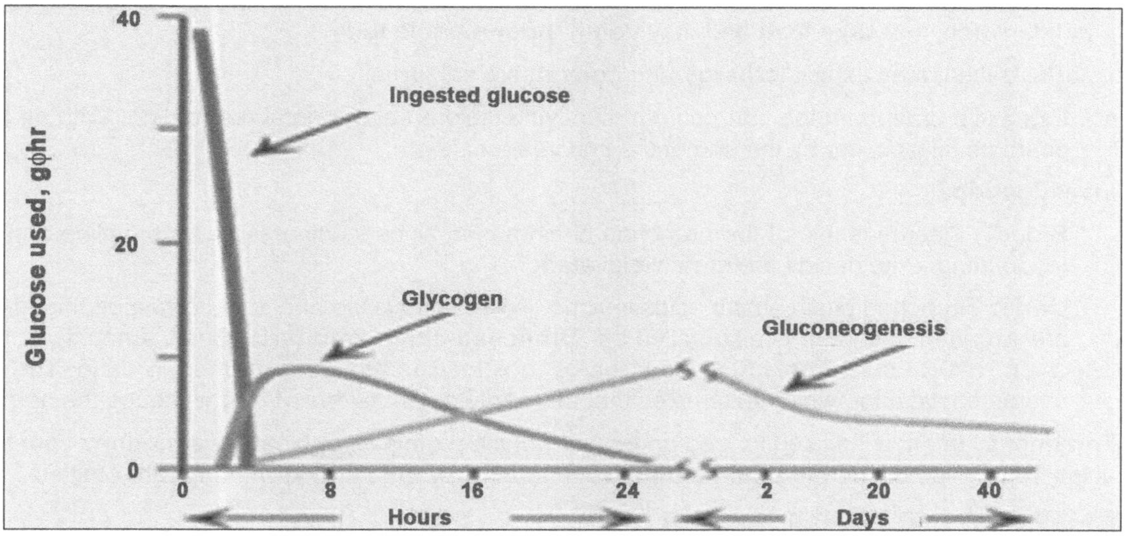

Substrates used in well fed state versus starvation

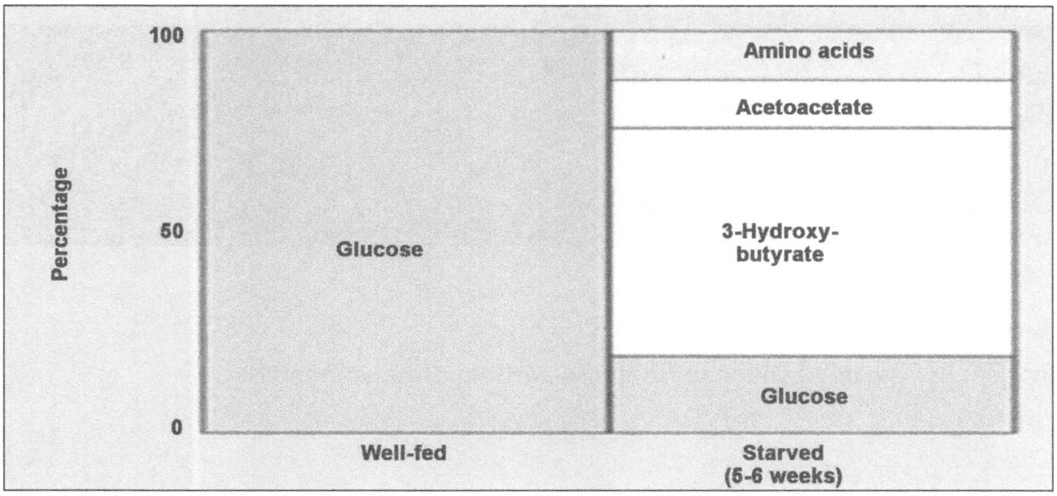

Ans: (d) Non-esterified Free fatty acid

Ref: *Lippincott's Illustrated Reviews, 5th Edition, Chapter 24, page 324-332*

5. A child presents with a history of irritability, developmental delay and urine with burnt sugar odor to a Pediatrics OPD. Which of the following is found to be reduced in blood?

(a) Valine (b) Leucine

(c) Isoleucine (d) Alpha ketoacid decarboxylase

Explanation:

Maple Syrup Urine Disease

- An inherited disorder of branched chain amino acids
- **Enzyme defect:** Absence of **alpha-ketoacid decarboxylase** (branched chain keto acid dehydrogenase complex) or greatly reduced activity of the enzyme. As a result, the conversion of all three branched chain α-ketoacids to CO_2 and acyl CoA-thioesters is interfered with

- **Clinical features:**
  - The disease is evident by the end of first week of extrauterine life
  - Infant does **not take feed** and may **vomit**, **poor muscle tone**
  - The patient may exhibit **lethargy** and **convulsive seizures**
  - Extensive brain damage can occur in surviving children and mental retardation. Without treatment, death usually occurs by the end of the first year of life
- **Investigations:**
  - **Blood:** Plasma levels of the branched chain amino acids leucine, isoleucine, valine and their corresponding α-ketoacids are greatly elevated
  - **Urine:** Branched chain amino acids leucine, isoleucine, valine and their corresponding α-ketoacids are excreted. Hence it is also called as **Branched-chain ketonuria**. Small amounts of branched-chain α-OH-acids, formed by reduction of α-ketoacids are also excreted in urine. The urine has characteristic odor, which resembles that of **maple syrup or burnt sugar**, hence the name
- **Treatment:** Infant is advised to feed on a diet in which protein is replaced by a mixture of purified amino acids from which **branched chain amino** acids **leucine, valine and isoleucine** are omitted

Ans: (d) Alpha ketoacid decarboxylase

Ref: *Textbook of Medical Biochemistry by MN Chatterjee, 8th Edition, Chapter 27, page 524-525*

6. All are features of gluconeogenesis *except:*

(a) Gluconeogenesis is synthesis of glucose from non-carbohydrate sources

(b) Mainly takes place in liver

(c) Seen in Fasting state

(d) Steps are simple reversal of glycolysis

Explanation:

Gluconeogenesis

- Definition: **Synthesis of Glucose from non-carbohydrate sources** like
  - Pyruvate
  - Lactate
  - Glycerol
  - Propionate
  - Amino acids (glucogenic)
- Site: Liver mainly; kidney; small amount epithelium of small intestine
- Sub cellular site: Partly mitochondrial and partly cytoplasmic
- **Salient features**
  - Not a reversal of glycolysis
  - Four key enzymes-pyruvate carboxylase, phosphoenol pyruvate carboxykinase, fructose 1,6 bisphosphatase, glucose 6 phosphatase
  - Continuous supply of glucose for brain, RBC, testes and kidney
  - Only source of energy to skeletal muscle, in anaerobic conditions
  - Maintains blood glucose in starvation
  - Intermediates of citric acid cycle
  - Removal of metabolites lactate, glycerol, propionate etc

- **Four major reactions:**
  - **Pyruvate Carboxylase** catalyzes:
    - **pyruvate + HCO_3^- + ATP → oxaloacetate + ADP + P_i**
  - **PEP Carboxykinase** catalyzes:
    - **oxaloacetate + GTP → PEP + GDP + CO_2**
  - **Fructose-1,6-bisphosphatase** catalyzes:
    - **fructose-1,6-bisP + H_2O → fructose-6-P + P_i**
  - **Glucose-6-Phosphatase** catalyzes:
    - **glucose-6-phosphate + H_2O → glucose + P_i**
- Other steps are reversal of glycolysis

Ans: (d) Steps are simple reversal of glycolysis

Ref: *Medical Biochemistry by Vasudevan, Chapter 9, page 118*

7. A patient report is as follows; FBS – 82; PPBS 140; Urine was found to be positive for benedict test. What is the probable diagnosis?

(a) Renal glycosuria (b) Transient glycosuria
(c) Alimentary glycosuria (d) DM

Explanation:

Glycosuria

- Definition: Glycosuria is defined as the excretion of glucose in urine which is detectable by **Benedict's Qualitative test**
- Glucose is present in the glomerular filtrate in the same concentration as in the blood plasma
- Under normal conditions, it undergoes practically complete reabsorption by the renal tubular epithelial cells and is returned to the blood stream
- In normal subjects, a very small amount less than 0.5 gm of glucose may escape reabsorption by tubules and be excreted by urine. But this amount is not detected by Benedict's qualitative test
- The reabsorption of glucose by tubular epithelial cells is an "active" process, by "carrier Protein" which is Na+ dependant and requires energy (similar to absorption of glucose by intestinal epithelial cells)
- Rate of glucose absorption is expressed as TmG (tubular maximum for glucose) which is 350 mg/min
- When the blood levels of glucose are elevated, the glomerular filtrate may contain more glucose than can be reabsorbed, the excess passes in urine to produce "glycosuria"
- In normal individuals, glycosuria occurs when the venous blood glucose exceeds 170 to 180 mg/100 ml. This level of the venous blood glucose is termed as the **renal threshold** for glucose
- Since the maximal rate of reabsorption of glucose by the tubule (TmG—the tubular maximum for glucose) is a constant, it is a more accurate measurement than the renal threshold, which varies with changes in the GFR

Mechanism of glycosuria

- Excretion of abnormal amounts of glucose in the urine may be due to two types of abnormalities: (a) Increase in the amount of glucose entering in the tubule/minute. (b) Decrease in the glucose reabsorption capacity of the renal tubular epithelium

Renal Glycosuria

- **Hereditary**: A milder glycosuria occurs spontaneously, as hereditary familial traits, persisting throughout life, due to absence of "carrier Protein" or altered kinetics of the carrier system due to failure of development

- **Acquired:** Diseases of renal tubules: In some cases of kidney diseases, the renal tubules may be grossly damaged, thus the tubules fail to reabsorb glucose producing glycosuria
- Due to heavy metal poisoning: The heavy metals like Lead (Pb), Cadmium (Cd), Mercury (Hg), etc. can damage the renal tubules thus interfering with the reabsorption of glucose, resulting to glycosuria
- **Lowering of renal threshold**: 15 to 20 per cent cases of Pregnancy may be associated with the physiological glycosuria with advancement of pregnancy, due to lowering of renal threshold. But Pregnancy may be associated with Diabetes mellitus in which there will be hyperglycaemic glycosuria. These two can be differentiated by performing a fasting plasma glucose level
- **Renal glycosuria**: It may also occur in association with evidences of other renal tubular transport defects, e.g. aminoacidurias, Renal tubular acidosis, hyperphosphaturia as in Fanconi syndrome
- '**Experimental' renal glycosuria**- "**phloridzin" glycosuria:** Phloridzin is a glycoside found in roots of apple tree; when hydrolysed it gives glucose and aglycone Phloretin. When phloridzin is administered subcutaneously, it gives rise to intense glycosuria. The dose given to dogs is 1 gm/day, in oil, SC. Mechanism: Phloridzin displaces sodium from the sodium binding site from "Carrier protein" and hence glucose cannot be bound to the glucose binding site, thus inhibiting glucose reabsorption. Mechanism: Phloridzin displaces sodium from the sodium binding site from "Carrier protein" and hence glucose cannot be bound to the glucose binding site, thus inhibiting glucose reabsorption

Diagnosis of Renal glycosuria:

- Fasting plasma glucose and postprandial blood sugar may be normal (<100 mg/dl and <140 mg/dl respectively) but Benedict's test for urine will be positive suggesting the inability of renal tubules to reabsorb glucose at a level, much below renal threshold (180 mg/dl)

Following table helps to differentiate below mentioned conditions

	Normal	**Impaired glucose tolerance**	**Diabetes mellitus**	**Renal glycosuria**
FBS (mg/dl)	<100	100-125	>126	<100
PPBS(mg/dl)	<140	140-199	>200	<140
Benedict's test	Negative	May be positive when glucose level is more than 180 mg/dl	Positive	Positive even when blood glucose is <180 mg/dl

Ans: (a) Renal glycosuria

Ref: *Textbook of Medical Biochemistry by MN Chatterjee, 8th Edition, Chapter 23, page 378*

8. Which of the following is a true statement?

(a) Glucokinase has high km as compared to hexokinase

(b) Hexokinase has high km compared to glucokinase

(c) Both the enzymes have equal Km

(d) Both the enzymes have equal affinity for glucose

Explanation:

- **Km and affinity bear** an **inverse relationship**
- Greater the Km, lesser is the affinity of the enzyme for its substrate. Glucokinase has higher Km and lesser affinity for glucose as compared to hexokinase
- Michaelis – Menten equation
  - $V0 = V_{max}[S] / k_m+[S]$
- V0 - the initial rate of the reaction

- V_{max} - the maximum rate (saturation)
- K_m – Michaelis menten constant
- The Michaelis constant:
- K_M = substrate concentration when reaction velocity is ½ V_{max}
- K_M is constant for any given enzyme
- Independent of substrate or enzyme concentration
- K_M provides a measure of the affinity of the enzyme for its substrate
- The higher is K_M, the higher is the concentration of the substrate required to reach ½ V_{max}
- That is: at a lower affinity, a higher concentration of substrate is required to reach ½ V_{max}
- ↓ Km ↑ affinity
- According to Michaelis theory, the formation of enzyme- substrate complex is a reversible reaction, while the breakdown of the complex to enzyme + product is irreversible. The lesser the numerical value of km, the affinity of the enzyme for the substrate is more. To cite an example, Km of glucokinase is 10 mmol/L and that of hexokinase is 0.05 mmol/L. Therefore, 50% molecules of hexokinase are saturated even at a lower concentration of glucose. In other words, hexokinase has more affinity for glucose than glucokinase
- Km is the signature of the enzyme

Ans: (a) Glucokinase has high km as compared to hexokinase

Ref: *Textbook of Medical Biochemistry by MN Chatterjee, 8th Edition, Chapter 9, page126*

9. Not true regarding procalcitonin:

(a) Precursor of calcitonin involved in calcium metabolism

(b) Half life is 25 to 36 hours

(c) Normal levels 0.1 – 1 ng/ml

(d) Increased in gut and lung inflammation

Explanation:

Procalcitonin

- Precursor of peptide hormone **calcitonin**
- Produced by **parafollicular of thyroid**
- It is a 116-amino-acid protein that is formed by cleavage of **preprocalcitonin** by **endopeptidase**.
- Its gene is located on **chromosome 11**
- The PCT plasma level in healthy individuals is low; usually below 0.1 ng/mL
- The levels have been shown to rise with severity of sepsis. Over the last decade, PCT has become increasingly popular as a novel marker of infection in the intensive care unit. It can be considered as acute phase protein
- PCT is markedly elevated in acute bacterial infections; but not in viral infections
- **Induction** time for procalcitonin is **4-12 hours** and **half life** is **22-36 hours**
- Procalcitonin (PCT) It is a relatively new marker that has been associated with inflammation and sepsis

Ans: (c) Normal levels 0.1 – 1 ng/ml

Ref: *Medical Biochemistry by Vasudevan, Chapter 39, page 507*

10. Heme synthesis is inhibited by all the following *except:*

(a) Heme (b) Glucose

(c) Succinyl CoA (d) Hematin

Explanation:

- **ALA synthase** is subject to end product repression and end product inhibition by **hematin** and **heme**
- Hematin and heme also **inhibit translocation of ALA synthase** from cytosol into mitochondria
- Glucose prevents depression when hematin and heme concentration is low. Therefore, has inhibitory effect on heme synthesis
- Heme concentration is decreased in case of alcohol, steroids or drug intake as it is being used for synthesis of cyt. P_{450}

	Heme synthesis
Heme, hematin	↓
Glucose	↓
Starvation	↑
Alcohol	↑
Drug intake	↑

Heme synthesis

- Site: All tissues except mature (mammal) erythrocytes, Prominent in liver and erythroid tissue of bone marrow
- Subcellular site: Partly mitochondrial, partly cytosolic
- Precursors: Glycine and Succinyl CoA
- A brief overview of heme synthesis and disorder associated with it is given below

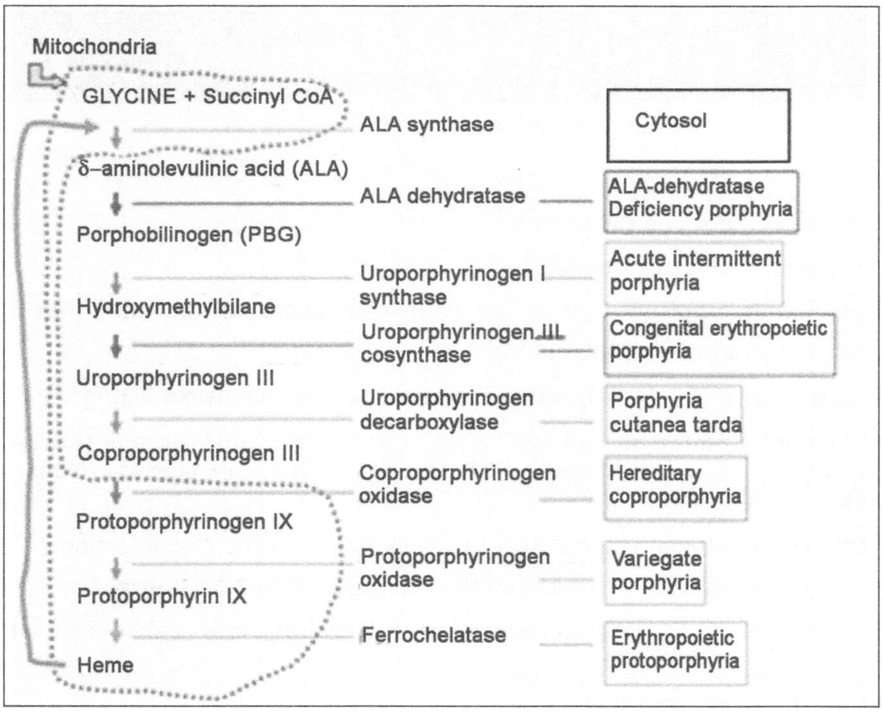

Ans: (c) Succinyl CoA

Ref: *Textbook of Medical Biochemistry by MN Chatterjee, 8th Edition, Chapter 30, page 543*

11. Ketone bodies are not utilized by:

(a) Brain
(b) RBC
(c) Heart
(d) Skeletal muscle

Explanation:

*"Unlike **fatty acids**, **ketone bodies** can be used by the **brain** (but **not** by cells, such as **red blood cells**, that **lack mitochondria**) and , thus are important **fuels** during a **fast**. The liver lacks the ability to degrade ketone bodies, and so synthesizes them specifically for the peripheral tissues"*

Ref: *Lippincott's Biochemistry, 3rd Edition, page 486*

Substrate utilized by various organs in different states

Organ	Fed State	Fasting	Starvation
Brain	Glucose	Glucose	Ketone bodies
Heart	Fatty acid	Fatty acid	Ketone bodies
Liver	Glucose	Fatty acid	Amino acid
Muscles	Glucose	Fatty acid	Fatty acid

Ketolysis

- Utilization of ketone bodies
- **Site**:
  - **Mitochondria**
  - **Extra hepatic tissue**
- Tissues
  - Heart
  - Brain (especially when starving)
  - Skeletal muscle
  - Renal cortex
- **Ketones** are **NOT** utilized by
  - **RBC** – Since it does **NOT** contain **Mitochondria**
  - **Liver** – Since it does **NOT** contain **thiophorase enzyme**

Note:

- **Liver** is the **ONLY organ** which produces **ketone bodies** and releases into **blood**, but it **lacks the enzyme** responsible (**Thiophorase**) for their degradration and utilization. This is the reason why liver does not utilize ketone bodies.

Ans: (b) RBC

Ref: *Harper's Illustrated Biochemistry, 27th Edition, page 190 and Lippincott's Biochemistry, 3rd Edition, page 486*

PHARMACOLOGY

1. Which of the following is not a peptide antimicrobial agent?

(a) Daptomycin (b) Cycloserine

(c) Colistin (d) Vancomycin

Explanation:

- Peptide antimicrobial agents (AMAs) are one, which contain protein(s) in their structure
- The therapeutically available peptide AMAs are:

Peptide AMAs	Chemical Nature
Vancomycin	Glycopeptide
Teicoplanin	
Bacitracin	Polypeptide(s)
Colistin	
Polymyxin B	
Daptomycin	Lipopeptide
Telavancin	Lipoglycopeptide
Dalbavancin	
Oritavancin	

- **Cycloserine:**
  - Antibiotic
  - Source: *S. orchidaceus*
  - Analogue of D-alanine
  - Second line antitubercular drug

Ans: (b) Cycloserine

Ref: *MacDougall C, Protein Synthesis Inhibitors and Miscellaneous Antibacterial Agents, In: Brunton LL, Hilal-Dandan R, Knollmann BC Editors, Goodman and Gilman's The Pharmacological Basis of Therapeutics, 13th Edition, New York, McGraw-Hill, 2018, page 1049-65*

2. Monoclonal antibody used in malignant ascites

(a) Panitumumab (b) Nivolumab

(c) Catumaxomab (d) Ramucirumab

(e) Trastuzumab

Explanation:

- **Catumaxomab:**
  - Monoclonal antibody against **CD3 and EpCAM**
  - Effective in the treatment of **neoplastic ascites**
- The therapeutically available monoclonal antibodies are:

Monoclonal Antibody	Target	Therapeutic Indication
Abciximab	GP IIb/IIIa	CVS disorders
Adalimumab	TNF -α	Rheumatoid Arthritis
Alemtuzumab	CD -52	CLL, Hematopoietic Transplantation
Basiliximab	IL -2	Transplant Rejection
Bevacizumab	VEGF	Colorectal Carcinoma
Cetuximab	EGFR	Colorectal Carcinoma
Daclizumab	IL -2	Transplant Rejection
Eculizumab	Complement (C5)	Inflammatory Disorders
Efalizumab	CD -11	Psoriasis
Gemtuzumab	CD -33	ALL
Ibritumomab	CD -20	Non-Hodgkin Lymphoma
Infliximab	TNF -α	Rheumatoid Arthritis
Muromonab	CD3	Organ Transplantation
Natalizumab	T cell VLA4 Receptor	Inflammatory Disorders
Nivolumab	PD -1	Colorectal Carcinoma, Renal Cell Carcinoma, Melanoma, Hepatocellular Carcinoma
Omalizumab	IgE	Inflammatory Disorders (Bronchial Asthma)
Panitumumab	EGFR	Colorectal Carcinoma
Palivizumab	F Protein of RSV	RSV Infection
Ramucirumab	VEGF	Solid tumors
Ranibizumab	VEGF	Macular Degeneration
Rituximab	CD -20	Resistant B Cell Follicular Lymphoma
Tositumomab	CD -20	Follicular and Non-Hodgkin's lymphoma
Trastuzumab	HER2/neu	HER2 receptor +ve cancers

Ans: (c) Catumaxomab

Ref: *Bellati F, Napoletano C, Gasparri ML, Visconti V, Zizzari IG, Ruscito I et al., Monoclonal Antibodies in Gynecological Cancer, A Critical Point of View, Clin Dev Immunol 2011, 1(1) :1-16*

3. Which drug dose should be reduced if taken along with allopurinol or febuxostat?

(a) Methotrexate (b) 6-Mercaptopurine

(c) 5- Fluorouracil (d) 6-Thioguanine

Explanation:

- **Allopurinol:**
  - Uric acid synthesis inhibitor
  - **MOA:**
    - Inhibits the xanthine oxidase enzyme, which is responsible for the synthesis of uric acid
  - **Pharmacokinetics:**
    - Oral absorption: 80%
    - Plasma $t_{1/2}$: 2 hours
  - **Drug Interactions:**

- Inhibits the metabolism of **Azathioprine** and **6-Mercaptopurine** and hence their doses should be reduced by one third
- **Along with probenecid:** Allopurinol (↑) the half life of probenecid, while probenecid (↓) half life of allopurinol
- Inhibits the metabolism of Warfarin and Theophylline

– **ADRs:**
  - Hypersensitivity reactions
  - GIT disturbances
  - Stevens-Johnson syndrome (*Rare*)
  - Hepatotoxicity (*Rare*)

- **Febuxostat**:
  – **MOA:**
    - Inhibits xanthine oxidase enzyme, which is responsible for the synthesis of uric acid
  – **Pharmacokinetics:**
    - Oral absorption: Good
    - Plasma $t_{1/2}$: 6 hours
  – **Drug Interactions:**
    - Inhibits the metabolism of **Azathioprine**, **6-Mercaptopurine and Theophylline**
  – **ADRs:**
    - GIT disturbances, hepatotoxicity (*Common*)
    - Hypersensitivity reactions (*Rare*)

Ans: (b) 6-Mercaptopurine

Ref: *Grosser T, Smyth EM, FitzGerald GA, Pharmacotherapy of Inflammation, Fever, Pain and Gout, In: Brunton LL, Hilal-Dandan R, Knollmann BC Editors, Goodman and Gilman's The Pharmacological Basis of Therapeutics, 13th Edition, New York, McGraw-Hill, 2018, page 685-709*

4. Hemodialysis is not effective in:

(a) Aminophylline/Theophylline (b) Carbamazepine
(c) Digoxin (d) Lithium

Explanation:

- ***Hemodialysis is effective in the poisoning of:***
  – Vancomycin
  – Gentamicin
  – Lithium
  – Aspirin
  – Theophylline/Aminophylline
  – Carbamazepine
  – Valproic acid
  – Metformin
  – Methotrexate

- ***Hemodialysis is not effective in digoxin toxicity due to following reasons:***
  - High volume of distribution (7 L/Kg)
  - Because of high volume of distribution, digoxin is highly concentrated in the tissues like heart, liver, skeletal muscle and kidney; This makes difficult to remove the drug from the body

Ans: (c) Digoxin

Ref: *Bunchman TE, Ferris ME, Management of Toxic Ingestions with the Use of Renal Replacement Therapy, Pediatr Nephrol 2011, 26: 535-41*

5. In which of the following the therapeutic dose of antidepressant drug is correctly matched

(a) Fluoxetine – 2.5-10 mg
(b) Fluvoxamine – 10-20 mg
(c) Amitriptyline – 75-200 mg
(d) Nortriptyline – 10-50 mg

Explanation:

- The therapeutic dose(s) of antidepressant drugs are as follows:

Antidepressant Drug(s)	Therapeutic Dose (mg)
Tricyclic Antidepressants (TCAs)	
Clomipramine	
Dothiepin	
Doxepin	50 -150
Nortriptyline	
Trimipramine	
Amitriptyline	50 -200
Imipramine	
Selective Serotonin Reuptake Inhibitors (SSRIs)	
Escitalopram	10 -20
Citalopram	
Fluoxetine	20 -40
Paroxetine	20 -50
Sertraline	50 -150
Fluvoxamine	50 -200
Serotonin and Noradrenaline Reuptake Inhibitors (SNRIs)	
Duloxetine	30 -80
Venlafaxine	75 -150
Atypical Antidepressants	
Mirtazapine	15 -45
Mianserin	30 -100
Trazodone	50 -200
Amoxapine	100 -300
Bupropion	150 -300

Ans: (c) Amitriptyline – 75-200 mg

Ref: *Tripathi KD, Essentials of Medical Pharmacology, 8th Edition, New Delhi, Jaypee Brothers Medical Publishers, 2019, page 486*

6. A patient on haloperidol developed ataxia, dystonia, muscle rigidity, akathisia and hyperprolactinemia. Which drug will be tolerated in this situation?

(a) Chlorpromazine
(b) Lurasidone
(c) Fluphenazine
(d) Lithium

Explanation:

- **Haloperidol:**
  - It is a antipsychotic drug
  - Acts by blocking **D_2 receptors** in the CNS
  - Most of the extrapyramidal side effects (Like *Parkinsonism, muscular dystonia, akathisia and hyper-prolactinemia*) are due to the blockade of D_2 receptors
- Drugs which blocks the D_2 receptors, are more commonly used as antipsychotic agents therapeutically and which in turn have more tendency to produce extrapyramidal side effects include:

Antipsychotic Drug(s)	
Phenothiazines	Chlorpromazine
	Fluphenazine
	Perphenazine
	Trifluoperazine
First-Generation Agents	Haloperidol
	Loxapine
	Thiothixene
Second-Generation Agents	Lurasidone
	Cariprazine
	Risperidone

- **Lithium:**
  - It is used in mania and bipolar disorders
  - It do not have any action on D_2 receptors and hence no extrapyramidal side effects

Ans: (d) Lithium

Ref: *Meyer JM, Pharmacotherapy of Psychosis and Mania, In: Brunton LL, Hilal-Dandan R, Knollmann BC Editors, Goodman and Gilman's The Pharmacological Basis of Therapeutics, 13th Edition, New York, McGraw-Hill; 2018, page 279-302*

7. Therapeutic range of phenytoin is:

(a) 10 -20 mcg/ml
(b) 20 to 40 mcg/ml
(c) 40 to 60 mcg/ml
(d) 20 to 40 ng/ml

Explanation:

- Clinically established therapeutic range of common anti-seizure drugs are as follows:

Anti-Seizure Drug(s)	Therapeutic Range
(In ng/mL)	
Clonazepam	10–70
(In μg/mL)	
Carbamazepine	4–12
Primidone	

Contd.

Contd.

Phenytoin	10–20
Lamotrigine	2.5–20
Gabapentin	2–20
Topiramate	
Oxcarbazepine	10–35
Phenobarbital	10–40
Zonisamide	
Felbamate	30–60
Levetiracetam	5–45
Ethosuximide	40–100
Valproic acid	50–125

Ans: (a) 10 -20 mcg/ml

Ref: *Lowenstein DH, Seizures and Epilepsy, In: Jameson JL, Kasper DL, Longo DL, Fauci AS, Hauser SL, Loscalzo J Editors, Harrison's Principles of Internal Medicine Vol II, 20th Edition, New York, McGraw-Hill, 2018, page 3050-68*

8. Time dependent pharmacokinetics is seen with:

(a) Aminoglycosides (b) Fluoroquinolones

(c) Metronidazole (d) β-Lactams

Explanation:

- The pharmacokinetic exhibition of Antimicrobial Agents (AMAs) is as follows:

Pharmacokinetic Profile	Examples
Concentration Dependent Killing (It is the ratio of peak concentration of AMA and MIC at the site of action)	Fluoroquinolones
	Aminoglycosides
	Metronidazole
Time Dependent Killing (It is the time of AMA concentration which remains higher to the MIC at the site of action)	Macrolides
	β-Lactams
	Glycopeptides

Ans: (d) β-Lactams

Ref: *Tripathi KD, Essentials of Medical Pharmacology, 8th Edition, New Delhi, Jaypee Brothers Medical Publishers, 2019, page 748*

9. Protein synthesis inhibitor used in CML:

(a) Omacetaxine (b) Panobinostat

(c) Bortezomib (d) Carfilzomib

Explanation:

- **Omacetaxine:**
  - **Protein translation inhibitor**: Inhibits total **protein biosynthesis** by binding to A-site cleft of ribosomes
  - Clinically used in **CML**

- FDA approved for **Philadelphia-positive CML** either in **chronic** or **accelerated** phase whose disease failed prior with TKIs (*Like Imatinib, dasatinib, nilotinib and ponatinib*)
- Route of administration: **Subcutaneous**
- Tmax (*Time taken to reach maximum plasma concentration at therapeutic doses*): 1 hour
- $t_{1/2}$: 7 Hours

- ***Other protein synthesis inhibitors studied for treatment of hematological malignancies:***
  - Silvestrol
  - Hippuristanol
  - Pateamine A
- **Panobinostat:**
  - Oral non-selective histone deacetylase inhibiotor
  - ***Clinical Indications:*** Multiple myeloma
- **Bortezomib:**
  - First therapeutic proteasome inhibitor tested in human clinical trials
  - ***Clinical Indications:*** Relapsed cases of multiple myeloma and mantle cell lymphoma
- **Carfilzomib:**
  - Selective proteasome inhibitor
  - ***Clinical Indications:*** Relapsed/Refractory cases of multiple myeloma

Ans: (a) Omacetaxine

Ref: *Gandhi V, Plunkett W, Cortes JE, Omacetaxine: A Protein translation Inhibitor for Treatment of Chronic Myelogenous Leukemia, Clin Cancer Res 2014, 20, 1735-40*

10. Most Common side effect of Bedaquiline is:

(a) QT prolongation (b) Rashes

(c) Hemoptysis (d) Arthralgia

Explanation:

Bedaquiline

- **MOA of Bedaquiline:** (–) Mycobacterial ATP synthase
- **Mechanism of Resistance:**
  - Mutation in the ATP synthase enzyme
  - Drug efflux
- **Pharmacokinetics:**
  - Good oral absorption
  - ***Plasma protein binding:*** High
  - ***Metabolism:*** Liver [CY3A4]
  - ***Terminal $t_{1/2}$:*** Long [160 days]
  - ***Excretion:*** Feces
- **Indications:**
  - Pulmonary MDR-TB in adults

- **Precaution:**
  - Always should be combined with at least three/four other susceptible antitubercular drugs as per culture sensitivity pattern to enhance the efficacy and reduce the resistance pattern
- **Dosage and Regimen:**
  - Initially 400 mg/day for 2 weeks
  - Then 200 mg three times/week for next 22 weeks
  - Total duration of therapy is 24 weeks
- **ADRs:**
  - **Mild:** Nausea (30%), headache (22%), arthralgia (26%), Anorexia (7%)
  - Hemoptysis (14%)
  - Chest pain (9%)
  - Rash (6%)
  - ECG changes: QTc prolongation
  - Hepatotoxicity

Ans: (d) Arthralgia

Ref: *Deoghare S, Bedaquiline: A New Drug Approved for Treatment of Multidrug-Resistant Tuberculosis, Indian J Pharmacol 2013, 45, 536-37*

11. Which of the following drug is not metabolized by plasma esterases?

(a) Esmolol (b) Clevidipine
(c) Mepivacaine (d) Remifentanil

Explanation:

Local Anaesthetics:

- ***Ester Linked Anaesthetics*** *(Undergo hydrolysis by plasma esterases):*
  - Cocaine
  - Procaine
  - Tetracaine
  - Benzocaine
  - Chloroprocaine
- ***Amide Linked Anaesthetics:***
  - **Includes:** Lignocaine, Dibucaine, Ropivacaine, Prilocaine, Bupivacaine, Mepivacaine
  - **Common Characteristics of Amide Linked Anaesthetics:**
    - Binds to plasma α-1 acid glycoprotein
    - Have longer lasting anesthesia
    - Hypersensitivity reactions (*Rare*)
    - No cross sensitivity with ester LAs
    - Do not undergo hydrolysis by plasma esterases
- **Drugs metabolized by plasma esterases:**
  - Esmolol
  - Clevidipine
  - Remifentanil

- Aspirin
- Heroin
- Rivastimine
- Carbimazole
- Enalapril
- *Ester linked local anaesthetics*

[**Note:** Amide Linked LAs contains (Two i) in their names; while Ester linked LAs contains only (Single i) in their names)]

Ans: (c) Mepivacaine

Ref: *Catterall WA, Mackie K, Local Anesthetics, In: Brunton LL, Hilal-Dandan R, Knollmann BC Editors, Goodman and Gilman's The Pharmacological Basis of Therapeutics, 13th Edition, New York, McGraw-Hill, 2018, page 405-19*

12. All the following β-2 agonists are approved in specified dosage(s) by the World Anti-Doping Agency (WADA) in athletes *except:*

(a) Inhaled salmeterol
(b) Inhaled formoterol
(c) Inhaled salbutamol
(d) Inhaled bambuterol

Explanation:

- *All selective and non-selective **beta-2 agonists**, including all **optical isomers**, are prohibited by the World Anti-Doping Agency (WADA) for use in athletes to enhance their athletic performance and the list is as follows:*
  - Fenoterol
  - Formoterol
  - Indacaterol
  - Olodaterol
  - Procaterol
  - Reproterol
  - Salbutamol
  - Salmeterol
  - Terbutaline
  - Tretoquinol
  - Tulobuterol
  - Vilanterol
  - Bambuterol
- **However the exception to the above list is:**
  - Inhaled **Salbutamol**: *Maximum 1600 micrograms over 24 hours; in divided doses not to exceed 800 micrograms over 12 hours starting from any dose*
  - Inhaled **Formoterol**: *Maximum delivered dose of 54 micrograms over 24 hours*
  - Inhaled **Salmeterol**: *Maximum 200 micrograms over 24 hours*

Ans: (d) Inhaled bambuterol

Ref: *World Anti-Doping Agency, Prohibited at All Times (Beta -2 Agonists) [webpage on internet] 2020 [cited on 2020 April 12] Available from: https://www.wada-ama.org/en/content/what-is-prohibited/prohibited-at-all-times/beta-2-agonists*

13. Which of the following is on WHO priority list while looking for formation of new antibiotics?

(a) MRSA
(b) VRE
(c) Carbapenem Resistant –*Acinetobacter baumannii*
(d) Ampicillin Resistant–*Haemophilus influenzae*
(e) Clarithromycin Resistant–*Helicobacter pylori*

Explanation:

- The WHO published the list of bacteria for which new antibiotics are urgently needed
- **WHO priority pathogens list for research and development of new antibiotics includes:**
  - **Priority 1: CRITICAL**
    - *Acinetobacter baumannii*, carbapenem-resistant
    - *Pseudomonas aeruginosa*, carbapenem-resistant
    - *Enterobacteriaceae*, carbapenem-resistant, ESBL-producing
  - **Priority 2: HIGH**
    - *Enterococcus faecium*, vancomycin-resistant
    - *Staphylococcus aureus*, methicillin-resistant, vancomycin-intermediate and resistant
    - *Helicobacter pylori*, clarithromycin-resistant
    - *Campylobacter* spp., fluoroquinolone-resistant
    - *Salmonellae*, fluoroquinolone-resistant
    - *Neisseria gonorrhoeae*, cephalosporin-resistant, fluoroquinolone-resistant
  - **Priority 3: MEDIUM**
    - *Streptococcus pneumoniae*, penicillin-non-susceptible
    - *Haemophilus influenzae*, ampicillin-resistant
    - *Shigella* spp., fluoroquinolone-resistant

Ans: (c) Carbapenem Resistant–*Acinetobacter baumannii*

Ref: *World Health Organization, WHO publishes list of bacteria for which new antibiotics are urgently needed [webpage on internet] 2020 [cited on 2020 April 12] Available from: https://www.who.int/news-room/detail/27-02-2017-who-publishes-list-of-bacteria-for which-new-antibiotics-are-urgently-needed*

14. Antimicrobial agent with MAO inhibitor activity is:

(a) Polymyxin B
(b) Linezolid
(c) Quinupristin
(d) Colistin
(e) Bacitracin

Explanation:

Linezolid:

- Synthetic oxazolidinone
- **Antimicrobial Spectrum:**
  - Resistant gram-positive coccal (*Aerobic and anaerobic*)
  - Bacillary infections
  - MRSA, VRSA, VRE
  - Penicillin-resistant *Strep. Pyogenes*

- *Strep. Viridians, Strep. Pneumoniae, M. tuberculosis*
- *Corynebacterium, Listeria*
- *Clostridia, Bact. fragilis*

- **Mechanism of Action:**
  - Inhibition of bacterial protein synthesis (*Binds at 50S ribosomal subunit*)
  - Bacteriostatic and can be cidal against few microorganisms
- **Pharmacokinetics:**
  - Good oral absorption (*Oral bioavailability =100%*)
  - Plasma $t_{1/2}$ =5 hours
  - Safe in renal failure
- **Adverse Drug Reactions (ADRs):**
  - GIT disturbances
  - Hypersensitivity reactions
  - ***Hematological:*** Neutropenia, anaemia and thrombocytopenia
  - Candidiasis (*Oral and vaginal*) on prolonged use
  - ***Ophthalmological (Optic neuropathy):*** On prolonged use for more than four weeks
  - ***Drug Interactions:***
    - Linezolid is a MAO inhibitor and hence interactions with adrenergic/serotonergic drugs (SSRIs, etc.) is possible

Ans: (b) Linezolid

Ref: *MacDougall C, Protein Synthesis Inhibitors and Miscellaneous Antibacterial Agents, In: Brunton LL, Hilal-Dandan R, Knollmann BC Editors, Goodman and Gilman's The Pharmacological Basis of Therapeutics, 13th Edition, New York, McGraw-Hill, 2018, page 1049-65*

15. False statement on dronabinol:

(a) Act as cannabinoid receptors -1 (CB_1) antagonist

(b) Used for treatment of nausea, vomiting due to cancer chemotherapy in cancer patients

(c) Appetite stimulant in AIDS patients

(d) Synthetic cannabinoid

Explanation:

Dronabinol (Δ-9-tetrahydrocannabinol):

- Natural cannabinoid and can be synthetic from the marijuana
- Cannabinoid receptor agonist (CB_1 and CB_2)
- **Antiemetic MOA:** CB_1 agonism in brain (CTZ and emetic centre)
- **Pharmacokinetics:**
  - Highly lipid soluble
  - Good oral absorption; However oral bioavailability is only (10 -20%) due to extensive first pass metabolism
  - ***Onset of action:*** Within an hour
  - ***Cmax:*** 2 -4 hours
  - ***Major route of excretion:*** Biliary-fecal

- *High plasma protein binding:* More than 95%
- *Avd:* Large

- **Clinical Indications:**
  - Chemotherapy induced nausea and vomiting
  - Appetite stimulant in AIDS and anorexia patients
- **Therapeutic Dose** *(As an antiemetic):*
  - Initial 5 mg/m^2 before 1–3 hour of chemotherapy and then every 2–4 hour afterwards for a maximum of 4 to 6 doses in 24 hours
- **Adverse Drug Reactions (ADRs):**
  - Central sympathomimetic action (*Palpitations, tachycardia*)
  - Later vasodilation, hypotension and bleeding into the conjunctiva
  - Marijuana-like effects (*Euphoria, somnolence, detachment, dizziness, anxiety, nervousness, panic attacks including paranoid reactions and abnormalities of thinking*)
  - Withdrawal syndrome (*Irritability, insomnia and restlessness*)
  - Protein displacement reactions due to its high nature of binding to plasma proteins

Ans: (a) Act as cannabinoid receptors -1 (CB1) antagonist

Ref: *Sharkey KA, MacNaughton WK, Gastrointestinal Motility and Water Flux, Emesis, and Biliary and Pancreatic Disease, In: Brunton LL, Hilal-Dandan R, Knollmann BC editors, Goodman and Gilman's The Pharmacological Basis of Therapeutics, 13th Edition, New York: McGraw-Hill, 2018, page 921-44*

16. Most potent and longest acting bisphosphonates is:

(a) Alendronate (b) Risedronate

(c) Pamidronate (d) Zoledronate

Explanation:

Bisphosphonates (BPNs):

- Group of drugs used for prevention of osteoporosis including in the management of hypercalcaemia and metabolic bone disorders
- Some of the BPNs with their potency is depicted in the following table:

Generation(s)	BPNs	Potency
1st	Etidronate	1
	Tiludronate	10
2nd	Pamidronate	10 -100
	Alendronate	10 -100
	Ibandronate	500 -1000
3rd	Risedronate	10000
	Zoledronate	10000

- **Therapeutic Uses:**
  - **Osteoporosis:**
    - Mainly 2nd and 3rd generation BPNs are preferred because of their additional mechanisms and higher efficacy

- **Hypercalcaemia:**
  - Etidronate, Zoledronate, Pamidronate
  - Pamidronate Dose: IV infusion of 60–90 mg over 2–24 hour
- **Paget's Disease:**
  - Tiludronate, Alendronate, Risedronate, Zoledronate

- **Standard Doses:**
  - ***Pamidronate:*** IV infusion of 60–90 mg over 2–24 hour (Hypercalcaemia)
  - ***Tiludronate:*** 400 mg/d orally for 3 months (*Hypercalcaemia*)
  - ***Ibandronate:*** 3 mg IV every 3 months (*Osteoporosis*)
  - ***Zoledronate:*** 5 mg IV every 12 months (*Osteoporosis*)
  - ***Zoledronate:*** Single 5-mg infusion, (↓) bone turnover markers for 6 months with no loss of therapeutic effect (*In Paget's disease*)

Ans: (d) Zoledronate

Ref: *Nolin TD, Friedman PA, Agents Affecting Mineral Ion Homeostasis and Bone Turnover, In: Brunton LL, Hilal-Dandan R, Knollmann BC Editors, Goodman and Gilman's The Pharmacological Basis of Therapeutics, 13th Edition, New York, McGraw-Hill, 2018, page 887-906*

17. True statement regarding bisphosphonates use in osteoporosis is:

(a) Inhibit farnesyl pyrophosphate synthetase (b) Reduce the effect of osteoprotegrin
(c) Causes apoptosis of osteoclasts (d) Stimulates osteoblasts

Explanation:

Bisphosphonates (BPNs):

- Group of drugs used for prevention of osteoporosis including in the management of hypercalcaemia and metabolic bone disorders
- **Mechanism of Action:**
  - BPNs have strong affinity for bone Ca^{2+} and undergo internalization within osteoclasts by process of endocytosis, resulting into apoptosis of osteoclasts
  - BPNs also disrupts the cytoskeleton structures including vesicle movement and membrane ruffling of the osteoclasts triggering their apoptosis
  - BPNs also inhibits the IL -6, which is an essential cytokine for differentiation of osteoclasts
  - BPNs also interferes in the process of lipid biosynthesis through affecting the mevalonate pathway; This action is mainly responsible for its antineoplastic activity specially in bony metastasis
- **Pharmacokinetics:**
  - Poor oral absorption
  - ***Oral Bioavailability <1%:*** Alendronate, Risedronate
  - ***Oral Bioavailability 6%:*** Etidronate, Tiludronate
  - Further oral bioavailability is hampered by food, divalent cations, iron and antacids
  - Hence BPNs ideally should be taken following overnight fasting and at least half an hour before the breakfast
- **Adverse Drug Reactions (ADRs):**
  - GIT (Gastritis, esophagitis, abdominal pain, loose stools./constipation)
  - ***On IV administration:*** Flushing, flue like symptoms, arthralgia, GIT upset

- Renal toxicity and hypocalcaemia (*Zoledronate*)
- Osteonecrosis of the jaw (*Rare; 2 in 1 Lakh Patient-Years*)
- Stress fractures in the lateral cortex of the femoral shaft (*Most common with Alendronate and least with Zoledronate*)

Ans: (c) Causes apoptosis of osteoclasts

Ref: *Nolin TD, Friedman PA, Agents Affecting Mineral Ion Homeostasis and Bone Turnover, In: Brunton LL, Hilal-Dandan R, Knollmann BC editors. Goodman and Gilman's The Pharmacological Basis of Therapeutics, 13th Edition, New York: McGraw-Hill, 2018, page 887-906,* (**NOTE:** Also refer previous MCQ No. 16)

18. Shortest acting Opioids is:

(a) Remifentanil (b) Sufentanil
(c) Alfentanil (d) Fentanyl

Explanation:

Opioid Analgesics:

- Used mainly as analgesics, as part of balanced anaesthesia
- Their use in anaesthesia reduces the total dose requirement of general anesthetics and hence further reduces their adverse effects
- Important parenteral opioid preparations used in perioperative period includes:
  - Fentanyl
  - Sufentanil
  - Alfentanil
  - Remifentanil
  - Meperidine (Pethidine)
  - Morphine
- **Mechanism of Action:** μ opioid receptors agonism
- The duration of action of commonly used opioids is as follows:

Opioid(s)	Duration of Action (min)
Remifentanil	< 10
Alfentanil	15
Sufentanil	20
Fentanyl	30
	(In Hours)
Pethidine	2 -4
Pentazocine	3 -5
Morphine	4 -6
Tramadol	
Methadone	
Buprenorphine	6 -8

Ans: (a) Remifentanil

Ref: *Patel HH, Pearn ML, Patel PM, Roth DM, General Anesthetics and Therapeutic Gases. In: Brunton LL, Hilal-Dandan R, Knollmann BC Editors, Goodman and Gilman's The Pharmacological Basis of Therapeutics, 13th Edition, New York: McGraw-Hill, 2018, page 387-404*

19. Anaerobes show intrinsic resistance to:

(a) Ampicillin + Clavulanate (b) Aminoglycosides
(c) Meropenem (d) Metronidazole

Explanation:

Aminoglycosides:

- Antimicrobial agents against gram negative aerobic microorganisms
- ***The available class of drugs include***:
  - Streptomycin, Tobramycin, Kanamycin, Neomycin, Paromomycin
  - Amikacin, Netilmicin, Sisomicin, Gentamicin
- **Mechanism of Action:**
  - Protein synthesis inhibition [*Binds to 30S ribosomal subunit (Streptomycin) and rest aminoglycosides at 30S -50S ribosomal interface*]
  - Misreading of mRNA
  - Bactericidal
  - The efficacy of aminoglycosides depends on the entry of the drug into the microorganism(s) and this entry requires oxygen molecule (*Oxygen dependent process*); Hence aminoglycosides have their intrinsic antimicrobial spectrum only against oxygen producing microorganisms (i.e aerobic microorganism);
- **Common ADRs:**
  - Ototoxicity (*Irreversible*)
  - Nephrotoxicity (*Reversible*)
  - Neuromuscular toxicity (*Due to inhibition of release of Ach from the presynaptic terminals*)
- **Drugs Effective Against Anaerobes Include:**

Drugs For Anaerobes	
Carbapenems	Imiprenem
	Meropenem
	Ertapenem
β-Lactams along with *β-Lactamase inhibitors*	Ampicillin/Ticarcillin + Clavulanate
	Amoxicillin + Sulbactam
	Piperacillin + Tazobactam
Others	Chloramphenicol
	Metronidazole
	Tigecycline
	Clindamycin

Ans: (b) Aminoglycosides

Ref: *MacDougall C. Aminoglycosides, In: Brunton LL, Hilal-Dandan R, Knollmann BC Editors, Goodman and Gilman's The Pharmacological Basis of Therapeutics, 13th Edition, New York, McGraw-Hill, 2018, page 1039-47*

20. Concentration dependent killing is seen with:

(a) β-Lactams (b) Fluoroquinolones
(c) Macrolides (d) Vancomycin

Explanation:

- The pharmacokinetic exhibition of Antimicrobial Agents (AMAs) is as follows:

Pharmacokinetic Profile	Examples
Concentration Dependent Killing (It is the ratio of peak concentration of AMA and MIC at the site of action)	Fluoroquinolones
	Aminoglycosides
	Metronidazole
Time Dependent Killing (It is the time of AMA concentration which remains higher to the MIC at the site of action)	Macrolides
	β-Lactams
	Glycopeptides

Ans: (b) Fluoroquinolones

Ref: *Tripathi KD, Essentials of Medical Pharmacology, 8th Edition, New Delhi, Jaypee Brothers Medical Publishers, 2019, page 748*

21. Proteasome inhibitor

(a) Romidepsin (b) Omacetaxine
(c) Panobinostat (d) Bortezomib

Explanation:

- **Bortezomib:**
  - First therapeutic proteasome inhibitor tested in human clinical trials
  - ***Clinical Indications:*** Relapsed cases of multiple myeloma and mantle cell lymphoma
- **Romidepsin:**
  - Natural compound obtained from *Chromobacterium violaceum* (Bacteria)
  - ***Mechanism of Action:*** Histone deacetylase inhibiotor
  - ***Clinical Indications:*** Cutaneous T–Cell lymphoma, Other peripheral T –Cell lymphomas
- **Omacetaxine:**
  - ***Protein Translation Inhibitor:*** Inhibits total protein biosynthesis by binding to A-site cleft of ribosomes
  - Clinically used in CML
  - FDA approved for Philadelphia-positive CML either in chronic or accelerated phase whose disease failed prior with TKIs (*like Imatinib, dasatinib, nilotinib and ponatinib*)
  - ***Route of administration:*** Subcutaneous
  - ***Tmax*** (Time taken to reach maximum plasma concentration at therapeutic doses): 1 hour
  - $t_{1/2}$: 7 Hours
- **Other protein synthesis inhibitors studied for treatment of hematological malignancies:**
  - Silvestrol
  - Hippuristanol
  - Pateamine A
- **Panobinostat:**
  - ***Mechanism of Action:*** Oral non-selective histone deacetylase inhibiotor
  - ***Clinical Indications:*** Multiple myeloma

(**NOTE:** Also refer previous MCQ No. 9)

Ans: (d) Bortezomib

Ref: *Kubiczkova L, Pour L, Sedlarikova L, Hajek R, Sevcikova S, Proteasome Inhibitors: Molecular Basis and Current Perspectives in Multiple Myeloma, J Cell Mol Med 2014, 18, 947-61*

22. A patient took excess metoprolol and developed bradycardia and hypotension. Which drug is used to reverse the overdose symptoms?

(a) Glucagon (b) Atropine

(c) Adrenaline (d) Noradrenaline

Explanation:

- **Atropine:**
  - Universal antimuscarinic drug
  - (↑) Heart rate
  - Little or no effect on BP
- **Isoproterenol (Isoprenaline):**
  - Non-selective β receptor agonist
  - (↑) Heart rate
  - (↓) Mean BP
- **Glucagon:**
  - Endocrinal hormone
  - (↑) Heart rate
  - (↑) Myocardial contractility
  - Improves atrioventricular conduction
- **Adrenaline (Epinephrine):**
  - Nonselective α and β receptor agonist
  - (↑) Heart rate
  - (↑) Mean BP
  - Associated with cardiac toxicity in higher doses
- **Noradrenaline (Norepinephrine):**
  - Nonselective α and β receptor agonist (Except at β_2)
  - (↑) Heart rate
  - (↑) Mean BP
  - Associated with cardiac toxicity in higher doses
- **Beta Blocker Toxicity:**
  - Associated with cardiovascular depression (*Hypotension, bradycardia, heart failure, impaired atrioventricular conduction*), bronchospasm and rarely seizures
  - Glucagon is the most safer and effective therapy in reversing the symptoms of beta blocker(s) toxicity and this action is independent of the β receptors

Ans: (a) Glucagon

Ref: *Peterson CD, Leeder JS, Sterner S, Glucagon Therapy for Beta-blocker Overdose, Drug Intell Clin Pharm 1984, 18, 394-98*

23. All the following are possible ADRs of dapsone *except:*

(a) Cardiotoxicity
(b) Nephrotoxicity
(c) Neurotoxicity
(d) Hepatotoxicity

Explanation:

Dapsone:

- First antimicrobial agent found effective against leprosy
- Chemically related to sulfonamides
- Generally safe and inexpensive, However it is associated with known reported ADRs in the literature and have been tabulated as follows:

Adverse Drug Reactions Associated with Dapsone	
Pharmacologic/Toxic	Hemolysis in G6PD or Glutathione reductase deficiency
	Methemoglobinemia
	Anemia
	Fatigue, anorexia
	Nausea and vomiting
	Headache and dizziness
Allergic/ Idiosyncratic	Hypersensitivity
	Steven-Johnson Syndrome (SJS)
	Toxic Epidermal Necrolysis (TEN)
	Photosensitivity
	Peripheral neuropathy
	Cholestatic hepatitis
	Nephritis and renal failure
	Hypoalbuminemia
	Hypothyroidism

- **Contraindications of Dapsone are tabulated as follows:**

Contraindications of Dapsone
Severe anemia
Porphyria
G6PD deficiency
Glutathione/*Methemoglobin reductase* deficiency
Allergy to sulfonamides
Liver disorders
Along with other hemolytics

Ans: (a) Cardiotoxicity

Ref: *Tripathi KD, Essentials of Medical Pharmacology, 8th Edition, New Delhi, Jaypee Brothers Medical Publishers, 2019, page 832*

PATHOLOGY

1. What is the shelf life of platelets that are not agitated?

(a) 4 hr
(b) 8 hr
(c) 24 hr
(d) 1 hr

Explanation:

- Platelet concentrate:
  - Should be stored At **22°C ± 2°C**
  - Continuous agitation of **60-70/min** or a rotor at **5-10 cycles/min**
  - Shelf life under agitation: **3-5 days***
- Shelf life of platelets that are not agitated **– 30 min*** (If no agitation, platelets must be transfused within half hour)
- Natural life span of platelets**: 7-10 days.**
- Lack of agitation leads to production of lactic acid and decreases pH
- Bacterial contamination is a complication with platelet concentrate

Ans: (d) 1 hr

Ref: *Transfusion Medicine – Technical Manual – Ministry of Health and Family Welfare, Government of India*

2. Which of the following is not an AIDS defining cancer?

(a) Cervical cancer
(b) Ovarian cancer
(c) CNS lymphoma
(d) Kaposi sarcoma

Explanation:

Table: AIDS-Defining Opportunistic Infections and Neoplasms Found in Patients with HIV Infection
Infections
Protozoal and Helminthic Infections
Cryptosporidiosis or isosporidiosis (enteritis)
Pneumocystosis (pneumonia or disseminated infection)
Toxoplasmosis (pneumonia or CNS infection)
Fungal Infections
Candidiasis (esophageal, tracheal or pulmonary)
Cryptococcosis (CNS infection)
Coccidioidomycosis (disseminated)
Histoplasmosis (disseminated)
Bacterial Infections
Mycobacteriosis ("atypical", e.g., *Mycobacterium avium-intracellulare*, disseminated or extrapulmonary; *Mycobacterium tuberculosis*, pulmonary or extrapulmonary)
Nocardiosis (pneumonia, meningitis, disseminated)
Salmonella infections, disseminated
Viral Infections
Cytomegalovirus (pulmonary, intestinal, retinitis, or CNS infections)
Herpes simplex virus (localized or disseminated infection)
Varicella-zoster virus (localized or disseminated infection)
Progressive multifocal leukoencephalopathy

Contd.

Contd.

Neoplasms
Kaposi sarcoma
Primary lymphoma of brain
Invasive cancer of uterine cervix

Patients with AIDS have a high incidence of certain tumors

- Kaposi sarcoma
- B-cell lymphoma
- Cervical cancer in women
- Anal cancer in men
- 25% to 40% of untreated HIV-infected patients develop malignancy
- A common feature of these tumors is that they are caused by oncogenic DNA viruses
  - Kaposi sarcoma: Herpesvirus
  - B-cell lymphoma: EBV
  - Cervica l and anal carcinoma: Human papillomavirus

Ans: (b) Ovarian cancer

Ref: *Robbins Basic Pathology, 9th edition, Elsevier, page 253*

3. Gene implicated in MEN 4 syndrome?

(a) Tyrosine kinase receptor (b) Menin
(c) CDKN1B (d) RET

Explanation:

MEN syndromes

- The MEN syndromes are a group of inherited diseases resulting in proliferative lesions of multiple endocrine organs.
- Distinct features of tumors in MEN:
  - Younger age
  - Arise in multiple endocrine organs, synchronously or metachronously
  - Multifocal
  - Preceded by an asymptomatic stage of hyperplasia
  - More aggressive and recur
  - Autosomal dominant
- **4 forms:**
  - MEN1 (Wermer syndrome): **Menin mutations**
  - MEN 2(previously MEN 2A/Sipple's syndrome): **RET mutation**
  - MEN 3 (previously MEN 2B): **RET mutations**
  - MEN 4 (MENX): **CDNK1B mutation**
- **Associated Tumors:**
  - **MEN1:** Parathyroid, pancreatic islet and anterior pituitary tumors (3Ps)
  - **MEN 2:** Medullary thyroid carcinoma, pheochromocytoma, parathyroid tumors

- **MEN 3:** Medullary thyroid carcinoma, pheochromocytoma, marfanoid habitus, mucosal neuromas, megacolon
- **MEN 4:** Parathyroid and anterior pituitary tumors with tumors of adrenals, kidneys and reproductive organs

Ans: (c) CDKN1B

Ref: *Robbins Basic Pathology, 9th edition, Elsevier, page 1136*

4. FGFR3 mutation is seen in:

(a) Osteopetrosis (b) Achondroplasia

(c) Osteogenesis imperfecta (d) Pagets disease

Explanation:

Achondroplasia

- Most common skeletal dysplasia and a major cause of dwarfism
- Autosomal dominant
- Retarded cartilage growth
- **Clinical features**
  - Shortened proximal extremities
  - Trunk of relatively normal length
  - Enlarged head
  - Bulging forehead
  - Depression of root of the nose
- Caused by gain-of-function mutations in the **FGF receptor 3 (FGFR3).**
- **Thanatophoric dysplasia** is the most common **lethal form of dwarfism**

Ans: (b) Achondroplasia

Ref: *Robbins Basic Pathology, 9th edition, Elsevier, page 1184*

5. Which is true regarding Langerhans Cell Histiocytosis?

(a) Positive for CD1a

(b) Large cells with non- grooved indented reniform nuclei

(c) Positive for CD 117

(d) Eosiniphic background in peripheral smear

(e) CD marker 110

Explanation:

Langerhans Cell Histiocytosis

- Spectrum of proliferations of a special type of immature dendritic cell called the Langerhans cell
- Most common mutation: **BRAF** *
- Features of Langerhans cells
  - Have abundant, often vacuolated cytoplasm
  - Vesicular nuclei containing linear grooves or folds

- **Birbeck granules** in the cytoplasm
- Express **HLA-DR, S-100, and CD1a***

- **Clinicopathologic entities:**
  - Multifocal multisystem Langerhans cell histiocytosis (**Letterer-Siwe disease**)
  - Unifocal and multifocal unisystem Langerhans cell histiocytosis (**eosinophilic granuloma**)
  - Pulmonary Langerhans cell histiocytosis
  - **Hand-SchüllerChristian triad**–Calvarial bone defects, Diabetes insipidus, and Exophthalmos.

Ans: (a) Positive for CD1a

Ref: *Robbins Basic Pathology, 9th edition, Elsevier, page 622*

6. A child presents with abdominal mass. Biopsy showed sheet of cells with irregular margin, scant cytoplasm, big nucleus. Which of the following feature will confirm the diagnosis?

(a) Pseudo rosettes
(b) PAS positivity
(c) WT1 mutation
(d) Abortive tubules

Explanation:

Wilms tumor

- Most common primary renal tumor of childhood
- Fourth most common pediatric malignancy
- Synchronous/metachronous
- **Associations**
  - **WAGR syndrome-** Wilms tumor, aniridia, genital anomalies, and mental retardation.
  - **Denys-Drash syndrome-** gonadal dysgenesis (male pseudohermaphroditism) and early-onset nephropathy leading to renal failure. Risk for developing germ cell tumors called gonadoblastomas.
  - **Beckwith-Wiedemann syndrome** - organomegaly, macroglossia, hemihypertrophy, omphalocele, adrenal cytomegaly
- Microscopy: **Classic triphasic combination** of blastemal, stromal, and epithelial cell types
- Mutations: **WT1 gene on chromosome 11**

Ans: (c) WT1 mutation

Ref: *Robbins Basic Pathology, 9th edition, Elsevier, page 479*

7. Marfan syndrome is associated with mutation seen in?

(a) Collagen
(b) Dystrophin
(c) Spectrin
(d) Fibrillin 1

Explanation:

Marfan syndrome

- Disorder of connective tissues
- Involves **skeleton**, **eyes**, and **cardiovascular** system
- Autosomal dominant inheritance
- Defect in **extracellular glycoprotein called fibrillin1***

- Skeletal abnormalities-most striking feature
- Ocular changes–**ectopia lentis**
- Cardiovascular lesions–**mitral valve prolapse** and **aortic dissection**
- Clinical diagnosis: **revised Ghent criteria***

Ans: (d) Fibrillin 1

Ref: *Robbins Basic Pathology, 9th edition, Elsevier, page 144*

8. PLAP and C kit positive testicular tumor in 40 year old male?

(a) Seminoma (b) Teratoma

(c) Embryonal cell tumor (d) Yolk sac tumor

Explanation:

Seminoma

- Most common type of germ cell tumor
- Male counterpart of dysgerminoma
- 25% have KIT activating mutations
- **Histological types**: classical, spermatocytic, anaplastic
- **Gross:**
  - Homogeneous
  - Graywhite
  - Lobulated cut surface
  - Devoid of hemorrhage or necrosis
  - Tunica albuginea is not penetrated
- **Microscopy**:
  - Sheets of uniform cells divided into lobules by delicate fibrous septa containing a lymphocytic infiltrate
  - Seminoma cells- large,round to polyhedral, distinct cell membrane; clear cytoplasm, large, central nucleus with prominent nucleoli
  - Cytoplasm contains glycogen
- **IHC**:
  - **cKIT***
  - **OCT4***
  - **Placental alkaline phosphatase (PLAP)***

Ans: (a) Seminoma

Ref: *Robbins Basic Pathology, 9th edition, Elsevier, page 976*

9. Which is not a Tumor marker for Fibrollamellar Liver Carcinoma?

(a) Vitamin B12 binding protein (b) AFP

(c) PIVKA (d) Glypican

(e) Neurotensin

Explanation:

Fibrollamellar Liver Carcinoma

- Variant of liver cell carcinoma
- In young patients without cirrhosis
- Favorable prognosis
- **Microscopy**:
  - Fibrosis in lamellar fashion around neoplastic hepatocytes
  - Tumor cells are polygonal and oncocytic, due to an increase in number of mitochondria
- **IHC**:
  - Cytokeratins **8 and 18**
  - **Glypican-3**
  - **Anterior gradient-2**
  - **Epidermal growth factor receptor**
- **Negative for alpha fetoprotein**

Ans: (b) AFP

Ref: *Rosai and Ackerman's Surgical Pathology, 10th edition, Vol 1, page 951*

10. Ovarian tumour derived from Walthard cell nest:

(a) Brenner's tumour (b) Clear cell Ca

(c) Serous cystadenoma (d) Yolk sac tumor

Explanation:

Brenner's tumour

- Constitute 1%-2% of ovarian neoplasms
- Average age: 50 years
- Symptom: postmenopausal bleeding
- Grossly: unilateral, firm, and white or yellowish white
- **Microscopy:**
  - Solid and cystic nests of epithelial cells resembling transitional epithelium
  - Stroma–fibroblastic
  - Grooved nucleus–**coffee bean** appearance
- Associations: **Mucinous tumors and Struma ovarii**
- 50% malignant transitional epithelium: considered as transitional cell carcinomas

Ans: (a) Brenner's tumour

Ref: *Rosai and Ackerman's Surgical Pathology, 10th edition, Vol 1, page 1574*

11. Which graft reaction can be reversed once it is established?

(a) Hyperacute rejection (b) Acute rejection

(c) Chronic rejection (d) Acute on chronic rejection

Explanation:

- **Types**:
  - T Cell–Mediated/ cellular
  - Antibody-Mediated Reactions
- **Acute cellular rejection:**
  - By CD8+ CTLs
- **Hyperacute rejection**:
  - **Preformed antidonor** antibodies are present in circulation of recipient
  - Within minutes or hours after transplantation
  - Fibrinoid necrosis occurs in arterial walls

Ans: (b) Acute rejection

Ref: *Robbins Basic Pathology, 9th edition, Elsevier, page 233*

12. In Cystic fibrosis, which type of mucins is formed in respiratory tract?

(a) MUC5A (b) MUC5B

(c) MUC2 (d) MUC6

Explanation:

Cystic fibrosis

- Inherited disorder of ion transport that affects fluid secretion in exocrine glands and in epithelial lining of the respiratory, gastrointestinal, and reproductive tracts
- Autosomal recessive
- Defect–in CFTR gene on chromosome 7q31.2
- Abnormal function of an epithelial chloride channel protein
- Functions of CFTR are tissue-specific
- CFTR regulates transport of bicarbonate ions
- **Clinical Features:**
  - Chronic sinopulmonary diseas
  - **Meconium ileus** in neonatal period
  - Pancreatic insufficiency
  - Biliary cirrhosis
  - Salt-loss syndromes
  - Obstructive azoospermia
- **Diagnosis:**
  - Abnormally salty sweat (normal-<60 mM/L)
  - Sequencing the CFTR gene-**Gold Standard**

Note:

- Trapping of foreign material such as particulates and baceteria is accomplished by mucins.
- Mucins are complex glycoproteins that form gels, exemplified by **MUC5A**, present in lung of humans
- Other mucins like **MUC5B** and **MUC7** become expressed in airway epithelial cells in diseases such as cystic fibrosis.

Ans: (b) MUC5B

Ref: *Robbins Basic Pathology, 9th edition, Elsevier, page 466*

13. True regarding type 1 Von Willebrand disease:

(a) Affects nearly 1% of the population
(b) Ristocetin induced aggregation is normal
(c) Factor VIII is increased
(d) X linked inheritence

Explanation:

Von Willebrand disease

- Type 1, 2A, 2B and 2M-Autosomal dominant
- Type 3 and 2N - Autosomal recessive
- Clinical picture:
  - Mucosal and cutaneous bleeding
- **Laboratory findings**
  - Hess test–positive
  - Bleeding lime–prolonged
  - APTT–prolonged
  - vWF assay–decreased
  - Ristocetin induced aggregation is defective
  - Genetic studies
- Acquired von Willebrand syndrome-antibody formation against vWF
- Management: DDAVP

Ans: (a) Affects nearly 1% of the population

Ref: *Dr. Tejindar Singh*, *Atlas and Text of Hematology, 4th edition, page 579*

14. True regarding Hairy cell leukaemia is:

(a) Characterized by mild splenomegaly
(b) Pancytopenia is the characteristic finding
(c) Monocytosis is seen
(d) Hairy cells are TRAP negative

Explanation:

Hairy cell leukaemia

- Rare chronic B-cell leukemia of elderly
- Hair like projections seen
- Clinical features:
  - Moderate to massive splenomegaly
- Hematological findings:
  - **Pancytopenia***
  - Monocytopenia
  - Hairy cells are TRAP +ve
  - NAP score is elevated

- Immunophenotype:
  - Annexin A1I, anti TRAP, DBA44, GD25, CD20O and CD2Q
  - CD25, CD103, CD123 and CD11c
- **BRAF v600E mutation**
- **Hairy cell leukemia variant:**
  - Not biologically related to HCL
  - Splenomegaly present
  - TLC is higher
  - Monocytopenia absent
  - Cells have more basophilic cytoplasm with or without hairy processes
  - TRAP negative

Ans: (b) Pancytopenia is the characteristic finding

Ref: *Dr. Tejindar Singh*, *Atlas and Text of Hematology, 4th edition, page 424*

15. Which is not a pathologic feature H.pylori chronic gastritis?

(a) Eosinophilic infiltrates (b) Intraepithelial neutrophil deposits

(c) Affects Intestinal gland formation in stomach (d) Subepithelial plasma cell deposits

Explanation:

H. pylori chronic gastritis

Morphology

- Organism is concentrated within the **superficial mucus** overlying epithelial cells
- H. pylori **tropism for gastric epithelia** (Not seen in gastric intestinal metaplasia or duodenal epithelium)
- H. pylori may be present in **foci of pyloric metaplasia** within **chronically injured duodenum** or **gastric-type mucosa** within **Barrett esophagus**
- In Stomach, H. pylori are typically found in the **Antrum**
- Although there is a good concordance between colonization of the antrum and cardia, infection of the cardia occurs at somewhat lower rates.
- H. pylori are **uncommon** in **oxyntic (acid-producing) mucosa of the fundus** and **body**
- **Antral biopsy** is **preferred** for evaluation of H. pylori gastritis.
- When viewed endoscopically, H. pylori–infected antral mucosa is usually **erythematous** and has a **coarse or even nodular appearance**.
- The inflammatory infiltrate generally includes variable numbers of **neutrophils** within the **lamina propria**, including some that cross the basement membrane to assume an intraepithelial location and accumulate in the lumen of gastric pits to create **pit abscesses.**
- Superficial lamina propria has large numbers of **plasma cells,** and increased numbers of **lymphocytes and macrophages**.
- **Intraepithelial neutrophils** and **subepithelial plasma cells** are **characteristic of H. pylori** gastritis.
- When intense, inflammatory infiltrates may create **thickened rugal folds**, mimicking **early infiltrative lesions.**
- Long-standing cases involve **body and fundus,** and the mucosa becomes **atrophic**.
- **Lymphoid aggregates**, some with germinal centers, are frequently present and represent an induced form of **mucosa-associated lymphoid tissue**, or **MALT**, that has the potential to transform into **lymphoma**.

Characteristics of *Helicobacter pylori*–Associated and Autoimmune Gastritis

	***H. pylori*–Associated**	**Autoimmune**
Location	Antrum	Body
Inflammatory infiltrate	• Neutrophils • Subepithelial plasma cells	• Lymphocytes • Macrophages
Acid production	Increased to slightly decreased	Decreased
Gastrin	Normal to decreased	Increased
Other lesions	Hyperplastic/inflammatory polyps	Neuroendocrine hyperplasia
Serology	Antibodies to *H. pylori*	Antibodies to **parietal cells** (**H^+, K^+-ATPase, intrinsic factor**)
Sequelae	• Peptic ulcer • Adenocarcinoma	• Atrophy • Pernicious anemia • Adenocarcinoma • Carcinoid tumor
Associations	• Low socioeconomic status • Poverty • Residence in rural areas	• Autoimmune disease • Thyroiditis • Diabetes mellitus • Graves disease

Note:

- **Eosinophilic infiltrates** of mucosa and submucosa of stomach is characteristically seen in **Eosinophilic gastroenteritis**

Ans: (a) Eosinophilic infiltrates

Ref: *Robbins Pathologic Basis of Disease, 8th edition, page 776*

16. Which of the following is a feature of anemia of chronic disease?

(a) Increased TIBC
(b) Increased serum iron
(c) Increased serum ferritin
(d) Increased Transferrin saturation

Explanation:

	Normal Values	**Iron deficiency anemia**	**Thalassemia**	**Sideroblastic anemia**	**Anemia of Chronic Disease**
Peripheral Smear		Microcytic Hypochromic	Microcytic Hypochromic	Microcytic Hypochromic	Normocytic normochromic > > Microcytic Hypochromic
Serum Iron	50–150 microg/dl	Low	Normal or ↑	Normal or ↑	↓
Total iron binding Capacity (TIBC)	300–600 microg/dl	High ↑↑	Normal	Normal or ↑	↓
% Transferrin Saturation	30–50%	<10 (↓)	Normal or ↑	Normal or ↑	↓
Serum Ferritin (microgram/L)	50–200	<15	↑	↑	Normal or ↑
Hemoglobin Pattern	HbA2 – 1.5 – 3.5% total Hb	Normal	Abnormal	Normal	Normal

Ans: (c) Increased serum ferritin

Ref: *Robbins Pathologic Basis of Disease, 9th edition*

MICROBIOLOGY

1. 1, 3 beta glucan indicates infection due to all except:

(a) Cryptococcus (b) Candida
(c) Aspergillus (d) Fusarium

Explanation:

- The polysaccharide beta (1,3)-D-glucan is a component of the **cell wall** of many **fungi**.
- Synthesis of the **linear polymer** is catalysed **by UDP-glucose beta (1,3)-D-glucan beta(3)-D-glucosyltransferase.**
- This enzyme has a key role in **fungal cell-wall synthesis**, in many organisms that are responsible for **human mycoses**.
- Beta (1,3)-D-glucan is produced by
  - *Candida albicans**
  - *Aspergillus fumigatus* *
  - *Cryptococcus neoformans**
- *These organisms* produce walls that are rich in beta (1,3)-glucan, which has been the main focus of intensive study and lab diagnosis.

Ans: (d) Fusarium

Ref: https://www.ncbi.nlm.nih.gov/pubmed/11800269

2. A patient presents with membrane on tonsil. Most appropriate media to be used for throat swab culture in this patient is:

(a) Chocolate agar (b) Blood agar
(c) Loeffler's Serum Slope (d) Potassium tellurite agar

Explanation:

Whenever a patient presents with membrane on tonsil, Diphtheria is the single most important DD to be ruled out.

Corynebacterium diphtheria

- Selective media **– Hoyle's potassium tellurite blood agar*/Tinsdale** media*
- Enriched media–**Loeffler's serum slope***
- **Loeffler's serum slope** is enriched media used for isolation as well for production of metachromatic granules by *Corynebacterium diphtheriae*

Clinical features of diphtheria
• Types of Diptheria – Faucial, Respiratory, Cutaneous and invasive form. It causes membrane over tonsil
• **Most common diphtheria** – Respiratory form
• Diphtheria is toxaemia not bacteremia–**Cardiotoxicity**
• **Pseudomembrane formation**–Leathery
• **Bull neck appearance*** of lymph nodes

Contd.

Contd.

Diagnosis
• **Albert/Neisser's/Ponders staining**
• **Toxigenic test**–In vivo: **Guinea pig inoculation** and in vitro: **Elek gel precipitation** test, Immunochromatographic strip test
• Test for immune status – **Schick test**
• Matrix assisted laser desorption/ionization time of light (MALDI-TOF) and PCR

Ans: (c) LSS

Ref: *Ananthanarayan and Paniker, 9th edition, page 242*

3. Autolysis is shown by which bacteria?

(a) S. pneumoniae *(b) S.equisumillis*

(c) S. pyogenes *(d) S. agalactiae*

Explanation:

Points to remember about *Streptococcus pneumoniae:*

B- **Bile solubility** (present)

I-**Inulin** fermenter

O- **Optochin** sensitivity

M- Morphology: flame shaped diplococci

C- Colony morphology: earlier **Draughtsman or Carrom coin** and later **autolysis**

Q- **Quellung** reaction positive

(Mnemonic: BIO MCQ)

Virulence factors
• **Capsular polysaccharide** – most virulent
• **Autolysin-** Amidase (autolytic in nature), Cleaves peptidoglycan layer, Responsible for Draughtsman colony (autolysis)
• **Pnuemolysin** – cytotoxin and immunogenic
• Extracellular protease – **Ig A1 protease** – establishes infection in upper respiratory tract
• **Raised CRP** detected by passive agglutination test

Ans: (a) *S. pneumoniae*

Ref: *Ananthanarayan and Paniker, 9th edition, page 225-226*

4. Aspiration of Amoebic liver abscess is done. What can be detected in microscopy?

(a) Cyst (b) Cyst and trophozoite

(c) Only trophozoite (d) Precyst

Explanation:

- Adherence of ***E. histolytica*** to colonic epithelial cells is thought to be through the **galactose/N-acetyl-galactosamine-specific lectin**.
- *E. histolytica* carries cytolytic capabilities and also kills mammalian cells through programmed apoptosis.
- Once *E. histolytica* trophozoites reach the liver, they create abscesses comprising well-circumscribed areas of **cellular debris, dead hepatocytes, and liquefied cells**.

- The lesion is surrounded by a rim of connective tissue with some **inflammatory cells and amebic trophozoites.**
- In humans, the small number of organisms compared to the actual dimensions of the abscess supports the concept that *E. histolytica* can destroy hepatocytes without contact with the cells.

Laboratory Diagnosis of Amoebic Liver Abscess

- **Microscopy and Histopathology of liver pus** shows **trophozoites*** but never **cyst**. This is specific but of low sensitivity (< 25%)
- Stool microscopy and culture is not useful.
- **Lectin antigen** is usually absent in stool but can be demonstrated in serum, liver pus and saliva.
- **Antibody detection**–Antibodies are often elevated and can be detected by ELISA and IHA. However, antibodies persist even after the cure, so it cannot differentiate recent and old infection.
- **PCR** done on amoebic liver pus
- USG of liver shows the site of the abscess and its extension

Ans: (c) Trophozoites

Ref: https://www.ncbi.nlm.nih.gov/books/NBK430832/; *Apurba Sastry Essentials of Medical Parasitology 2nd edition, page 30-35*

5. Most common organism in epidural abscess:

(a) *Staphylococcus aureus* (b) Meningococcus
(c) *Streptococcus pneumoniae* (d) Micrococci

Explanation:

Brain abscesses:

Site	Source of infection	Organism involved	Clinical presentation
Frontal lobe	Paranasal sinusitis, Dental infection	Streptococci, Anaerobes	Hemiparesis, Personality changes
Temporal lobe	Middle ear infection	Streptococci, Enterobacteriaceae	Dysphasia, Upper homonymous hemianopia
Cerebellum	Sphenoid sinusitis, Mastoiditis and Middle ear infection	Pseudomonas, Anaerobes	Nystagmus Ataxia
Epidural abscess	Spinal procedures, Trauma and RTA	Staphylococcus aureus	Raised ICT and neck stiffness

- Epidural abscess of the spinal column is a rare condition that can be fatal if left untreated.
- **Risk factors for epidural abscess**: immunocompromised states such as diabetes mellitus, alcoholism, cancer, and acquired immunodeficiency syndrome (AIDS), as well as spinal procedures including epidural anesthesia and spinal surgery.
- **The signs and symptoms of epidural abscess**: nonspecific and can range from low back pain to sepsis.
- **The treatment of choice** in most patients is surgical decompression followed by four to six weeks of antibiotic therapy.
- Nonsurgical treatment may be appropriate in selected patients.
- The most common causative organism in spinal epidural abscess is ***Staphylococcus aureus***.

Ans: (a) *Staphylococcus aureus*

Ref: *Harrison's Infectious Disease, 2nd edition, page 406, 430, 500; Ananthanarayan and Paniker, 9th edition, page 204; https://www.aafp.org/afp/2002/0401/p1341.html*

6. Hot air oven is used for:

(a) Vaccine
(b) Culture medium
(c) Serum
(d) Liquid paraffin

Explanation:

HOT AIR OVEN

- This method was introduced by Louis Pasteur.
- **Denaturation of protein**, drying effect
- **Use:** Powders and non-aqueous **liquids like paraffin or vaseline, oils, grease, petroleum jelly**; **metallic instruments** (like forceps, scalpels, scissors), **glass wares** (such as petri-dishes, pipettes, flasks, all-glass syringes), swabs.
- **Temperature and time relation:**

160°C	120 min
170°C	60 min
180°C	30 min

Note:

Materials sterilized by **hot air oven**	• **Powders and non-aqueous** liquids like paraffin or vaseline, oils, grease, fat, dusting powder and petroleum jelly • **Metallic instruments** (like forceps, scalpels, scissors), **Glass wares** (such as petri-dishes, pipettes, flasks, all-glass syringes) • Swabs
Sterilization Control used in hot air oven	• **Clostridium tetani** (non-toxigenic strain) • Browne's tube • Thermocouple

Ans: (d) Liquid paraffin

Ref: *Ananthanarayan and Paniker, 9th edition, page 35-38*

7. Not a mode of transmission of toxoplasma:

(a) After solid organ transplant
(b) Transplacental / Vertical transmission
(c) Inoculation of saliva
(d) Bradyzoite with sporulated oocyst/Bradyzoite deposition in subcutaneous tissue

Explanation:

Toxoplasma has been reported to be **transmitted by the following ways** in man and animals:

- (a) **Through cat:**
  - The cat is the only **definitive host** of the parasite. Infected cats **shed large number of oocysts** in the faeces. Stray cats contaminate the soils around the human habitations and thus play a vital role in the **transmission of toxoplasmosis**.

- **Meat and meat products:**
  - Consumption of **raw or under cooked meat** or meat products are important source of toxoplasmosis.
- **Congenital infection:**
  - From **infected mother** to the fetus
- **Other methods:**
  - **Blood transfusion** and ingestion of infected milk may transmit the infection.
  - Infection has been traced to be transmitted through semen.
- **Experimental transmission (accidental inoculation)** can be made by intramuscular, subcutaneous or intraperitonial inoculation of infected materials.

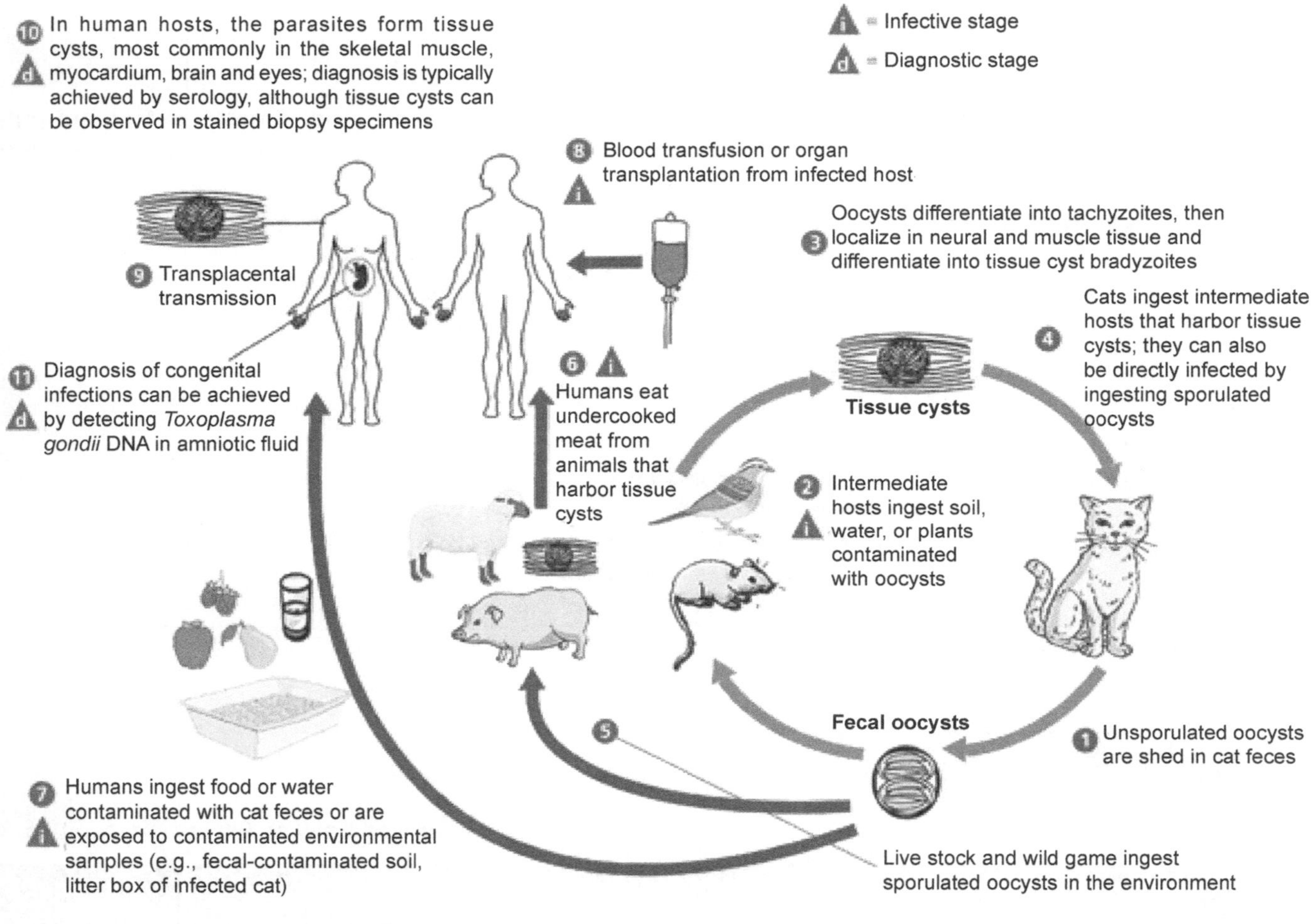

Ans: (c) Inoculation of saliva

Ref : https://www.cdc.gov/parasites/toxoplasmosis/epi.html

8. Yellow colour hair is caused by:

(a) *Corynebacterium minutissimum*
(b) *Clostridium tetanus*
(c) *Corynebacterium tenuis*
(d) *Corynebacterium ulcerans*

Explanation:

- **Trichomycosis axillaris** is a superficial bacterial infection of underarm hair.

- The disease is characterised by yellow, black or red granular nodules or concretions that stick to the hair shaft. It can also affect pubic hair (when it is called trichomycosis pubis), scrotal hair, and intergluteal hair.
- The name is misleading because "trichomycosis" is bacterial in origin rather than a fungal infection.
- Trichomycosis axillaris is caused by the overgrowth of Corynebacterium ***(Corynebacterium tenuis, C propinguum, C flavescens)*** and ***Serratia marcescens***.
- The concretions consist of tightly packed bacteria. The bacteria proliferate in moist areas of the body, thus mainly affect underarm hairs, and to a lesser extent, pubic hair.

Ans: (c) *Corynebacterium tenuis*

Ref: https://dermnetnz.org/topics/trichomycosis-axillaris/

9. True about Nipah virus are all *except*:

(a) Fruits bats are amplifying
(b) Can be spread by aerosol
(c) Category C bioterrorism
(d) Herring bone appearance on electron microscopy

Explanation:

- **Herring bone appearance on electron microscopy is seen *in Canine distemper viruses and in NIPAH VIRUS.***

Transmission of NIPAH virus:

- Transmission of Nipah virus to humans may occur after direct contact with **infected bats, infected pigs, or from other NiV infected people.**
- In Malaysia and Singapore, humans were apparently infected with Nipah virus only through **close contact with infected pigs.** The NiV strain identified in this outbreak appeared to have been transmitted initially **from bats to pigs**, with subsequent spread within pig populations. **Incidental human infections** resulted after exposure to infected pigs. **No occurrence of person-to-person** transmission was reported in this outbreak.
- Conversely, **person-to-person transmission of Nipah virus in Bangladesh and India is regularly reported**. This is most commonly seen in the family and caregivers of Nipah virus-infected patients. Transmission also occurs from **direct exposure to infected bats**. A common example is **consumption of raw date palm sap contaminated with infectious bat excretions.**

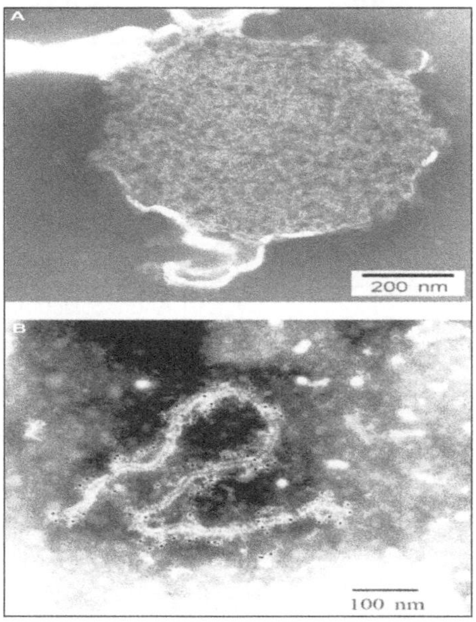

Structure of the Nipah virus virion core. Notes: (A) Nucleocapsid core with residual envelope; **(B) Herringbone-shaped fragment** of the nucleocapsid with immuno-gold labeling of P proteins

Category A	Category B	Category C
Anthrax	Brucellosis (*Brucella* species)	Emerging infectious diseases (e.g., *Nipah virus, Hanta virus*)
Botulism	Epsilon toxin of *Clostridium perfringens*	
Plague	Food safety threats (e.g., *Salmomella* species)	Emerging future toxins
Smallpox	Glanders (*Burkholderia mallei*)	
Tularemia	Melioidosis (*Burkholderia pseudomallei*)	
Viral hemorrhagic fevers	Psittacosis (*Chlamydia psittaci*) Q fever (*Coxiella burnetii*) Ricin toxin from *Ricinus communis* Staphylococcal enterotoxin B Typhus fever (*Rickettsia prowazekii*) Viral encephalitides (*alphaviruses*) Water safety threats (e.g., *Vibrio cholerae*)	

Classification of Bioterrorism Agents Centers for Disease Control and Prevention Categories of Bioterrorism Agents/Diseases

Ans: (b) Can be spread by aerosol

Ref: https://www.cdc.gov/vhf/nipah/transmission/index.html

10. Cause of hemorrhagic cystitis:

(a) Corona virus
(b) Adenovirus type 11, 21
(c) Ebola virus
(d) Dengue virus

Explanation:

Disease spectrum of adenovirus:

System	Serotype	Disease pattern
Respiratory system	3, 7	Atypical pneumonia Pharyngitis
	4, 7, 21	ARDS
	3, 7, 14	Pharyngoconjunctival fever
Eye	8	Epidemic keratoconjunctivitis
	3, 4, 11	Acute follicular conjunctivitis
Intestine	40, 41	Diarrhea
Bladder	**11, 21**	**Acute hemorrhagic cystitis**
Skin	12	Generalized exanthema

Ans: (b) Adenovirus type 11, 21

Ref: *Ananthanarayan and Paniker, 9th edition, page 487,488*

11. Which of the following causes toxic form of food poisoning?

(a) *Staphylococcus aureus* (b) *Campylobacter jejuni*
(c) *Bacillus anthracis* (d) *Bordetella pertussis*

Explanation:

Bacterial food poisoning: Toxin mediated

Time period	Organism involved
1 – 6 hours	***Staphylococcus aureus*** (Heat stable toxin) *Bacillus cereus* (Heat stable toxin)
8 – 16 hours	*Clostridium perfringens* (Heat labile toxin) *Bacillus cereus* (Heat labile toxin)
>16 hours	*Vibrio cholerae* ETEC and EHEC strains of *E.coli* *Salmonella spp.* *Shigella spp.* *Campylobacter jejuni* *Vibrio parahemolyticus*

Ans: (a) *Staphylococcus aureus*

Ref: *Ananthanarayan and Paniker, 9th edition, page 204-206*

12. True statement regarding a 14-year-old boy with EBV infection are all *except*:

(a) Downey cell (b) Spontaneous recovery
(c) It's a cause of CLL (d) Sore throat and hepatosplenomegaly

Explanation:

Epstein Barr virus:

- Member of Herpesviridae (HHV-4); sub family gammaherpesviridae
- Primarily infects B cells, which carry CD 21 receptors
- **EBV associated conditions: Lymphocytosis** with atypical lymphocytes, **Infectious mononucleosis, X-linked Lymphoproliferative syndrome, Burkitt's lymphoma, Nasopharyngeal carcinoma**, Gastric carcinoma, Peripheral neuritis, T cell lymphoma, **Oral hairy leukoplakia**, Leiomyosarcoma, Hodgkin's lymphoma, CNS lymphoma, Guillain Barre syndrome, Chronic fatigue syndrome, Acute transverse myelitis.
- **Lab diagnosis: EBNA** (EBV nuclear antigens), **NAAT**, Isolation, Heterophile antibody test (**Paul-Bunnell**), EBV specific antibodies, antibodies to Viral core antigen (**VCA IgG and IgM**), **EBNA Ig**
- **Reactive lymphocytes** or **variant lymphocytes** are cytotoxic ($CD8^+$) lymphocytes that become large as a result of antigen stimulation. Typically, they can be more than 30 μm in diameter with varying size and shape.
- The nucleus of a reactive lymphocyte can be round, elliptic, indented, cleft, or folded. The cytoplasm is often abundant and can be basophilic. Vacuoles and/or azurophilic granules are also sometimes present. Most often, the cytoplasm is gray, pale blue, or deep blue in colour.
- The distinctive cell associated with EBV or CMV is known as **Downey cells,** after Hal Downey, who contributed to the characterization of it in 1923

Ans: (c) It's a cause of CLL

Ref: https://en.wikipedia.org/wiki/Reactive_lymphocyte; *Ananthanarayan and Paniker, 9th edition, page 481-483*

13. Which of the following is a dimorphic fungus?

(a) Rhizopus
(b) Sporothrix schenckii
(c) Tinea versicolor
(d) Microsporum

Explanation:

- Dimorphic fungi can occur as ***filaments or as yeasts***, depending on the conditions of growth.
- In **host tissues or cultures** at **37°C** they occur as **yeasts**, while in the **soil and in cultures** at **22°C** they appear as **moulds**.
- Most fungi causing systemic infections are dimorphic fungi.
- **List of dimorphic fungi**
  - ***Systemic dimorphic fungi***
    - *Histoplasma capsulatum*
    - *Blastomyces dermatitidis*
    - *Coccidiodes immitis*
    - *Paracoccidiodes brasiliensis*
  - ***Subcutaneous dimorphic fungus*** – *Sporothrix schenckii*
  - ***Opportunistic fungus*** – *Penicillium marneffei*

Ans: (b) Sporothrix schenckii

Ref: *Ananthnarayan R, Paniker CKJ, Textbook of Microbiology, 8th Edition, Hyderabad, Universities Press, 2009, page 601-15*

FORENSIC MEDICINE

1. Pyrogallol test is used to diagnose:

(a) Fat embolism
(b) Air embolism
(c) Stillbirth
(d) Pneumothorax

Explanation:

Pyrogallol test

- Used to diagnose **Air embolism**
- It differentiates gas present in the **heart** from gas formed due to **decomposition**
- **Oxygen** present in **air** turns 2% freshly prepared pyrogallol solution **brown**.
- **Procedure:** A 2% pyrogallol solution mixed with sodium hydroxide is taken in a syringe. Gas is then aspirated from the right side of the heart and then shaken. The mixture will turn brown, if air is present. In the absence of air, the solution stays clear (indicating gas production by bacteria).

Ans: (b) Air Embolism

Ref: *KSN Reddy, The Essentials of Forensic Medicine and Toxicology, 34th edition, page 104*

2. Studying Sweat gland ridges from fingerprints:

(a) Poroscopy
(b) Rugoscopy
(c) Dactyloscopy
(d) Edgescopy

Explanation:

- Poroscopy is study of pores of sweat glands present on the ridges on fingers and hands
- Devised by **Edmund Locard** (Also known for **Locard's principle** of **exchange**)

Poroscopy

- Described by Edmund Locard (in 1912) - consists of study of microscopic pores of ridges formed by the mouths of ducts of sub- epidermal sweat glands
- Each mm of a ridge contains **9 to 18 pores**.
- Pores are permanent and vary in size, shape, position and no. over a given length in each individual
- Useful when only fragments of fingerprints or partial prints are available.

Methods of Identification based on Prints

System of Identification	Method	Devised by
Fingerprint/Dactylography	Study of ridge patterns in skin	Sir Francis Galton
Poroscopy	Study of pores of sweat glands on fingers and hands	Edmund Locard
Rugoscopy/Palatoprint	Study of rugae on anterior part of palate	Harrison Allen
Edgeoscopy	Study of edges of friction ridges	Salil K Chatterjee
Cheiloscopy	Study of lip prints	

Ans: (a) Poroscopy

Ref: *KSN Reddy, The Essentials of Forensic Medicine and Toxicology, 34th edition, page 83*

3. Bhilawanol is derived from:

(a) Ricinus communis (b) Semecarpus anacardium

(c) Nerium odorum (d) Abrus precatorius

Explanation:

Vegetable Poisons	Active Principle
Ricinus communis	Ricin (Toxalbumen)
Croton tiglium	Crotin (Toxalbumen)
Abrus precatorius	Abrin (Toxalbumen)
Semecarpus anacardium	Bhilawanol
Calotropis	Calotropin, calotoxin
Datura	Hyoscine
Cannabis	Tetrahydrocannabinol (THC)
Nerium odorum	Nerin, oleandrin
Cerbera thevetia	Thevetin
Cerbera odallam	Cerberin, odollin

Ans: (b) Semecarpus anacardium

Ref: *KSN Reddy, The Essentials of Forensic Medicine and Toxicology, 34th edition, page 517*

4. Which is not seen in sulphuric acid poisoning?

(a) White colorization of teeth (b) Black colorization of stomach

(c) Perforation of stomach (d) Grey colorization of stomach and intestine

Explanation:

Sulphuric Acid

- Odourless, colourless, oily liquid having painful burning taste.
- Teeth are chalky white and brittle
- Skin, Stomach walls shows blackening and excoriation
- Perforation of stomach is common compare to other acids
- FD: 5 – 10 ml. FP: 12-24 hours.

Treatment:

- Gastric lavage - contraindicated.
- Weak solutions of non-carbonate alkalies e.g. calcium oxide, magnesium oxide
- PM appearances: Blotting paper appearance of stomach

Vitriolage:

- Throwing of sulphuric acid to someone's body particularly face to disfigure
- May involve any other acid or agents
- **326A IPC** – voluntarily causing grievous hurt by use of acid : imprisonment of minimum 10 years upto life sentence fine of Rs 10 lakhs (cognizable)
- **326B IPC** – voluntarily throwing or attempting to throw acid : 5 to 7 years

Ans: (d) Grey colorization of stomach acid poisoning

Ref: *KSN Reddy, The Essentials of Forensic Medicine and Toxicology, 34th edition, page 493-94*

5. Which can be used as an ecbolic?

(a) Estrone
(b) Castor oil
(c) Ergot
(d) Potassium permanganate

Explanation:

Abortifacient Drugs

Acting on Uterus		Genitourinary Irritants	Gastrointestinal Irritants
Ecbolics (↑ uterine contraction)	**Emmenagogues (↑ menstrual flow)**		
• Ergot (Most common) • Hydrastis canadensis • Quinine • Lead (lead oleate) • Pituitary extract	• Savin • Borax • Oestrogen • Sanguinarin	• Turpentine oil • Cantharides • Pot. permanganate	• Mag. sulphate • Castor oil

Ans: (a) Ergot

Ref: *KSN Reddy, The Essentials of Forensic Medicine and Toxicology, 34th edition, page 376*

6. Keraunoparalysis is seen in:

(a) Electrocution
(b) Lightning strike
(c) Cold immersion
(d) Mercury poisoning

Explanation:

- **Keraunopathology** is study of **pathology of lightening**
- **Keraunoparalysis**, (**Lightning paralysis**) is a transient paralysis of lower limb
- Associated with extreme vasoconstriction and sensory disturbances of one or more extremities

LIGHTENING INJURY – Due to electrical discharge from clouds

Filigree or **Arborescent burns /Lichtenberg's flower – Pathognomonic**

- Superficial, thin, irregular and tortuous marking over skin mainly over shoulders and flanks.
- Resembles branches of a tree (**Fern like pattern**) of erythema
- Not associated with burning
- May be caused by slight staining of tissue by hemoglobin from lysed RBCs along path of current.
- Indicates the path taken by current but does not corresponds to vascular channels
- Disappears in 1 or 2 days if survives.

Ans: (b) Lightening strike

Ref: *Andrews et al., Lightening Injuries – Electrical, Medical and Legal Aspects, CRC Press, 1st edition, page 86*

7. Mercury poisoning: Pharaoh serpent is:

(a) Mercuric iodide
(b) Mercuric chloride
(c) Mercury thiocyanate
(d) Mercuric sulphide

Explanation:

- **Mercury thiocyanate** is used in Diwali as it produces a large winding snake when set on fire. This is known as **Pharaoh snake/serpent**.
- Named after Biblical story when Pharaoh of Egypt calls his magicians who turned their staffs into snakes.

MERCURY (Hg; Quick silver)

- Toxicity - Organic Mercury > Mercuric compounds > mercurous compounds
- Important toxic compounds: mercuric chloride (corrosive sublimate), mercuric cyanide, mercuric oxide, methyl mercury (most toxic) etc

MOA - Inactivates sulfhydryl enzymes and thus interferes with cellular metabolism and functions.

Sign and symptoms:

- Acrid, metallic taste,
- A feeling of constriction or choking sensation in throat, hoarse voice
- Mouth, tongue and esophagus become corroded, swollen, and coated with greyish white coating.

If survive initial stage:

- Glossitis and ulcerative gingivitis (in 24-36 hrs) followed by loosening of teeth and necrosis of jaw
- Renal tubular necrosis and gangrenous colitis

Treatment

- Stomach wash and chelating agents
- Haemodialysis if required

Chronic Hg poisoning - HYDRARGYRISM

- **Hatter's shake** or **Glass blower's shakes**: Coarse with jerky movements; Involvement – Hands → lips and tongue → arms and legs
- **Mercurial erethism** (personality disorder)- excitability, memory loss, insomnia, timidity, sudden attacks of anger and later delusions and hallucinations – Mad as a hatter
- **Mercuria lentis** – deposition of Hg on the anterior lens capsule, bilateral and has no effect on visual acuity
- **Acrodynia - Pink disease or Swift's disease**
  - Mercurous Cl – given to children as tooth powder.
  - Characterized by – Pink, puffy, painful, parestethic, peeling and perspiring hands and feet (6Ps)
- **Minimata Bay epidemic**: Due to chronic organic Hg poisoning (1955) – Methyl mercury

Treatment–N-acetyl penicillamine/BAL

Ans: (c) Mercury thiocyanate

Ref: *Anil Aggarwal, Forensic Medicine and Toxicology for MBBS, 1st edition, APC, page 522*

8. Enblock dissection of organs:

(a) Letulle (b) Ghon

(c) Rokitansky (d) Virchow

Explanation:

Methods of Organ Dissection

Method	Technique	Remarks
M. Letulle (lEtulle – En-mass)	En masse dissection and organ separation + dissection	Ideal because it preserves connection between organs
R. Virchow (vIrchOw – Individual Organs)	Individual organ removal + dissection	Most common
A. Ghon (ghOn – Organ block/ Enblock)	Separate block dissection and organ separation + dissection	
C. Rokitansky (rokItanSky – In-Situ)	In-situ organ dissection	Preferred in children and infected bodies

Ans: (b) Ghon

Ref: *KSN Reddy, The Essentials of Forensic Medicine and Toxicology, 34th edition, page 104-105*

9. Drooling of saliva is pathagnomonic of:

(a) Postmortem hanging
(b) Antemortem hanging
(c) Strangulation/ Homicidal hanging /throttling
(d) Suicidal hanging

Explanation:

*" Normally **salivary** secretion is a **constant phenomenon** in life, however, it is being **swallowed** continuously. When death takes place the **deglutition also stops**, while the local pressure and irritation exerted by the ligature on submandibular salivary glands continues and this results in secretion of saliva. This can **flow passively** through the lower angle or **dependent parts** of the **mouth**, and is suggestive of **antemortem hanging**." **Ref: NG Rao***

*"**Dribbling of saliva** is the **surest sign** of **antemortem hanging.**" **Ref: KS Narayan Reddy***

Diagnosis of Hanging

- Ligature mark around the neck
- Presence of abrasions, ecchymoses and redness about the ligature mark
- Trickling of saliva from the mouth
- Ecchymoses of the larynx or epiglottis
- Rupture of the intima of the carotid, and
- Postmortem signs of asphyxia.

Note:

- **Dribbling of saliva/semen/urine** is a sure sign of antemortem hanging, while others can be seen in postmortem hanging as well.
- **La facies sympathique** is when the ligature knot presses on the cervical sympathetic chain, the eye on the same side may remain open with its pupil fully dilated.
- **Ligature mark**, **cartilage #** and **Tardieu spots** can also be seen in strangulation.

Sure signs of antemortem hanging

a. Dribbling of Saliva
b. Ecchyomosis of Ligature mark
c. Rupture of Intimae of carotid

Differences between Antemortem and Postmortem Hanging

Sl No	Features	Antemortem Hanging	Postmortem Hanging
1	**Motive**	Usually suicidal. Homicidal only in cases of lynching	Motive to disguise as suicide
2	**Ligature Mark**	Ligature mark well developed, base is parchment like and is yellow or brown	No such features seen
3	**Saliva**	Dribbling of saliva may be seen	Absent
4	**Injuries**	No other injuries may be seen	Other injuries which causes death may be seen
5	**Asphyxial features**	Will be seen in the body	No asphyxia signs present
6	**Circumstantial evidence**	Closed room. No signs of struggle may be seen	Signs of struggle may be seen
7	**Drag marks on the body**	Not present	May be seen
8	**Suicide Note**	May or may not be present	Never present
9	**Rope fibres**	Maybe seen in the hands	Not seen

Ans: (b) Antemortem hanging

Ref: *The Essentials of Forensic Medicine and Toxicology by KS Narayan Reddy, 29th edition, 2010 and Textbook of Forensic Medicine and Toxicology NG Rao, page 199*

PSM

1. Human anatomical waste is discarded in which of the following colour bins?

(a) Yellow (b) Red

(c) White (d) Blue

Explanation:

According to Biomedical Waste Management Rules (BMW) 2016

Schedule I, Part I: Biomedical wastes, categories and their segregation, collection, treatment, processing and disposal options:

Category	Type of bag/container used	Type of waste	Treatment/disposal options
Yellow 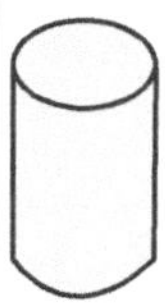	Non-chlorinated plastic bags	Human anatomical waste Animal anatomical waste Soiled waste Expired or discarded medicines Chemical waste Chemical liquid waste Discarded linen, mattresses, beddings contaminated with blood or body fluids Microbiology biotechnology and other clinical laboratory waste	Incineration/plasma pyrolysis/ deep burial
Red 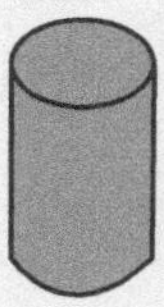	Non-chlorinated plastic bags or containers	Contaminated waste (recyclable) tubing, bottles, intravenous tubes and sets, catheters, urine bags, syringes (without needles and fixed needle syringes) and gloves	Autoclaving/microwaving/ hydroclaving and then sent for recycling. Not to be sent to landfill
White 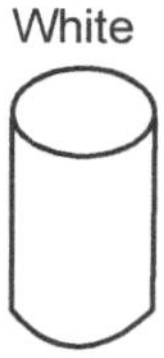	Puncture, leak, tamper proof containers (Translucent)	Waste sharps including Metals: Needles, syringes with fixed needles, needles from needle tip cutter or burner, scalpels, blades or any other contaminated sharp object that may cause puncture and cuts. This includes both used, discarded and contaminated metal sharps	Autoclaving or dry heat sterilisation followed by shredding or mutilation or encapsulation
Blue 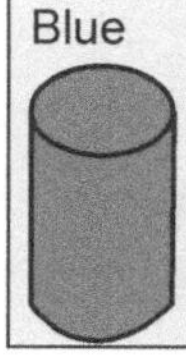	Cardboard boxes with blue coloured marking	Glassware: Broken or discarded and contaminated glass including medicine vials and ampoules except those containing cytotoxic wastes Metallic body implants	Disinfection or autoclaving/ microwaving/hydroclaving and then sent for recycling

Schedule II: STANDARDS FOR TREATMENT AND DISPOSAL:

Standards for:

- Incinerators

- Waste autoclave
- Liquid waste
- Microwaving
- Deep burial
  - Waste treatment facility should be available within a distance of seventy-five kilometers.
  - Occupier shall hand over segregated waste to common bio-medical waste treatment facility.
  - The biomedical waste shall be segregated into containers or bags at the point of generation.
  - The Occupier or Operator of a common bio-medical waste treatment facility shall maintain a record of recyclable wastes.

SCHEDULE – IV Part A: label for BMW Container/Bags

BIOHAZARD SYMBOL CYTOTOXIC HAZARD SYMBOL

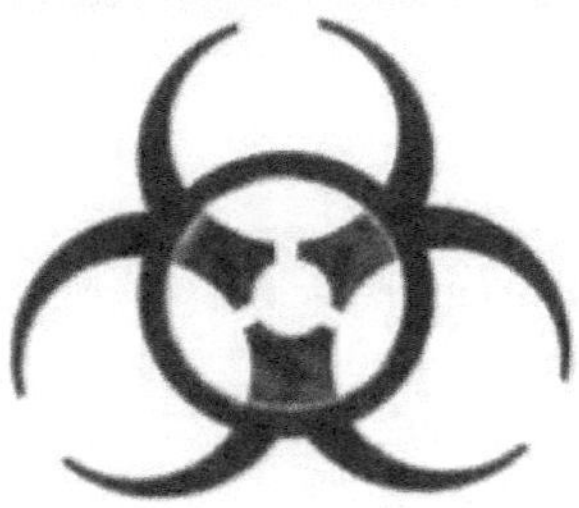

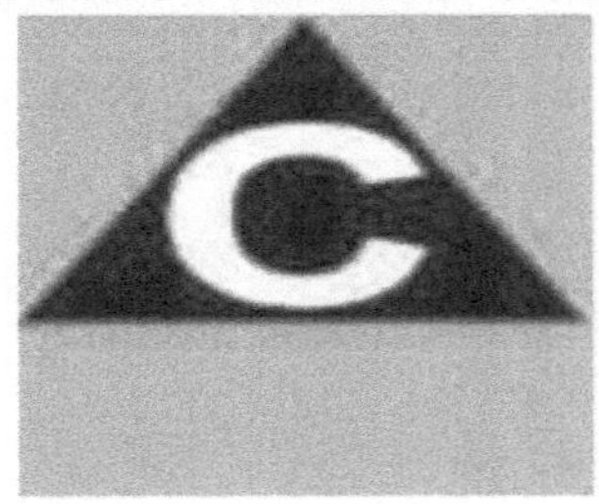

BIOHAZARD CYTOTOXIC

HANDLE WITH CARE

Note : Label shall be non-washable and prominently visible.

Ans: (a) Yellow

Ref: *Park's Textbook of Preventive and Social Medicine, 24th edition, page 829-831*

2. The result of a randomized trial was that the mortality rate in treatment group was 20% and the mortality rate in placebo group was 25%. Calculate NNT.

(a) 15 (b) 25

(c) 20 (d) 10

Explanation:

The results of randomized trials (RCT) can be expressed in number of ways such as:

- Calculate the risk of death or risk of developing the disease/complication after exposure to risk factor
- Calculate the reduction of risk/disease after treatment with drug/vaccine i.e. efficacy of drug or vaccine
- Calculate the ratio of the risks in the two treatment groups (the relative risk)
- Compare the survival curves for each of the groups
- To estimate the number of patients who would need to be treated (NNT) to prevent one adverse outcome such as one death
- To estimate the risk of side effects by calculating the number needed to harm (NNH) to cause one additional person to be harmed.

NNT (Number of patients who would need to be treated): $\dfrac{1}{\text{Rate in untreated group–Rate in treated group}}$

Here the rate of mortality in untreated group (placebo) is 25% and rate of mortality in treated group is 20%

$$NNT = \frac{1}{25\% - 20\%} = \frac{1}{0.05} = 20$$

Thus, NNT 20 means that 20 patients are needed to be treated to prevent one death.

Ans: (c) 20

Ref: *Book Epidemiology, Leon Gordis, Fifth edition, page 161-162*

3. More people seem to be affected by leukemia in town A than in town B. Which of the following study designs would be best suited to determine if there is a difference between prevalence of leukemia in these two towns?

(a) Case - control (b) Cross - sectional

(c) Clinical trial (d) Cohort

Explanation:

Cross-sectional study

- **Cross-sectional study** also called **Prevalence** study.
- Here both the exposure and disease outcome are determined simultaneously for study subjects at a certain point of time.
- The prevalent cases of the disease existed at the time of the study.
- Here we do not know the duration of disease.
- This study can only suggest the possible risk factor or risk factors for a disease.

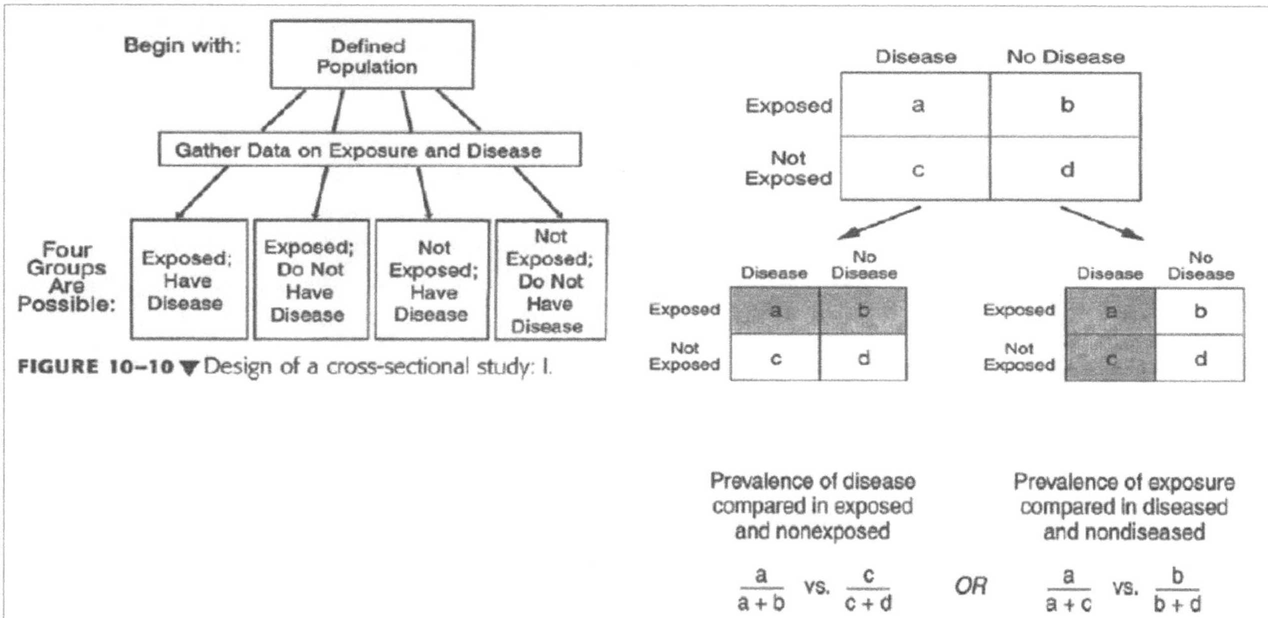

FIGURE 10–10 ▼ Design of a cross-sectional study: I.

Drawback of cross-sectional study:

- Calculates only the prevalent cases and excludes those who died due to disease before the study was conducted. The association of exposure and the disease is observed with survived patients rather than with the risk of developing the disease.

- Not possible to establish the temporal relationship between the exposure and the onset of disease.

Ans: (b) Cross-sectional study

Ref: *Book Epidemiology, Leon Gordis, fifth edition, page 210-212*

4. In a randomized trial study to test a new drug, 36 deaths were reported out of sample of 120 in placebo group. With the new treatment, 26 deaths were reported from a sample size of 130. How many patients should be treated to avert 1 death?

(a) 100 (b) 10

(c) 250 (d) 160

Explanation:

- Mortality rate of disease by pre-existing drug = 36/120*100 = 30%
- Mortality rate of disease by new drug = 26/130*100 = 20%

NNT (Number of patients needed to be treated): $\frac{1}{\text{Rate in untreated group} - \text{Rate in treated group}}$

Here the rate of mortality in untreated group (placebo) is 30% and rate of mortality in treated group is 20%

$$NNT = \frac{1}{30\% - 20\%} = \frac{1}{0.01} = 100$$

Thus, 100 patients are needed to be treated to prevent one death.

Ans: (a) 100

Ref: *Book Epidemiology, Leon Gordis, fifth edition, page 161-162*

5. What happens to the sensitivity and specificity when two screening tests are done in series?

(a) Sensitivity decreases specificity increases (b) Both increased

(c) Both decreased (d) None of the above

Explanation:

- **Validity** of a test is defined as its ability to distinguish between who has a disease and who does not.
- **Sensitivity** of the test is defined as the ability of the test to identify correctly those who have the disease i.e. the proportion of diseased people who were correctly identified as "positive" by the test.
- **Specificity** of the test is defined as the ability of the test to identify correctly those who does not have the disease i.e. proportion of non-diseased people who are correctly identified as "negative" by the test.

Note: To calculate the sensitivity and specificity of a test, we should know who really have the disease i.e. compare the test results with any gold standard test.

Results of Screening	Have the disease	Do not have the disease	Totals
Positive	80 True positive (TP) Have the disease and test positive	100 False positive (FP) Donot have the disease but test positive	**180**
Negative	20 False negative (FN) Have the disease but test negative	800 True negative (TN) Do not have the disease and test negative	**820**
Totals	100	900	**1000**

Sensitivity= TP/TP+FN = 80/100 = 80%

Specificity= TN/TN+FP = 800/900 = 89%

For a **continuous variable**, such as blood pressure or blood glucose level, there is no positive or negative result. The decision is therefore made by establishing the cut off level for the disease above which the test result is considered positive and below which a result is considered negative.

Below the figure shows a population of 20 diabetic and 20 nondiabetics who are screened using a blood sugar test whose scale is shown along the vertical axis from high to low.

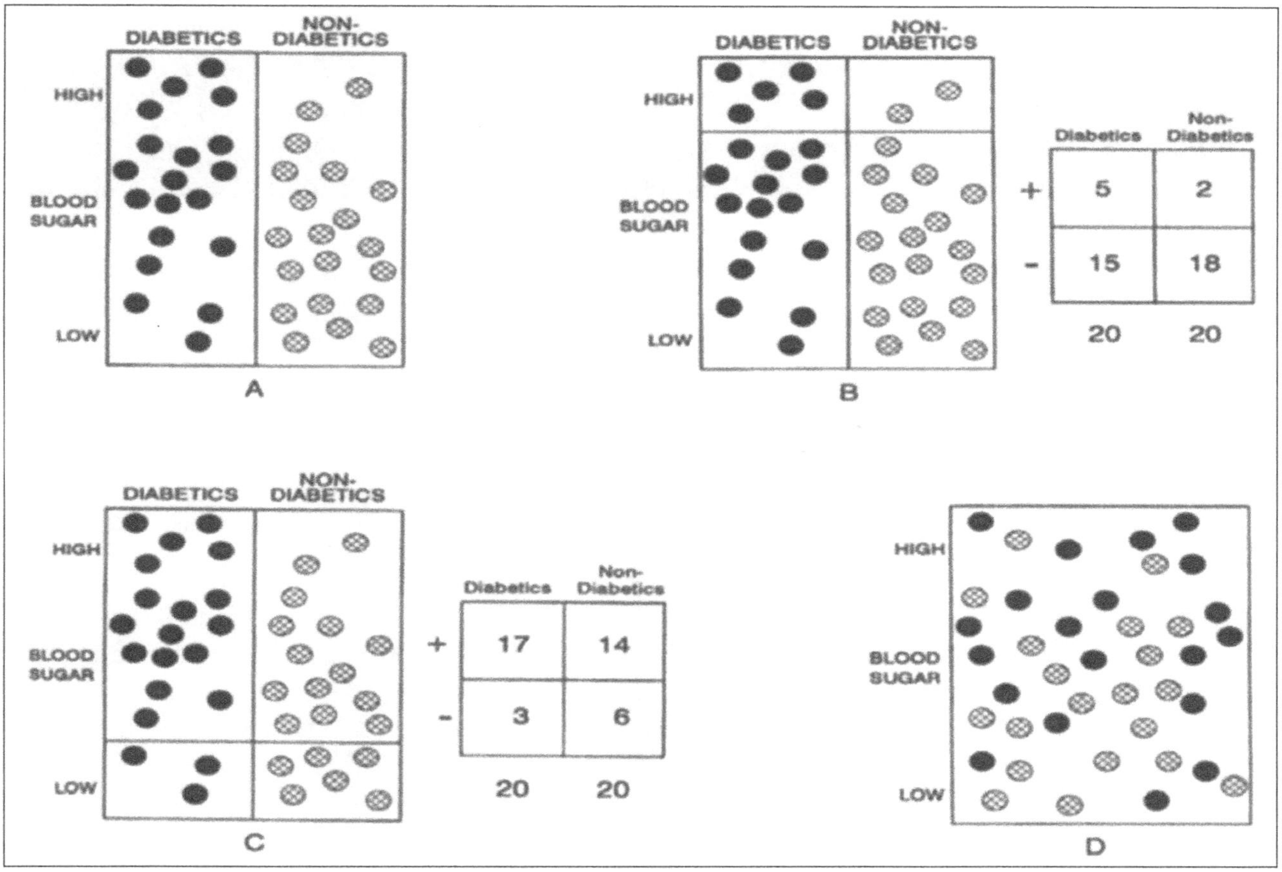

In figure B

- High cut off level is chosen.
- Clearly many diabetics will not be identified (FN increases and TP decreases, thus sensitivity of test will be low).
- Here, most of non-diabetics will be correctly identified as negative (TN increases and FP decreases, thus specificity of test increases).
- The sensitivity of test using this cut off will be 25% (5/20) and specificity will be 90% (18/20).
- The consequence of this is that the person with false negative result will be told that they do not have the disease and will not be followed.
- So, serious disease might be possibly missed at an early treatable stage.

In figure C

- Low cut off level is chosen.
- Very few diabetics will be misdiagnosed (TP increases and FN decreases, thus sensitivity of test will be high).
- Here, large numbers of non-diabetics are now identified as positive (TN decreases and FP increases, thus specificity of test decreases).

- The sensitivity of test using this cut off will be 85% (17/20) and specificity will be 30% (6/20).
- The consequence of this is that the person with false positive result will be brought back for further testing which is more expensive and thus burden on the health care system will increase. Anxiety and worry will be induced in person who has been told that they have tested positive.

Thus, if the sensitivity of a test increases specificity decreases and vice versa.

Ans: (a) Sensitivity decreases specificity increases

Ref: *Book Epidemiology, Leon Gordis, fifth edition, page 89-95*

6. Which one of these sampling methods is a probability sampling method?

(a) Snowball Method (b) Quota Method
(c) Lottery Method (d) Convenience Method

Explanation:

- Sampling is selection of a small number of elements from a larger defined target group of elements.
- Information from the small group will allow judgments to be made about the larger groups.

Types of sampling

A. Probability/Random sampling	B. Non-Probability sampling	C. Mixed sampling
a. Simple Random b. Systematic Random c. Stratified Random d. Cluster Sampling	a. Convenience b. Quota c. Purposive/Judgement d. Snowball/ Referral	a. Multistage b. Multiphase c. Lot quality assurance (LQA) sampling

A. PROBABILITY/RANDOM SAMPLING

Probability means chance - element of the population has **known** chance of being selected in the sample. Results are more accurate and reliable

Eg. If a sample of 100 students is to be selected from a population of 1000 students, then it is known to every one that each student has 100/1000 i.e., 1 in10 chance of being selected.

a. Simple random sampling

- All items selected independently.
- At each selection, all remaining items have same chance of being selected.
- **Done by:** (a) Random number tables (b) Lottery Method

Lottery method:

- With replacement
  - Probability each item: 1/N
- Without replacement
  - **Probability 1st draw: 1/N**
  - Probability 2nd draw**:** 1/N-1
- **Merits**
  - Known chance of selection.
  - No personal bias.
  - Easy method when there is an electronic database.

- **Demerits**
  - Complete accounting of population needed.
  - Cumbersome to provide unique designations to every population member.
  - Very inefficient when applied to skewed population distribution (over- and under-sampling problems).

b. **Systematic sampling:**

The procedure begins with finding out the sample interval

k=N/nk=sampling interval

N =universe size
n= sample size

Afterwards a random number is selected from the sample interval Selecting other units at evenly spaced intervals

Merits

- Easy and convenient.Less time consuming

Demerits

- Sample may be biased if hidden periodicities of the population coincide with that of selection.

c. **Stratified Random Sampling**

- Universe sub divided into mutually exclusive groups. A simple random sample is then chosen independently from each group.

Sample size within strata:

1. Proportional (proportionate in each stratum)
2. Disproportional (equal no. in each stratum)

d. **Cluster Sampling**

- Both simple random and stratified random sampling are not suitable while dealing with large and geographically scattered populations
- Therefore, large-scale sample surveys are conducted on cluster sampling basis.
- Entire population of interest divided into groups (clusters). Random sample of these clusters is then selected.
- In cluster sampling, the clusters are the primary sampling unit (PSU's).
- Units within the clusters are the secondary sampling units (SSU's)

B. **NON-PROBABILITY SAMPLING**

a. **Convenience**

- Sample selected neither by probability nor by judgment.
- Merit – Useful in pilot studies.
- Demerit – Results usually biased and unsatisfactory.

b. **Quota sampling**

- Most commonly used NPS.
- Quotas set up according to some specified characteristics.
- Within the quota, selection depends on personal judgment.
- Merit–Used in public opinion studies
- Demerit – personal prejudice and bias

c. **Purposive/Judgement/Deliberate sampling**
- Depends exclusively on the judgment of investigator.
- Sample selected which investigator thinks to be most typical of the universe.
- **Merits**
  - Small no. of sampling units
  - Urgent public policy and business decisions
- **Demerits**
  - *Personal prejudice and bias
  - No objective way of evaluating reliability of results
  - Proceeds on the belief that researcher knows enough about the population and its element to handpick the sample

d. **Snowball sampling**
- Used when the desired sample characteristic is rare
- When locating respondents is extremely difficult or cost prohibitive.
- Snowball sampling relies on referrals from initial subjects to generate additional subjects
- Make contact with one or two cases in the population.
- Ask these cases to identify further cases.
- Ask these new cases to identify further new cases.
- Stop when either no new cases are given or the sample is as large as is manageable.
- Merit
  - For difficult to reach populations (other methods may not yield any results).
- Demerit
  - Not representative of the population and will result in a biased sample as it is self-selecting.

Ans: (c) Lottery Method

Ref: *Methods in Biostatistics by BK Mahajan, 9th edition, page 125-138*

7. What does Correlation co-efficient of 0.5 indicate:

(a) Confidence interval of 95% (b) Weak association
(c) Not statistically significant (d) Good association

Explanation:

Correlation coefficient (r)
- Correlation coefficient lies between -1 to 1.
- How to interpret (r)
  - r=0 means no correlation.
  - r=-1 means perfect negative correlation
  - r=1 is perfect positive correlation
  - If 0>r>1 then it shows moderately positive correlation
  - If -1>r>0 suggests moderately negative correlation.
- The most accurate option here is c.
- r, >0.8- excellent, 0.6-0.8 is good , 04.-0.6 is fair, and <0.4 is poor.

- 95% confidence interval refers to range of results if the same study was done on 100 such sample, 95% of time results would lie in that range.

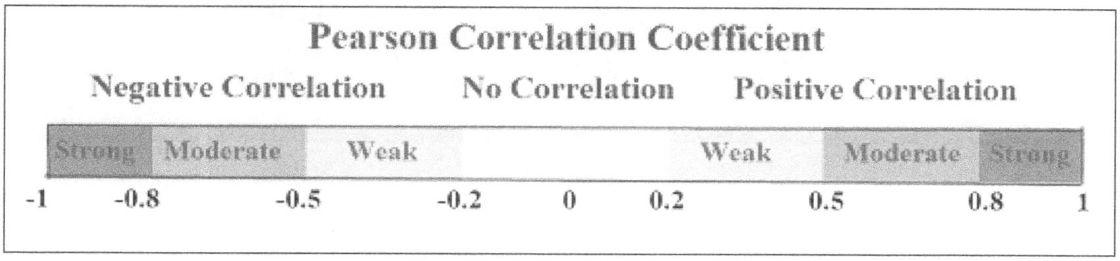

Ans: (b) Weak association

Ref: *Methods in Biostatistics by Mahajan 7th edition, page 196-200*

8. A patient with cervical cancer is missed by a screening test and later diagnosed to have advanced disease. This time interval is called:

(a) Lead time
(b) Screening time
(c) Serial interval
(d) Generation time

Explanation:

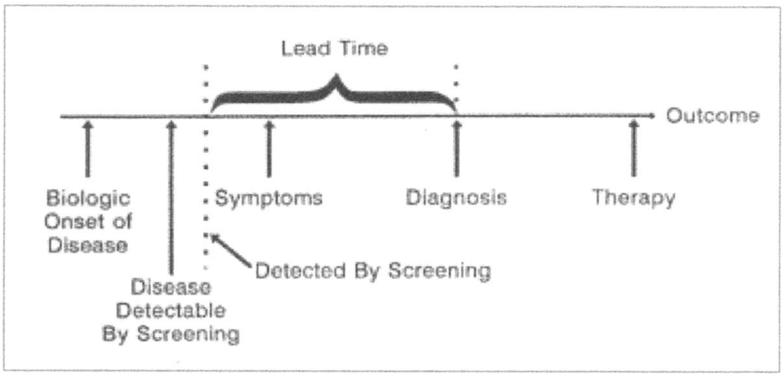

Lead time:

- Lead time is defined as the interval between the point a condition is detected through screening and the time it would normally have been detected due to appearance and reporting of signs and symptoms.
- It is the advantage gained by screening

Screening time:

- The time interval between the point a condition is detected through screening and final critical diagnosis by other means before usual time of diagnosis.

Serial Interval:

- The gap in time between the onset of the primary case and the secondary case is called the "serial interval".

Generation time:

- It is defined as "the interval of time between receipt of infection by a host and maximal infectivity of that host"

Ans: (a) Lead time

Ref: *K Park, Parks Textbook of Preventive and Social Medicine, 22th edition, page 127; Textbook of Public Health and Community Medicine, Armed Force Medical College, Pune, First edition 2009, page 136, 224*

9. A study is planned to check stool occult blood positivity using Hemooccult test among a group of participants aged 50 – 75 years. The second test is done if result is positive. No further testing if the test is negative. What is the effect of sensitivity and specificity for second test?

(a) ↑ specificity ↓ sensitivity
(b) ↓ specificity ↑ sensitivity
(c) ↑ specificity ↑ sensitivity
(d) No effect

Explanation:

- **The sequential/ serial testing-** two sequential tests are used and those who **test positive by the first test** are brought in for the second test. When we retest those who tested positive on the first test, there is a **loss in net sensitivity and a gain in net specificity**.
- The **simultaneous testing**, because an individual who tests positive on any one or multiple tests is considered positive, there is a **gain in net sensitivity and net loss in specificity**.

Basic measures used in evaluation of a diagnostic test are:

a. Sensitivity and specificity

b. Predictive values – positive predictive value and negative predictive value

Sensitivity: Ability of the test to identify **true positives** (TP)
Specificity: Ability of the test to identify **true negatives** (TN)
Positive predictive value: Probability that a patient with positive test result truly has the disease
Negative predictive value: Probability that a patient with negative test result truly does not have the disease

Ans: (a) ↑ specificity ↓ sensitivity

Ref: *Leon Gordis, Epidemiology, Fifth edition, page 99*

ENT

1. Which sinus is not seen on X-ray of 5 years old child?

(a) Sphenoid sinus
(b) Maxillary sinus
(c) Posterior ethmoid sinus
(d) Frontal sinus

Explanation:

Sinus	Status at birth	Growth	First radiological evidence
Maxillary	Present	Rapid growth from birth to 3 years and 7-12 years. Reaches adult size by 15 years	4-5 months after birth
Ethmoid	Present	Reaches adult size by 12 years	1 year
Frontal	Absent	Invades frontal bone by age of **4 years** and increases till teens	6 years
Sphenoid	Absent	Reaches sella turcica by age of 7 years, dorsum sellae by late teens and basisphenoid by adult age and reaches full size between 15 years to adult age.	4 years

Ans: (d) Frontal sinus

Ref: *Diseases of the Ear, Nose and Throat by PL Dhingra, 7th edition, page 211*

2. Which does not drain into middle meatus?

(a) Frontal Sinus
(b) Maxillary Sinus
(c) Posterior ethmoid
(d) Anterior Ethmoid

Explanation:

Openings of meatus (lateral walls) of nasal cavity

Sphenoethmoidal recess	Sphenoid sinus
Superior meatus	Posterior ethmoidal sinus*
Middle meatus	Maxillary sinus* Anterior and middle ethmoidal sinus* Frontal sinus*
Inferior meatus	Nasolacrimal duct*

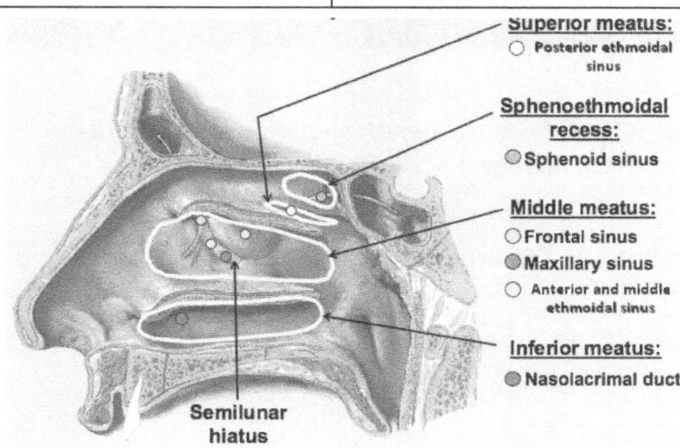

Ans: (c) Posterior ethmoid

Ref: *Diseases of the Ear, Nose and Throat by PL Dhingra, 7th edition, page 151*

3. Schwartz sign is seen in:

(a) Meniere's disease
(b) Acoustic neuroma
(c) Otosclerosis
(d) Otitis media with effusion

Explanation:

Otosclerosis

- Irregular spongy bone replaces the dense endochondral layer of the **bony labyrinth**
- Hereditary
- Associated with ***Van der hoove's*** **syndrome***
  - Osteogenesis imperfecta
  - Otosclerosis and
  - Blue sclera
- More common in **females**
- Hearing loss worsens during **pregnancy**
- **Cochlear type** presents with **Sensorineural Hearing loss**
- **Stapedial type** has **Conductive hearing loss** and may have anterior (most common) posterior, circumferential, biscuit or obliterative focus
- Clinical features: Hearing loss, **Paracusis willisi*** and tinnitus (indicates an active focus)
- O/E **Schwartz sign***- reddish hue over the promontory because of increased vasculature in active lesions
- PTA will show the type of hearing loss and **Carhart's notch*** which is a dip in the bone conduction at **2kHz**
- **Impedance audiometry** will show a **As type** curve
- Medical treatment with **sodium fluoride** can be tried
- **Surgery** is the **treatment of choice** and includes **stapedotomy or stapedectomy** followed by replacement with a **piston** made of **Teflon** or stainless steel or titanium

Ans: (c) Otosclerosis

Ref: *Diseases of the Ear, Nose and Throat by PL Dhingra, 7th edition, page 96*

4. Which of the following muscles of larynx and actions are correctly matched?

(a) Thyroarytenoid – Relaxes VC
(b) Cricothyroid – Tensor
(c) Lateral cricoarytenoid – abductor
(d) Posterior cricoarytenoid – adductor

Explanation:

- Please remember there is only one muscle which **abducts** the **vocal cords** and that is the **posterior cricoarytenoid***. It is supplied by the **recurrent laryngeal nerve***
- The muscles of the larynx are divided into
- **Intrinsic muscles** – They act on the structures inside the larynx like vocal cord. They are of the following types

Intrinsic muscles of the larynx

Those acting on the vocal cord	**Abductors**	Posterior cricoarytenoid
	Adductors	Lateral cricoarytenoid Interarytenoid Thyroarytenoid
	Tensors	External – Cricothyroid Internal – Vocalis
Those acting on the laryngeal inlet	**Opening the inlet**	Thyroepiglottis (part of thyroarytenoid)
	Closing the inlet	Interarytenoid (oblique part) Aryepiglottic (posterior oblique part of interarytenoid)

- All the **intrinsic muscles** of the larynx are supplied by **recurrent laryngeal nerve** except **cricothyroid** which is supplied by the **external laryngeal branch** of **superior laryngeal nerve**
- **Extrinsic muscles**–These connect the larynx to surrounding structures and are divided into

Extrinsic muscles of the larynx

Elevators	Primary	**Stylopharyngeus** **Salphingopharyngeus** **Palatopharyngeus** **Thyrohyoid**
	Secondary	**Mylohyoid** **Stylohyoid** **Digastric** **Geniohyoid**
Depressors	**Sternohyoid** **Sternothyroid** **Omohyoid**	

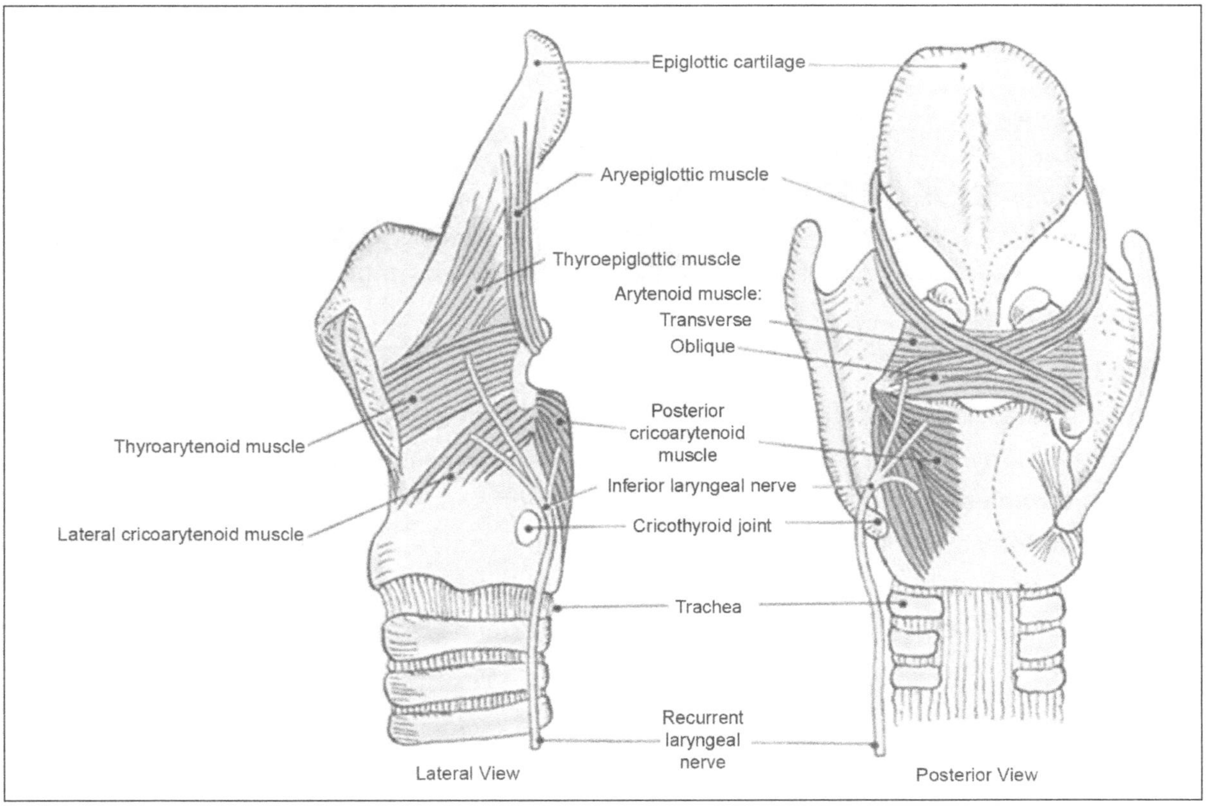

Ans: (b) Cricothyroid - Tensor

Ref: *Diseases of the Ear, Nose and Throat by PL Dhingra, 7th edition, page 320*

5. Muller's maneuver for:

(a) Eustachian tube (b) Vocal cord
(c) Dysphagia (d) OSA

Explanation:

Muller's maneuver

- The patient is asked to perform **forced inspiration** against **closed mouth and nose**
- It is a **reverse of Valsalva maneuver**
- Helps to **dynamically evaluate the upper airway** including nasopharynx, oropharynx and hypopharynx
- Main advantage is that **no sedation is required** as it can be safely performed in awake patient with minimal discomfort
- It helps us to evaluate the **level and degree of upper airway narrowing** and it has also been shown to be a **predictive value for the OSAS surgery**
- The level of collapse is classified according to the **VOTE criteria*** which includes:
  (1) Velum (soft palate and uvula)
  (2) Oropharyngeal lateral walls
  (3) Tongue base
  (4) Epiglottis
- It helps in deciding the type of surgery procedure which we use in OSAS patients.
- It is also used to terminate supraventricular tachycardia in an acute primary care setting.

Ans: (d) OSA

Ref: *Diseases of the Ear, Nose and Throat by PL Dhingra, 7th edition, page 315*

6. A patient sustains injury at carotid triangle during surgery and presents with weak voice postoperatively. Which nerve is likely affected?

(a) Ansa cervicalis (b) RLN
(c) Internal laryngeal nerve (d) External laryngeal nerve

Explanation:

Carotid triangle

- Muscular triangle in the neck bounded
  - **Posteriorly** by the anterior border of the **Sternocleidomastoid**
  - **Anteroinferiorly**, by the superior belly of the **Omohyoid**
  - **Superiorly** by the posterior belly of the **digastric muscle**
- **Contents** of the Carotid triangle include:
  - **Arteries** – External and internal carotid arteries, external carotid gives branches like superior thyroid artery, lingual artery, facial artery, occipital artery and ascending pharyngeal artery

- **Veins** – Internal jugular vein and veins draining into it namely superior thyroid vein, lingual veins, common facial vein, occipital vein and ascending pharyngeal vein
- **Nerves** – Hypoglossal nerve, Ansa cervicalis, Vagus nerve and its branches the superficial laryngeal nerve [internal and external branches], cervical sympathetic chain and spinal accessory nerve
- **Others** – deep cervical lymph nodes, carotid sinus and carotid body

Please Remember

- In **bilateral recurrent laryngeal nerve palsy** the vocal cords will be in the midline, this causes **respiratory distress** and stridor, however the vo**ice will be good**.
- In **unilateral recurrent laryngeal nerve palsy** all the ipsilateral internal laryngeal muscles are paralyzed except the cricothyroid (supplied by external laryngeal nerve); the vocal cord assumes a **median or Para median position** which results in hoarseness of voice. Since the other nerve is intact, the other side muscles work properly and the vocal cord can abduct. Therefore there will be **no stridor.**
- The internal branch of superior laryngeal nerve is purely sensory and its palsy will not cause much symptoms or mild aspiration
- The external branch of superior laryngeal nerve is motor to the cricothyroid muscle [external tensor] and therefore palsy will lead to weakness of voice and examination will reveal a drooped and shortened vocal cord

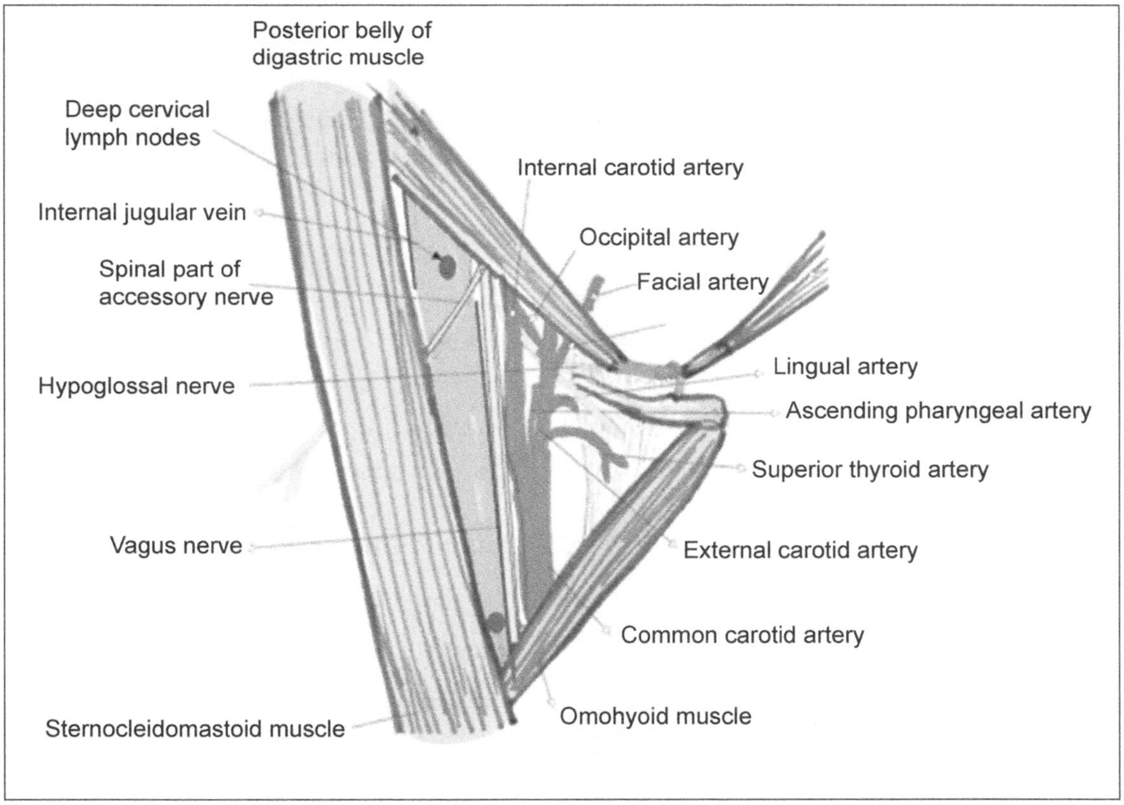

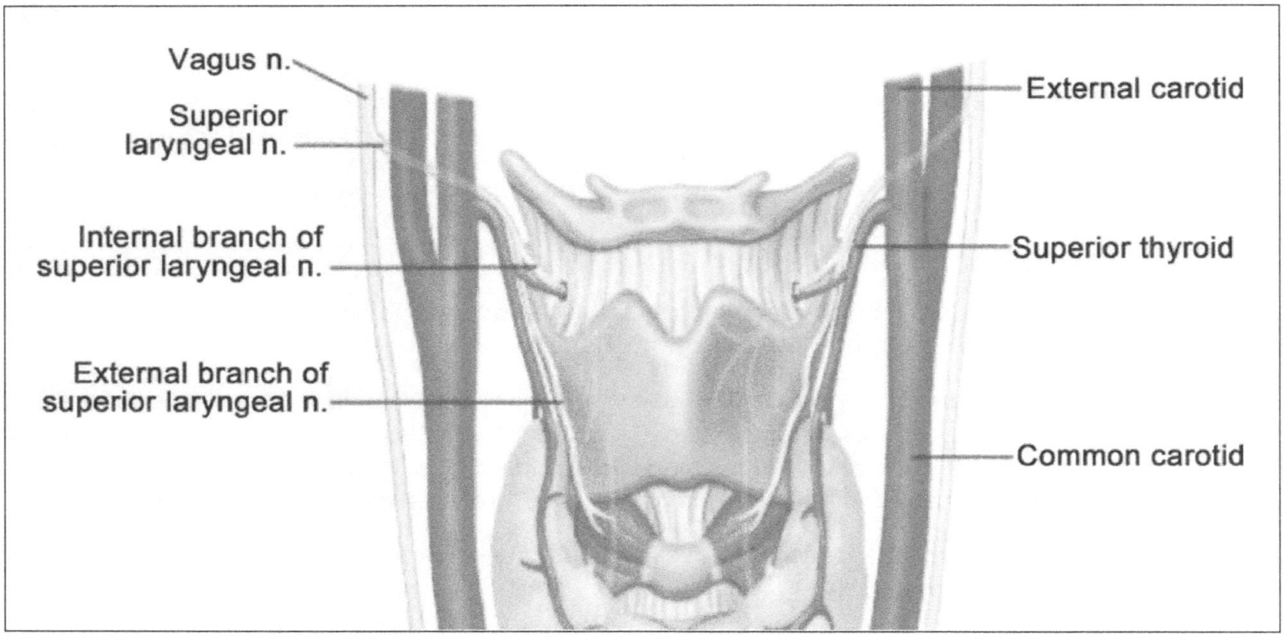

Ans: (d) External laryngeal nerve

Ref: *Diseases of the Ear, Nose and Throat by PL Dhingra, 7th edition, page 339*

7. Young's operation done in:

(a) Rhinophyma
(b) Atrophic rhinitis
(c) Rhinitis sicca
(d) Hypertrophic rhinitis

Explantation:

Young's operation

- It is done as a treatment of ***atrophic rhinitis***
- It involves ***closure of the nasal cavity*** affected with atrophic rhinitis by creating ***mucocutaneous flaps***
- These flaps are sutured together in two layers: first the mucosal layer, then the skin layer.
- The ***nasal cavity*** is kept ***closed for a period of 9 months***
- Re-examination is done after 9 months - if the crusts have disappeared, a revision surgery is performed and the nasal cavity is reopened.
- The theory behind this procedure is that the closed nasal cavity has time to heal

Ans: (b) Atrophic rhinitis

Ref: *Diseases of the Ear, Nose and Throat by PL Dhingra,7th edition, page 170*

8. A Patient with Peritonsillar abscess presents with ear pain. Most likely nerve responsible for this symptom is:

(a) Trigeminal nerve
(b) Glossopharyngeal nerve
(c) Mandibular nerve
(d) Auriculotemporal nerve

Explanation:

Referred otalgia: Pain in the ear due to lesions in distant regions.

Cranial Nerve	Nerve	Conditions
Via V Nerve (Trigeminal Nerve)	**Auriculo** temporal nerve	**Dental** • Caries • Apical abscess
		Oral cavity • Benign/malignant ulcers on tongue
		Temporomandibular joint disorder
		Sphenopalatine neuralgia
Via IX Nerve (Glossopharyngeal nerve)	**Jacobson's** nerve (tympanic branch)	**Oropharynx** • Acute tonsillitis • Peritonsillar abscess • Ulcer in soft palate • Post tonsillectomy
		Base of tongue • Malignancy • Ulcer
		Enlarged styloid process
Via X Nerve (Vagus Nerve)	**Arnold's nerve**	**Ulcer/malignancy of** • Vallecula • Epiglottis • Larynx • Oesophagus
Via C2 and C3 spinal nerves		• **Cervical spondylosis** • **Cervical injury**

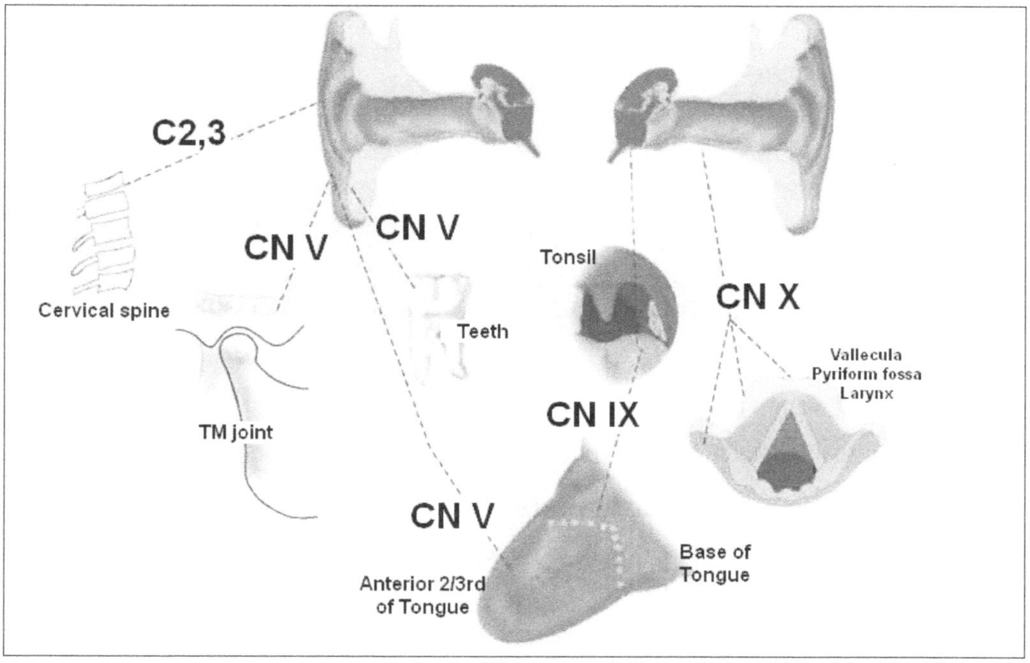

Figure: Schematic of Referred Otalgia

Ans. (b) Glossopharyngeal nerve

Ref: *Diseases of the Ear Nose and Throat by PL Dhingra, 6th edition, 2014, page 128*

OPHTHALMOLOGY

1. Axial proptosis is seen in:

(a) Hyperthyroidism (b) Optic nerve meningioma
(c) Orbital floor fracture (d) Lacrimal gland tumor

Explanation:

Axial Proptosis

	Causes
AXIAL PROPTOSIS	• **Intraconal Lesions**–Optic nerve glioma • **Thyroid Ophthalmopathy***
ECCENTRIC PROPTOSIS	
Lateral displacement	• **Medially placed masses**–Ethmoidal sinus mucocele / tumour • Sub-periosteal collection or pus
Medial and down	• Lacrimal gland tumour • Dacryoadenitis
Inferior displacement	• **Frontal sinus mucocele** • Encephalocele • Sphenoid wing meningioma • Orbital roof fracture
Superior displacement	• **Maxillary sinus tumour** • lymphoproliferative disorders

Ans: (a) Hyperthyroidism

Ref: *A.K. Khurana's Comprehensive Ophthalmology, 7th edition, page 422*

2. Rhegmatogenous retinal detachment is seen in which of the following conditions?

(a) Accelerated hypertension (b) Diabetes
(c) Myopia (d) Complicated cataract

Explanation:

RETINAL DETACHEMENT (RD):

- Separation of Neurosensory retina from Retinal Pigmentary epithelium.

Rhegmatogenous Retinal Detachment (RRD):

- RHEGMA means Break. Retinal detachment due to the **break in the neurosensory retina** is known as Rhegmatogenous Retinal detachment.
- **Pathological or Degenerative or Progressive Myopia is a** rapidly progressive refractive error resulting in high myopia (>-6 D) and is usually associated with degenerative changes in the peripheral retina.
- **Myopic Fundus**
- **Optic disc:** Large pale myopic disc with temporal myopic crescent and nasal supertraction crescent. Tilted optic disc can also occur.

- **Macula:** Foster - **Fuch's spots** (subretinal neovascularization and choroidal hemorrhage) and chorio retinal atrophic patches.
- **Tigroid Fundus: Tesselated** background.
- Peripheral retinal degenerations like Lattice, Cystoid, etc. will lead to retinal hole/tear and then retinal detachment.
- Posterior staphyloma due to ectasia of the sclera.
- Vitreous degeneration and liquefaction.

Mechanism of RRD:

Peripheral retinal degenerations → Retinal thinning → atrophic holes in the retina → vitreous seep into the hole → Retinal detachment

- **Accelarated hypertension** causes **Exudative RD***.
- **Diabetes:** Most common–**Tractional RD**. Combined Tractional and Rhegmatogenous RD can also occur.

RETINAL DETACHMENT

- Retinal detachment is defined as **separation of inner neurosensory retina** from the outer retinal pigment epithelium.
- It is classified as **rhegmatogenous, tractional and exudative**.

	Rhegmatogenous RD	Tractional RD	Exudative RD
Mechanism	Due to break or hole	Fibrovascular proliferation → pulls the neurosensory retina from the RPE	Due to accumulation of fluid (exudation)
Causes	• Myopia • Old age • Trauma	• DR • CRVO • PVR	From inflammatory process or neoplasm of retina/choroid/sclera
Symptoms	• Sudden painless loss of vision • **3 F's** - floaters, flashes of light, field loss	• Gradual loss of vision • Field loss	Defective vision depending on the cause
Configuration of retina	Convex	Concave	Bullous
Management	**3 S** • See the hole • Seal the hole • Drain the Subretinal fluid	• Vitrectomy • Endolaser photocoagulation	Treat the primary cause

Ans: (c) Myopia

Ref: *Parson's Diseases of the Eye, 22nd edition, page 331*

3. "a"wave in ERG is due to:

(a) Rods and cones (b) Bipolar cells

(c) RPE activity (d) Muller cells

Explanation:

The normal ERG is predominantly biphasic.

- **a wave–negative wave–**arising from the **rods and cones*.**
- **b wave–large positive wave–**generated by **Muller cells*** but represents the activity of the **bipolar cells*.**
- **c wave–positive wave–**representing the **metabolic activity** of the **RPE** seen* only in **dark adapted** state*.

ERG is very useful in detecting functional abnormalities in the outer retina upto Bipolar cell.

It is normal in diseases involving ganglion cells and the higher visual pathway such as Optic atrophy

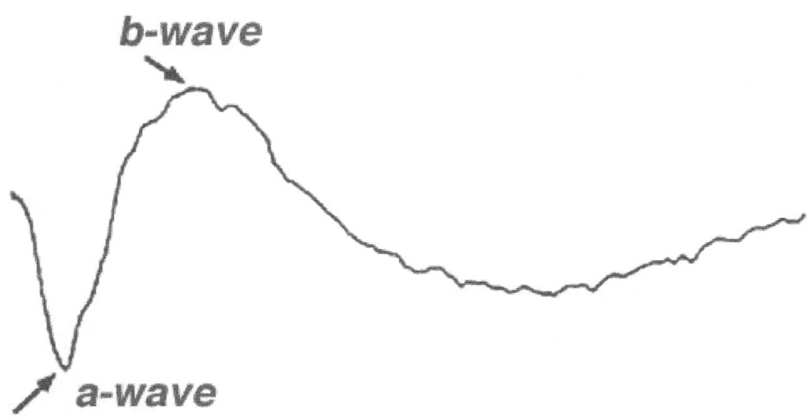

The biphasic waveform of the ERG of a normal patient.

- In standard full-field ERG, five recordings are taken during diffuse stimulation of the entire retinal area, and is used to assess generalized retinal disorders but may not detect localized pathology.
- **SCOTOPIC RESPONSES** depict the function of RODs. It is elicited after 30 minutes of dark adaptation.
- **PHOTOPIC RESPONSES** depict the function of cones and it is taken after 10 minutes of adaptation to moderately bright diffuse illumination.

Interpretation	
Non recording ERG	Leber congenital Amaurosis End Stage Retinitis pigmentosa Total RD Retinal Aplasia
Abnormal or non recordable photopic ERG	Gene degenerations Achromatopsia X-linked blue cone monochromatism X-linked cone dystrophy

Ans: (a) Rods and cones

Ref: *Parson's Diseases of the Eye, 22nd edition, page 109-111*

4. Levator palpebrae superioris is supplied by:

(a) 2nd CN (b) 3rd CN
(c) 4th CN (d) 6th CN

Explanation:

Nerve supply of ocular muscles

Extrinsic Muscles	Nerve Supply
Levator palpebrae superioris	3rd Cranial nerve
Orbicularis oculi	7th Cranial nerve
Lateral rectus	6th Cranial nerve
Remaining recti muscles	3rd Cranial nerve
Superior oblique	4th Cranial nerve
Inferior oblique	3rd Cranial nerve

Mnemonic: LR_6 SO_4 (Lateral rectus–6th CN and Superior oblique – 4th CN)

Intrinsic Muscles	Nerve Supply
Ciliary muscle	3rd Cranial nerve
Sphincter Pupillae	Parasympathetic supply along the 3rd Cranial nerve
Dilator pupillae	Sympathetic supply

Ans: (b) 3rd CN

Ref: *Parson's Diseases of the Eye, 22nd edition, page 408*

5. Most sensitive to radiation is:

(a) Retina (b) Optic nerve
(c) Lens (d) Cornea

Explanation:

Radiation induced changes in Eye

- The most radioresistant part in the retina is layer of rods and cones. Cones are more resistant than rods.
- The most radiosensitive part in the retina is vascular endothelium
- The most radiosensitive part of the eye is the **lens***.
- The **germinal layer of the lens** located at the equator is the layer most sensitive to radiation.
- The most radioresistant part of the eye is the **sclera**
- RT may cause acute ophthalmic complications such as **dry eye syndrome** (also known as "**ocular surface disorder**" and/or "**keratoconjunctivitis sicca**"), conjunctivitis, keratitis or chronic complications such as cataract, secondary glaucoma, radiation optic neuropathy, **retinopathy**, maculopathy, retinal vascular occlusions, and chorioretinal atrophy.
- Orbital bones, muscle, and fat can tolerate relatively high doses; the lens, eyelashes, retina, and lacrimal system are more radiosensitive.

Radiation Retinopathy

- Delayed retinal microvascular changes with endothelial cell loss, capillary occlusion and microaneurysm formation.
- Changes are directly proportional to the radiation dose.

CF:

- Presents commonly between 6 months and 3 years.

RETINA:

- Capillary occlusion with the development of telangiectasis and microaneurysms → retinal ischemia → **PROLIFERATIVE RETINOPATHY***
- Retinal oedema, exudate, cotton wool spots and haemorrhages
- Radiation optic neuropathy

TREATMENT: Usually unsatisfactory.

- Pan Retinal photocoagulation, intravitreal steroids and anti – VEGFs might help.

Ans: (c) Lens

Ref: *Ryan's Retina, Third edition, Vol. 2, page 1509*

MEDICINE

1. Not a feature of cauda equina syndrome:

(a) Asymmetric involvement
(b) Bladder and bowel spared
(c) Impaired Erection and ejaculation
(d) Absent Knee jerk

Explanation:

Cauda equina syndrome

- The **conus medullaris** is the tapered caudal termination of the spinal cord, comprising the sacral and single coccygeal segments
- The distinctive **conus syndrome** consists of **bilateral saddle anesthesia (S3-S5)**, prominent bladder and bowel dysfunction (urinary retention and incontinence with lax anal tone) and impotence
- The **bulbocavernosus** (S2-S4) and **anal** (S4-S5) reflexes are **absent***
- By contrast, lesions of the cauda equina, the nerve roots derived from the lower cord, are characterized by low back and radicular pain, asymmetric leg weakness and sensory loss, variable areflexia in the lower extremities, and relative sparing of bowel and bladder function

	Features	Cauda equina syndrome	Conus medullaris lesion
1.	Onset	Gradual and unilateral (or asymmetrical involvement of both lower limbs)	Sudden and bilateral
2.	Aetiology	PID, metastases	Intramedullary SOL (e.g., glioma)
3.	Root pain	Severe low backache	Usually absent
4.	Motor involvement	Asymmetric limb weakness	Muscle changes are not marked
5.	Sensory loss	Asymmetric sensory loss (i.e, unilateral saddle anaesthesia)	Bilateral saddle anaesthesia
6.	Bladder and bowel function	Late and less marked	Early and marked
7.	Anal reflex ($S_{3,4}$)	Areflexia if roots are involved	Anal reflex absent
8.	Deep reflexes	Ankle and knee jerks are lost	Ankle and knee jerks are usually preserved
9.	Trophic changes	Less	Early
10.	Plantar response	Flexor or no response	Extensor (not always)

* Cauda equina lesion usually gives rise to LMN signs whereas conus medullaris lesion have UMN signs

Ans: (c) Impaired erection and ejaculation

Ref: *Harrison Principles of Internal Medicine, 20th Edition, page 3173*

2. A patient of Pheochromocytoma presents with hypertension, hypokalemia and metabolic alkaloids. BP normalized after administration of a drug. Which drug was probably given?

(a) Spironolactone
(b) Clonidine
(c) Propanalol
(d) Hydrchlorothiazide

Explanation:

- Clinical presentation is so variable that pheochromocytoma has been termed "the great masquerader"
- The dominant sign is **hypertension**
- **Catecholamine crises*** can lead to **heart failure, pulmonary edema, arrhythmias, and intracranial hemorrhage**

- The diagnosis is based on documentation of
  - **Catecholamine excess** by biochemical testing and
  - Localization of the **tumor** by **imaging**
- Histologically the tumors often show a characteristic "**Zellballen" pattern**, consisting of nests of neuroendocrine chief cells with peripheral glial-like sustentacular cells
- **Complete tumor removal**, the ultimate therapeutic goal, can be achieved by partial or total adrenalectomy
- **Preoperative preparation** of the patient has to be considered, and blood pressure should be consistently <160/90 mm Hg. Classically, blood pressure has been controlled by α-adrenergic blockers (oral phenoxybenzamine, 0.5–4 mg/kg of body weight)
- Since patients are volume-constricted, liberal salt intake and hydration are necessary to avoid severe orthostasis
- **Oral prazosin** or **intravenous phentolamine** can be used to manage paroxysms while adequate alpha blockade is awaited
- **Beta blockers** (e.g.,10 mg of propranolol three or four times per day) can then be added
- The β-adrenergic antagonist should be administered only after α-adrenergic blockade is effective because with β-adrenergic blockade alone, severe hypertension or cardiopulmonary decom-pensation may occur as a result of the unopposed α-adrenergic stimulation
- Other antihypertensives, such as **calcium channel blockers or angiotensin-converting enzyme inhibitors**, have also been used effectively

Clinical Features Associated with Pheochromocytoma, Listed by Frequency of Occurrence	
1. Headaches	10. Weight loss
2. Profuse sweating	11. Paradoxical response to antihypertensive drugs
3. Palpitations and tachycardia	12. Polyuria and polydipsia
4. Hypertension, sustained or paroxysmal	13. Constipation
5. Anxiety and panic attacks	14. Orthostatic hypotension
6. Pallor	15. Dilated cardiomyopathy
7. Nausea	16. Erythrocytosis
8. Abdominal pain	17. Elevated blood sugar
9. Weakness	18. Hypercalcemia

Orally Administered Drugs Used to Treat Pheochromocytoma		
Drug	**Initial Dosage, mg/day[a] (Maximum)**	**Side Effects**
α-Adrenergic Blocking Agents		
Phenoxybenzamine	10[b] (100)[b]	Postural hypotension, tachycardia, miosis, nasal congestion, diarrhea, retrograde ejaculation, fatigue
Prazosin	1 (20)[c]	First-dose effect, dizziness, drowsiness, headache, fatigue, palpitations, nausea
Terazosin	1 (20)[b]	First-dose effect, asthenia, blurred vision, dizziness, nasal congestion, nausea, peripheral edema, palpitations, somnolence
Doxazosin	1 (20)	First-dose effect orthostasis, peripheral edema, fatigue, somnolence
Combined α-Adrenergic and β-Adrenergic Blocking Agent		
Labetalol	200[b] (1200)[b]	Dizziness, fatigue, nausea, nasal congestion, impotence

Contd.

Contd.

Calcium Channel Blocker		
Nicardipine sustained-release	30[b] (120)[b]	Edema, dizziness, headache, flushing, nausea, dyspepsia
Catecholamine Synthesis Inhibitor		
α–Methyi-p-L-tyrosine (metyrosine)	1000[c] (4000)[c]	Sedation, diarrhea, anxiety nightmares, crystalluria, galactorrhea, extrapyramidal symptoms
[a]Given once daily unless otherwise indicated [b]Given in two doses daily [c]Given in three or four doses daily		

Ans: (c) Propranolol

Ref: *Harrison Principles of Internal Medicine, 20th Edition, page 2740 and Williams Textbook of Endocrinology, 13th Edition, page 556*

3. Which parameter is last to decrease in sick euthyroid syndrome?

(a) t4 (b) t3

(c) tsh (d) rt3

Explanation:

- The most common hormone pattern in **sick euthyroid syndrome (SES),** also called **nonthyroidal illness (NTI),** is a
  - ***Decrease in total and***
  - ***Decrease in unbound T3 levels (low T3 syndrome) with***
  - ***Normal levels of T4 and TSH***
- Very sick patients may exhibit a dramatic fall in **total T4 and T3 levels (low T4 syndrome)**
- Fluctuation in TSH levels also creates challenges in the interpretation of thyroi nod function in sick patients. TSH levels may range from <0.1 mIU/L in very ill patients, especially with dopamine or glucocorticoid therapy, to >20 mIU/L during the recovery phase of SES

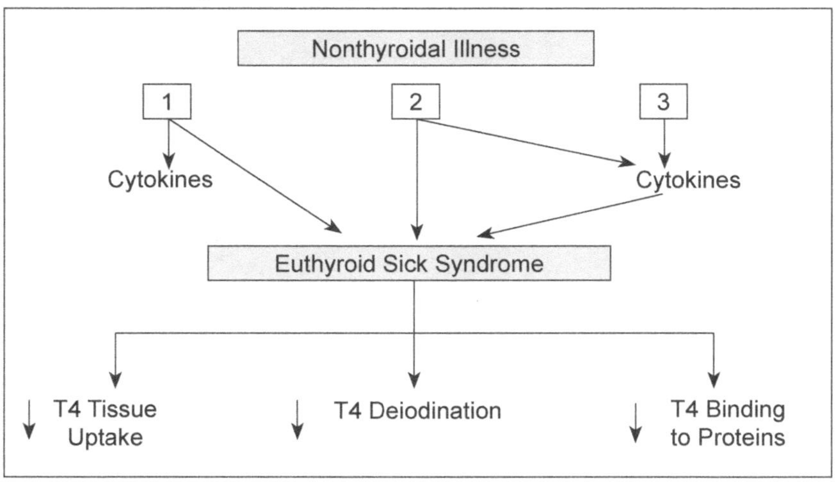

Figure: Relationship between ESS and cytokines

Ans: (c) TSH

Ref : *Harrison Principles of Internal Medicine, 20th Edition, page 2709*

4. Sodium content in hypertonic saline is:

(a) 90 (b) 154

(c) 513 meq/L (d) 130

Explanation:

- There are two types of IVFs:
  - Crystalloid and
  - Colloid solutions
- Crystalloid solutions are used to treat most patients with shock from **dengue**, while colloids are reserved for patients with profound or **refractory shock**

Crystalloid solutions

- Isotonic plasma volume expanders that contain electrolytes
- They can increase the circulatory volume without altering the chemical balance in the vascular spaces. This is due to their isotonic properties, meaning their components are close to those of blood circulating in the body
- Crystalloid solutions are mainly used to increase the intravascular volume when it is reduced. This reduction could be caused by haemorrhage, dehydration or loss of fluid during surgery

Crystalloid solutions and the concentrations of electrolytes:

Solution	Glucose (g/L)	Na^+	K^+	Ca^{+2}	Cl^-	Lactate	PO_4^{-3}	Mg^{+2}
5% Dextrose (D_5W)	50	0	0	0	0	0	0	0
10% Dextrose ($D_{10}W$)	100	0	0	0	0	0	0	0
Normal Saline (NS)	0	154	0	0	154	0	0	0
D_5NS	50	154	0	0	154	0	0	0
$D_{5½}NS$	50	77	0	0	77	0	0	0
0.2% NS	0	31	0	0	31	0	0	0
3% NaCl	0	513	0	0	513	0	0	0
Ringer's Lactate (LR)	0	130	4	3	109	28	0	0

Colloids:

- Colloids are gelatinous solutions that maintain a high osmotic pressure in the blood. Particles in the colloids are too large to pass semi-permeable membranes such as capillary membranes, so colloids stay in the intravascular spaces longer than crystalloids
- Examples of colloids
  - ***Albumin***
  - ***Hydroxy ethyl starch***
  - ***Dextran***
  - ***Gelatin***

Comparative summary of crystalloid and colloid solutions	
Crystalloid solution	**Colloid solution**
Half-life of 30-60 minutes	Half-life of several hours or days
Three times the volume needed for replacement	Replaces fluid volume for volume
Excessive use can cause peripheral and pulmonary oedema	Excessive use can precipitate cardiac failure

Contd.

Contd.

Molecules small enough to freely cross capillary walls, so less fluid remains in the intravascular spaces	Molecules too large to cross capillary walls, so fluid remains in intravascular spaces for longer
Inexpensive	More expensive than crystalloids
Non-allergenic	Risk of anaphylactic reactions
Suitable for vegetarian or vegan patients	Some preparations unsuitable for vegetarian or vegan patients

Ans: (c) 513 meq/L

Ref: *Harrison Principles of Internal Medicine, 20th Edition, page 513*

5. A patient with history of 10 years alcohol intake and 2 years history of IV drug abuse. Lab results reveal AST - 257 and ALT- 70. What is the diagnosis?

(a) Viral hepatitis (b) Alcoholic liver disease

(c) Autoimmune hepatitis (d) Drug Induced Liver Injury (DILI)

Explanation:

Drug-induced liver injury (DILI)

- Commonly categorized as either
  - **Intrinsic** (liver injury that is dose dependent and predictable due to the on-target, pharmacological activity of the drug) or
  - **Idiosyncratic** (liver injury that is unexpected or not readily anticipated based on pharmacological principles alone)
- DILI is also a leading cause of acute liver failure (ALF)
- Generally, the first indicator of DILI is detection of raised serum alanine aminotransferase (ALT) and/ or aspartate aminotransferase (AST) levels in patients with acute hepatocellular injury and of alkaline phosphatase in cholestatic injury
- **Alcohol** is the commonest cause of cirrhosis in the Western world
- Serum transaminase levels rarely exceed 300 IU/L. The aspartate aminotransferase (AST; serum glutamic oxaloacetic transaminase) level is usually higher than that of alanine aminotransferase (ALT; serum glutamic pyruvate transaminase), with the **AST: ALT ratio** usually exceeding **2:1**
- **Serum γ-GT** is a widely used **screening test** for hazardous drinking
- Serum alkaline phosphatase may be markedly **increased** (greater than **four times normal**) especially in those with **severe cholestasis** and **alcohol-related hepatitis. Serum IgA** values may be very high

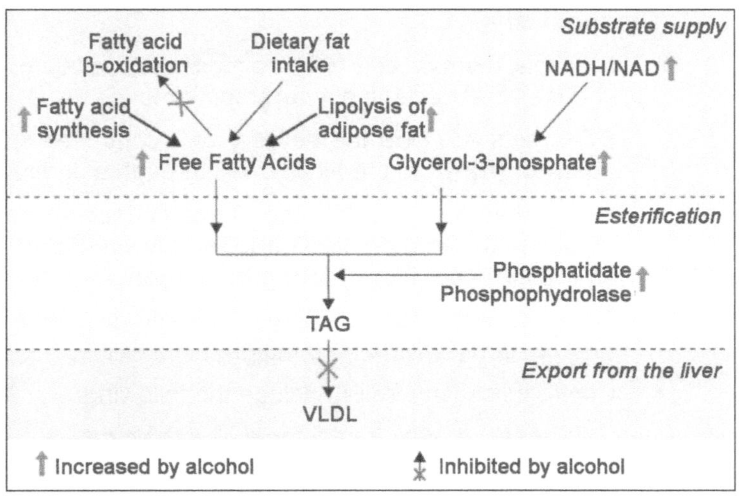

- International Serious Adverse Events Consortium (iSAEC) recommended in 2011 the modified biochemical criteria for the identification of **DILI** is as follows :
  - ALT ≥5 ULN

- ALP ≥2 ULN, especially in patients with elevated 5′-nucleotidase or GGT, and without bone-diseases-related ALP elevation
- ALT ≥3 ULN and T Bil ≥2 ULN.

Alcoholic liver disease (ALD)

- Has 3 stages of liver damage:
  - Fatty liver (steatosis)
  - Alcoholic hepatitis (inflammation and necrosis)
  - Alcoholic liver cirrhosis.
- All are caused by chronic heavy alcohol ingestion

Laboratory Diagnosis of Alcoholic Fatty Liver and Alcoholic Hepatitis	
Test	**Comment**
AST	Increased two- to sevenfold, <400 iU/L, greater than ALT
ALT	Increased two- to sevenfold, <400 iU/L
AST/ALT	Usually > 1
GGTP	Not specific to alcohol, easily inducible, elevated in all forms of fatty liver
Bilirubin	May be markedly increased in alcoholic hepatitis despite modest elevation in alkaline phosphatase

Ans: (b) Alcoholic liver disease

Ref: *Harrison, 20th Edition, Sherlock, page 494*

6. Thermoplasty is used in which condition?

(a) COPD (b) Asthma
(c) Bronchiectasis (d) Carcinoma lung

Explanation:

Thermoplasty

- Bronchial thermoplasty (BT) is a modality for treating **asthma** and is thought to prevent the chronic structural changes that occur in airway smooth muscle (ASM) in individuals with asthma
- BT targets ASM via the delivery of a controlled specific amount of **radiofrequency (RF) energy (RF ablation [RFA]**) to the airway wall through a dedicated catheter
- Candidates for bronchial thermoplasty include **adults** with **severe persistent asthma** who require regular **maintenance medications of inhaled corticosteroids** (>1000 μg/day of beclomethasone or the equivalent) and a **long-acting beta agonist** (≥100 μg/day of salmeterol or the equivalent)
- These patients would have received add-on therapies such as **leukotriene modifiers**, **omalizumab**, or **oral corticosteroids** (≤10 mg/day)
- Contraindications for BT include the following:
  - Presence of an implantable electronic device
  - Known hypersensitivity to drugs used during bronchoscopy
  - Severe comorbid conditions that would increase the risk of adverse events

Ans: (b) Asthma

Ref: *Medscape, Bronchial Thermoplasty by Said A Chaaban*

7. A 18-year-old male presented with recurrent urinary tract infection and dribbling of urine and secondary enuresis.What is the investigation used to diagnose the above mentioned condition?

(a) Urinalysis (b) Cystourethrogram

(c) IVP (d) Renal scintigraphy

Explanation:

Voiding cystourethrography (VCUG)

- Primarily used to establish the **presence** and **severity** of **vesicoureteral reflux (VUR)**
- VCUG is also used to diagnose
  - **Posterior urethral valves** and
  - To provide information on **bladder shape** and **function** in children with **bladder dysfunction**
- A voiding cystourethrogram (VCUG) is a contrast study that involves urethral catheterization and evaluates the bladder during both the filling and voiding phases
- **Reflux nephropathy** is the consequence of **vesicoureteral reflux (VUR**) or other urologic anomalies in early childhood. It was previously called **chronic pyelonephritis** because it was believed to result from **recurrent urinary tract infections (UTIs)** in childhood.
- VUR stems from abnormal retrograde urine flow from the bladder into one or both ureters and kidneys because of mislocated and incompetent ureterovesical valves
- Affected adults are frequently asymptomatic, but may give a history of **prolonged bed-wetting** or **recurrent UTIs during childhoo**d, and exhibit **variable renal insufficiency**, **hypertension**, mild to moderate **proteinuria**, and unremarkable urine sediment.

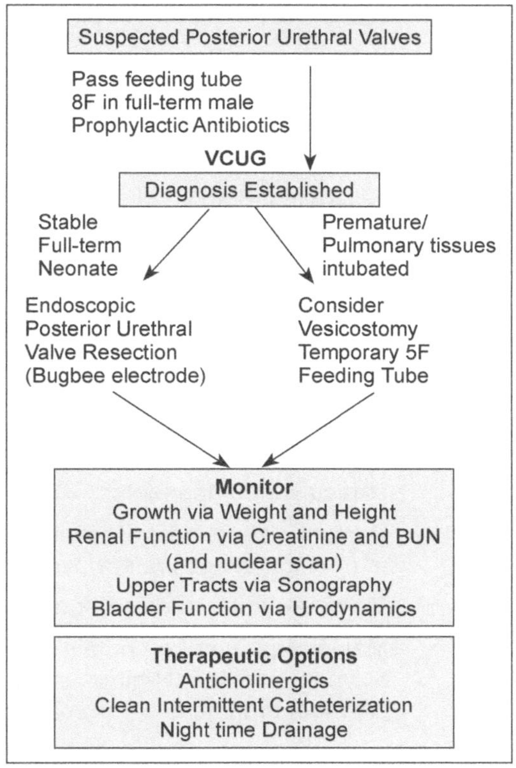

Figure: Treatment algorithm for patients with posterior urethral valves

Ans: (b) Cystourethrogram

Ref: *Harrison Principles of Internal Medicine, 20th Edition, page 2160*

8. Smoking is not a risk factor for:

(a) Respiratory bronchiolitic associated pneumonia (b) Sarcoidosis

(c) Desquamative interstitial pneumonia (d) Langerhan cell histiocytosis

Explanation:

- Although smoking-related ILDs including **respiratory bronchiolitis with interstitial lung disease (RB-ILD**), and **DIP** are frequently subclassified with the IIPs, these disorders (along with **Pulmonary Langerhans cell histiocytosis**, an **ILD** with unique clinical, imaging and histopathologic manifestations) are commonly felt to be the result of **active or prior tobacco smoke exposure**
- **Smokers**, particularly elderly smokers, frequently have radiologic (centrilobular) interstitial abnormalities
- Dyspnea and cough are relatively common
- HRCT Image Findings Prominent and common findings in RB-ILD include central bronchial wall thickening, peripheral bronchial wall thickening, centrilobular nodules, and ground-glass opacities

- Common features of RB-ILD include the accumulation of pigmented macrophages within the lumens of respiratory bronchioles and alveolar ducts, accompanied by chronic inflammation of the respiratory bronchiolar walls and both bronchiolar and peribronchiolar alveolar fibrosis causing architectural distortion
- All patients with smoking-related ILD should be counseled to discontinue smoking and/or encouraged to enroll in a formal smoking cessation program. Small studies have evaluated, and patients are often treated with immunosuppressive (e.g., prednisone) and cytotoxic (e.g., azathioprine, and cyclophosphamide) agents and in some cases with bronchodilators

Smoking

- Cigarette smoke is a complex aerosol composed of gaseous and particulate compounds
- Smoke consists of 2 components
  - Mainstream smoke
  - Sidestream smoke
- **Mainstream smoke** is produced by inhalation of air through the cigarette and is the primary source of smoke exposure for smokers
- **Sidestream smoke** is produced from smouldering of the cigarette between puffs and is the major source of environmental tobacco smoke or second-hand smoke
- There are more than 4000 chemical constituents of cigarette smoke: 95% of the weight of mainstream smoke comes from more than 400 gaseous compounds; rest of the weight is made up of more than 3500 particulate components
- Primary determinant of tobacco addiction is nicotine; tar is the total particulate matter of cigarette smoke after nicotine and water have been removed
- Exposure to tar seems to be a major component of lung cancer risk
- Mainstream smoke contains many potential carcinogens, including polycyclic aromatic hydrocarbons, aromatic amines, N-nitrosamines and other organic and inorganic compounds, such as benzene, vinyl chloride, arsenic and chromium

Diseases caused/worsened by smoking

- **Cancers**: Lung, oropharynx, oesophagus, stomach, pancreas, bladder, kidney, cervix, possibly colon and acute myeloid leukaemia
- **Respiratory diseases**: COPD, ILDs, chronic cough and infections
- **Cardiovascular diseases**: Coronary artery disease, cerebrovascular disease, peripheral artery disease, abdominal aortic aneurysm
- **Reproductive**: Miscarriage, prematurity, low birth weight
- **Gastrointestinal**: Gastro-oesophageal acid reflux, peptic ulcer and Crohn's diseases
- **Others**: Poor oral and skin health, cataract, fire-related injuries

Ans: (b) Sarcoidosis

Ref: *Harrison Principles of Internal Medicine, 20th Edition, page 2002*

9. All these management prolongs life in a COPD patient *except:*

(a) Long term O2 keeping pO_2 >95% (b) Bullectomy

(c) Smoking cessation (d) Steroids

Explanation:

- The two main goals of therapy are:
  - To provide symptomatic relief (reduce respiratory symptoms, improve exercise tolerance, improve health status) and

- To reduce future risk (prevent disease progression, prevent and treat exacerbations, and reduce mortality)

- Only three interventions have demonstrated to improve survival of patients with **COPD**. They are:
  - ***Smoking cessation***
  - ***Oxygen therapy in chronically hypoxemic patients***
  - ***Lung volume reduction surgery (LVRS) in selected patients with emphysema***

Ans: (d) Steroids

Ref: *Harrison Principles of Internal Medicine, 20th Edition, page 1996*

10. Diagnostic criteria for HHS:

(a) HCO_3 <15; Glucose > 600 and pH > 7.3
(b) HCO_3 >15; Glucose > 600 and pH > 7.3
(c) HCO_3 <15 Glucose > 600 and pH<7.3
(d) HCO_3 >15 Glucose >600 and pH< 7.3

Explanation:

Hyperglycemic hyperosmolar state (HHS)

- The prototypical patient with HHS is an **elderly individual** with **type 2 DM,** with a several-week history of **polyuria**, **weight loss**, and **diminished oral intake** that culminates in **mental confusion, lethargy, or coma**
- The physical examination reflects **profound dehydration**, **hyperosmolality** and **reveals hypotension**, **tachycardia, and altered mental status**
- HHS is often precipitated by a serious, concurrent illness such as myocardial infarction or stroke. Sepsis, pneumonia, and other serious infections are frequent precipitants and should be sought

Laboratory Values in Diabetic Ketoacidosis (DKA) and Hyperglycemic Hyperosmolar State (HHS) (Representative Ranges at Presenation)		
	DKA	**HHS**
Glucose,[a] mmol/L (mg/dL)	13.9-33.3 (250-600)	33.3-66.6 (600-1200)
Sodium, meq/L	125-135	135-145
Potassium[a,b]	Normal to ↑	Normal
Magnesium[a]	Normal	Normal
Chloridea	Normal	Normal
Phosphate[a,b]	Normal	Normal
Creatinine	Slightly ↑	Moderately ↑
Osmolality (mosm/mL)	300–320	330–380
Plasma ketones[a]	++++	+/–
Serum bicarbonate,[a] meq/L	<15	Normal to slightly ↓
Arterial pH	6.8-7.3	>7.3
Arterial PCO_2,[a] mm Hg	20-30	Normal
Anion gap[a] (Na – [cl + HCO_3])	↑	Normal to slightly ↑

[a]Large changes occur during treatment of DKA
[b]Although plasma levels may be normal or high at presentation, total body stores are usually depleted

- Most notable features of HHS are:
  - **Marked hyperglycemia (plasma glucose may be >55.5 mmol/L [1000 mg/dL])**
  - **Hyperosmolality (>350 mosmol/L)**
  - **Prerenal azotemia**

- The measured serum sodium may be normal or slightly low despite the marked hyperglycemia. The corrected serum sodium is usually increased (add 1.6 meq to measured sodium for each 5.6-mmol/L [100-mg/dL] rise in the serum glucose). In contrast to DKA, acidosis and ketonemia are absent or mild. A small anion-gap metabolic acidosis may be present secondary to increased lactic acid. Moderate ketonuria, if present, is secondary to starvation
- As in DKA, rehydration and volume expansion lower the plasma glucose initially, but insulin is also required. A reasonable regimen for HHS begins with an IV insulin bolus of 0.1 unit/kg followed by IV insulin at a constant infusion rate of 0.1 unit/kg per hour

Ans: (b) HCO_3>15; Glucose > 600 and pH > 7.3

Ref: *Harrison Principles of Internal Medicine, 20th Edition, page 2870*

11. Which of the following is false about Amoebic dysentery?

(a) Liver abscess is MC extraintestinal feature
(b) Most common site of ulcer is rectum
(c) Pus is due to liquefactive necrosis of liver
(d) Ulcer is punched put and in submucosa

Explanation:

Amebiasis

- Infection caused by Entamoeba **histolytica**, an intestinal protozoan.
- Its spectrum of clinical syndromes ranges from
  - Asymptomatic colonization (90% of cases) to
  - Invasive amebiasis, which accounts for 10% of affected individuals
- **Invasive amebiasis** frequently presents as **intestinal colitis** (dysentery or diarrhea) or as extraintestinal amebiasis, in which abscesses of the liver are more commonly found than involvement of the lungs or brain
- The earliest intestinal lesions are **micro-ulcerations** of the mucosa of the **cecum, sigmoid colon, or rectum** that release erythrocytes, inflammatory cells, and epithelial cells
- Rarely, intestinal infection results in the formation of a mass lesion, or ameboma, in the bowel lumen.
- The necrotic contents of a liver abscess are classically described as "**anchovy paste**,"
- Extraintestinal infection by E. histolytica most often involves the liver
- **Painful genital ulcers**, characterized by a punched-out appearance and profuse discharge, may develop secondary to extension from either the intestine or the liver
- Stool examinations, serologic tests, and noninvasive imaging of the liver are the most important procedures in the diagnosis of amebiasis

Indication	Therapy
Asymptomatic carriage	Luminal agent: Iodoquinol (650 mg tablets), 650 mg tid for 20 days; *or* paromomycin (250 mg tablets), 500 mg tid for 10 days
Acute colitis	Metronidazole (250 or 500 mg tablets), 750 mg PO or IV tid for 5-10 days; *or* tinidazole, 2 g/d PO for 3 days ***plus*** Luminal agent as above
Amebic liver abscess	Metronidazole, 750 mg PO or IV 5-10 days; or tinidazole, 2 g PO once; *or* ornidazole, 2 g PO once ***plus*** Luminal agent as above

Ans: (b) Most common site of ulcer is rectum

Ref: *Harrison Principles of Internal Medicine, 20th Edition, page 1568*

12. Which of the following causes toxic form of food poisoning?

(a) Staph aureus (b) Campylobacter jejuni
(c) Streptococcus (d) Pseudomonas

Explanation:

Staphylococcal food poisoning

- Results from the inoculation of **toxin-producing S. aureus** into food by colonized food handlers
- Toxin is then elaborated in such growth-promoting food as **custards**, **potato salad, or processed meats**
- The onset of illness is **rapid**, occurring within **1–6 hours of ingestion**
- The illness is characterized by **nausea and vomiting**, although **diarrhea, hypotension**, and **dehydration** also may occur
- Symptoms generally **resolve within 8–10 hours**
- The diagnosis can be established by the **demonstration of bacteria** or the documentation of **enterotoxin** in the implicated food. Treatment is entirely **supportive**

Campylobacter jejuni food poisoning

- Can be considered the prototype, in part because it is by far the most common enteric pathogen in the group.
- A prodrome of fever, headache, myalgia, and/or malaise often occurs 12–48 hours before the onset of diarrheal symptoms
- The most common signs and symptoms of the intestinal phase are **diarrhea, abdominal pain and fever**
- The degree of diarrhea varies from several loose watery stools to visibly bloody stools (~10% of cases in adults); most patients presenting for medical attention have ≥10 bowel movements on the worst day of illness
- Abdominal pain usually consists of cramping and may be the most prominent symptom. Pain is usually generalized but may become localized
- C. jejuni infection may cause **Pseudoappendicitis***
- Organisms which cause toxin induced diarrhoea are:
  - Campylobacter
  - Staphylococcus aureus
  - Salmonella
  - Shiga toxin-producing E. coli
  - Shigella
  - Vibrio
  - Yersinia
  - Listeria
  - Cyclospora
  - E.coli
  - Clostridium difficile
  - C. jejuni

Extra Edge

CAUSES OF SECRETORY DIARRHEA

Activation of Cyclic AMP
- **Bacterial toxins: Enterotoxins of cholera, *Escherichia coli (heat-labile), Shigella, Salmonella, Campylobacter jejuni, Pseudomonas aeruginosa***
- **Hormones: Vasoactive intestinal peptide, gastrin, secretin**
- **Anion surfactants: Bile acids, ricinoleic acid**

Activation of Cyclic GMP
- **Bacterial toxins: *E.coli* (heat-stable) enterotoxin, *Yersinia enterocolitica toxin***

Calcium-Dependent
- **Bacterial toxins: *Clostridium difficile enterotoxin***
- **Neurotransmitters: Acetylcholine, serotonin**
- **Paracrine agents: Bradykinin**

Ans: (a) Staph aureus

Ref: *Harrison Principles of Internal Medicine, 20th Edition, page 1076*

13. A Girl presents with history of ecchymosis and bleeding manifestations. Her CT, BT and platelets normal. Her Aptt is– 40. What's the most probable diagnosis?

(a) VWF deficiency
(b) Factor 5 deficiency
(c) Factor 9 deficiency
(d) Factor 11 deficiency

Explanation:

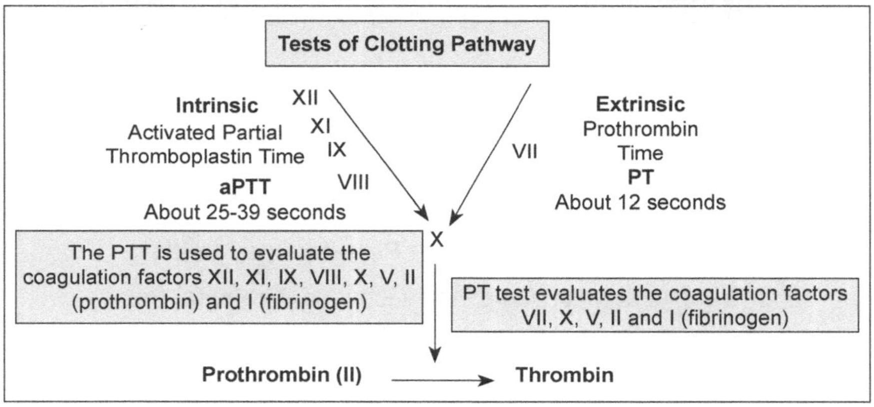

Von Willebrand Disease

- **VWD** is the most common inherited bleeding disorder
- VWD has been classified into three major types, with four subtypes of type 2
- VWF serves two roles:
  - As the major **adhesion molecule** that tethers the platelet to the exposed **subendothelium;** and
  - As the **binding protein for factor VIII (FVIII),** resulting in significant prolongation of the FVIII half-life in circulation.
- Patients with type O blood have VWF protein levels of approximately one-half that of patients with AB blood type; and, in fact, the normal range for patients with type O blood overlaps that which has been considered diagnostic for VWD
- **Acquired VWD**
- Rare disorder, most commonly seen in patients with underlying **lymphoproliferative** disorders, including:
  - **Monoclonal gammopathies of underdetermined significance (MGUS**),
  - **Multiple myeloma**, and
  - **Waldenström's macroglobulinemia**.
- Individuals with VWD may have a **normal** or **prolonged activated partial thromboplastin time (aPTT**), depending on the degree of reduction of the factor VIII level. The **prothrombin time (PT)** is normal in **VWD**.

- Individuals with VWD generally will have a normal CBC and a normal platelet count, with the exception of those with **type 2B VWD**, most of whom will have **mild thrombocytopenia**

Also Note:

- **Causes of prolonged APTT**
  - **Inherited**
    - Deficiency of factor VIII, IX, or XI
    - Deficiency of factor XII, prekallikrein, or HMW kininogen (not associated with a bleeding diathesis)
    - von Willebrand disease (variable)
  - **Acquired**
    - Heparin, dabigatran, argatroban, direct factor Xa inhibitors (variable)*
    - Acquired inhibitor of factor VIII, IX, XI, or XII
    - Acquired von Willebrand syndrome
    - Lupus anticoagulant (more likely to be associated with thrombosis than bleeding)

Ans: (a) VWF deficiency

Ref: *Harrison Principles of Internal Medicine, 20th Edition, page 828*

14. In Criggler Najjar syndrome, which drug should be avoided:

(a) Irinotecan (b) Topotecan
(c) Cefotaxime (d) Thiazides

Explanation:

- **Crigler-Najjar Syndrome, Type I** CN-I is characterized by striking **unconjugated hyperbilirubinemia** of about 340–765 μmol/L (20–45 mg/dL) that appears in the **neonatal period** and **persists for life**
- **Bilirubin glucuronides** are virtually **absent** from the bile, and there is **no detectable constitutive expression** of **UGT1A1 activity** in **hepatic tissue**
- The majority of patients (type IA) exhibit defects in the **glucuronide conjugation** of a spectrum of substrates in addition to bilirubin, including various drugs and other xenobiotics

Principal Differential Characteristics of Gilbert's and Crigler-Najjar Syndromes		
	Crigler-Najjar Syndrome	
Feature	**Type I**	**Type II**
Total serum bilirubin, mmol/L (mg/uL)	310-755 (usually >345) (18-45 [usually > 20])	100-430 (usually ≤ 345) (6-25 [usually ≤ 20])
Routine liver tests	Normal	Normal
Response to phenobarbital	None	Decreases bilirubin by > 25%
Kernicterus	Usual	Rare
Hepatic histology	Normal	Normal
Bile characteristics Color Bilirubin fractions	 Pale or colorless >90% unconjugated	 Pigmented Largest fraction (mean: 57%) monoconjugates
Bilirubin UDP-glucuronosyl transferase activity Inheritance (all autosomal)	Typically absent; traces in some patients Recessive	Markedly reduced: 0-10% of normal Predominantly recessive

- **Irinotecan** is Converted to SN-38 active metabolite; SN-38 is subsequently conjugated predominantly by the enzyme **UDP-glucuronosyl transferase 1A1 (UGT1A1)** to form a **glucuronide metabolite**
- UGT1A1 activity is reduced in individuals with genetic polymorphisms that lead to reduced enzyme activity such as the UGT1A1*28 polymorphism
- Adverse effects of **irinotecan** treatment include **severe diarrhea, myelosuppression and neutropenia**. These effects are likely induced by inefficient metabolism and excretion of SN-38, which undergoes glucuronidation primarily in the liver by UGT1A1 prior to excretion through the kidneys
- The UGT1A1 isoform is solely responsible for the metabolism of bilirubin, numerous endogenous hormones, and numerous pharmacologic compounds, including irinotecan. Thus, genetic variation in UGT1A correlates with adverse events caused by irinotecan toxicity

Ans: (a) Irinotecan

Ref: *Harrison Principles of Internal Medicine, 20th Edition, page 2344*

15. A patient with carcinoid syndrome is on long term octreotide therapy. This patient can develop which of the following vitamin deficiency?

(a) Vitamin B_6 (b) Vitamin B_{12}

(c) Vitamin B_1 (d) Vitamin C

Explanation:

Octreotide

- This synthetic octapeptide surrogate of somatostatin is 40 times **more potent in suppressing GH secretion** and **longer acting (t½ ~90 min),** but only a weak inhibitor of insulin secretion
- It is preferred over somatostatin for
  - **Acromegaly**
  - **Secretory diarrhea** associated with **carcinoid**
  - AIDS
  - Cancer chemotherapy
  - Diabetes
- Control of diarrhoea is due to suppression of hormones which enhance intestinal mucosal secretion.
- Somatostatin analog;
  - **Decreases** GH secretion, secretion of gastrin, VIP, glucagon, secretin, serotonin release and pancreatic polypeptide;
  - In **acromegaly**, octreotide decreases **growth hormone and IGF-1 secretion**;
  - Suppresses **LH response** to **GnRH secretion** and
  - **Decreases splanchnic blood flow**.
- **Adverse effects**
  - *Pancreatitis*
  - *Cholelithiasis*
  - *Vitamin B_{12} deficiency*
  - *Hypothyroidism*
  - *QT prolongation*

Established, Probable and Unestablished Indications for the Use of Somatostatin Analogues
Established indications
Pituitary adenomas secreting growth homone or thyrotropin that recur after surgery
Metastatic islet-cell tumors, especially vipomas and glucagonomas
Metastatic carcinoid tumors
Somatostatin-receptor scintigraphy of somatostatin-receptor-positive diseases
Probable indications
Acute esophageal variceal bleeding, especially if sclerotherapy is not available or has failed
Pancreatic and enteric fistulas
Prevention of complications after elective pancreatic surgery
Secretory diarrhea
AIDS-related diarrhea
Unestablished indications
Other somatostatin-receptor–positive neuroendocrine tumors and adenocarcinomas
Upper gastrointestinal bleeding
Pancreatitis induced by endoscopic retrograde cholangiopancreatography

Ans: (b) Vitamin B_{12}

Ref: *Essentials of Medical Pharmacology, Tripathi 8th Edition, page 238*

16. Prophylactic cranioradiation is given for which tumor?

(a) Small cell lung CA (b) NHL

(c) AML (d) CLL

Explanation:

- The WHO classification system divides **epithelial lung cancers** into four major cell types:
  - Small-cell lung cancer **(SCLC)**
  - Adenocarcinoma
  - Squamous cell carcinoma
  - Large-cell carcinoma
- Small-cell carcinomas consist of **small cells with scant cytoplasm**, **ill-defined cell borders**, **finely granular nuclear chromatin, absent or inconspicuous nucleoli, and a high mitotic count**

Management of Small Cell Lung Cancer

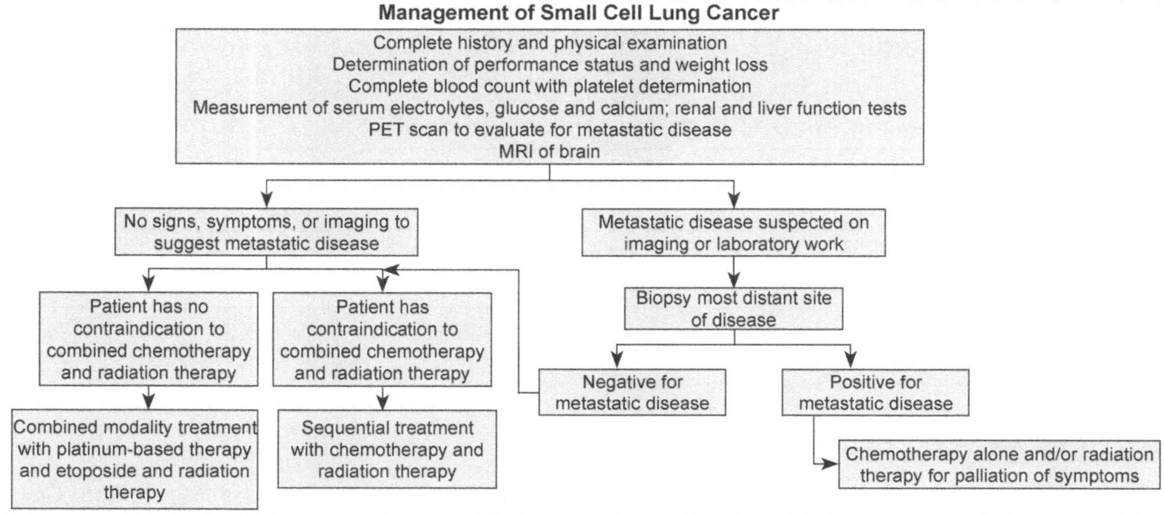

Note: Regardless of disease stage, patients who have a good response to initial therapy should be considered for prophylactic cranial irradiation after therapy is completed

Figure: Algorithm for management of small-cell lung cancer, MRI, magnetic resonance imaging; PET, positive emission tomography

Prophylactic Cranial Irradiation (PCI)

- Prophylactic cranial irradiation (PCI) should be considered in all patients with either **Limited disease – Small cell lung cancer (LD-SCLC) or Extensive disease – Small cell lung cancer (ED-SCLC)** who have responded well to initial therapy. Limited disease (LD-SCLC) is defined as local and regional disease stage and extensive disease (ED-SCLC) is defined as distant disease stage
- There is a significant rate of occult brain metastases even in patients who are diagnosed with SCLC (small cell lung cancer) but do not have neurologic symptoms, and patients who have a good response of their other disease to initial treatment will often develop brain metastases as the sole site of relapse
- Prophylactic cranial irradiation (PCI) has been extensively studied as a way **to decrease the incidence of brain metastases following chemotherapy** and to prevent the associated morbidity and mortality associated with brain metastases
- **PCI** both **increases overall survival** and decreases the incidence of brain metastases in patients who have responded to initial treatment for limited-stage (LS)-SCLC
- **Extensive-stage SCLC** — PCI decreases the incidence of **symptomatic brain metastases** in patients with ES-SCLC who have a response to systemic chemotherapy, although its effect on overall survival is uncertain
- Higher doses of radiation are associated with **better control of brain metastases**, although this benefit must be weighed against the risks of toxicity

Ans: (a) Small cell lung CA

Ref: *Harrison Principles of Internal Medicine, 20th Edition, page 538*

17. ARDS diagnostic criteria:

(a) PaO_2/FiO_2 less than 200 mm Hg
(b) PaO_2/FiO_2 less than 300 mm Hg
(c) PaO_2/FiO_2 more than 200 mm Hg
(d) PaO_2/FiO_2 more than 300 mm Hg

Explanation:

Berlin definition, ARDS is defined as a syndrome characterized by:

(1) Onset within 1 week of a known clinical insult
(2) Bilateral radiographic opacities, not fully explained by pleural effusions, atelectasis, or nodules
(3) Respiratory failure not fully explained by cardiac failure or fluid overload, and
(4) Poor systemic oxygenation, with a $PaO_2/FiO_2 \le 300$ and a PEEP or CPAP $\ge$ 5 cm H_2O

Clinical Variable	Mild ARDS	Moderate ARDS	Severe ARDS
Onset	Onset within 1 week of clinical insult known to cause ARDS		
Hypoxemia	$PaO_2/FiO_2 \le$ 300 mm Hg PEEP or CPAP $\ge$ 5 cm H_2O	$PaO_2/FiO_2 \le$ 200 mm Hg	PaO_2/FiO_2 $\le$ 100 mm Hg
Chest radiograph	Bilateral radiographic opacities, not fully explained by pleural effusions, atelectasis, or nodules		
Non Cardiac etiology	Respiratory failure not fully explained by cardiogenic pulmonary edema or fluid overload		

Ans: (b) PaO_2/FiO_2 less than 300 mm Hg

Ref: *Fishmans Pulmonary Disease and Disorders, 5th Edition, Chapter 141; Harrisons Principles of Internal Medicine, 19th Edition, page 1736*

18. True statement regarding Aplastic anemia:

(a) Bone marrow biopsy confirmatory test
(b) Electrophoresis is diagnostic
(c) Flow cytometry is the best test
(d) Pancytopenia with cellular marrow

Explanation:

- **Hypocellular** and **fatty bone marrow** is virtually diagnostic of Aplastic anemia

Aplastic Anemia:

- Aplastic anemia is characterized by **diminished or absent hematopoietic precursors** in the bone marrow, most often due to **injury to the pluripotent stem cell**
- **Causes of Aplastic anemia**

Idiopathic
Cytotoxic drugs and radiation
Cancer treatment (anticipated effect)
Drug reaction
Anticonvulsants: Carbamazepine, Hydantoins, Phenacemide ***Antibiotics***: Sulfonamides, Chloramphenicol **NSAIDs**: Phenylbutazone, Indomethacin **Anti-thyroid medications**: Carbimazole, Methimazole, Propylthiouracil Gold Arsenicals
Toxic chemicals
Benzene Solvents Glue vapors
Viral infections
Epstein-Barr virus Seronegative (non-A through -G) hepatitis Human immunodeficiency virus (HIV) Other herpes viruses
Immune disorders
Eosinophilic fasciitis Systemic lupus erythematosus Graft versus host disease
Miscellaneous
Paroxysmal nocturnal hemoglobinuria Thymoma Pregnancy Anorexia nervosa

- The diagnosis of Aplastic anemia should be considered in every patient presenting with **pancytopenia** - the simultaneous presence of:
  - ***Anemia***
  - ***Thrombocytopenia***
  - ***Neutropenia***
- Most common presentation of aplastic anemia is **Bleeding***
- **Examination** of the peripheral blood smear reveals

- **Normocytic or macrocytic red cells** with a marked **reduction** in **polychromatophilia** (**Reticulocytes**).
- **Neutrophils and platelets** are **decreased**
- Abnormal circulating white blood cells are **NOT present**

- The bone marrow **biopsy** is **diagnostic**
  - Profoundly hypocellular with a decrease in all elements
  - The marrow space is replaced with fat cells and marrow stroma
  - **Residual hematopoietic cells are morphologically normal**
  - Infiltration with **malignant cells or fibrosis** is **NOT** present
- **Flow cytometry** is important to rule out **Hypocellular MDS** (which may **mimic Aplastic anemia**)
- Chromosomal abnormalities are characteristic of **MDS** but absent in Aplastic anemia
- The **differential diagnosis of Aplastic anemia** includes **other causes of bone marrow failure**

Inherited bone marrow failure syndromes
• Fanconi anemia • Dyskeratosis congenita • Shwachman-Diamond syndrome • Amegakaryocytic thrombocytopenia • Reticular dysgenesis
Acquired causes of bone marrow failure
• Acquired aplastic anemia caused by drugs, chemicals, or radiation • Acquired aplastic anemia associated with viral infection or immune disorder • Myelodysplastic syndromes • Paroxysmal nocturnal hemoglobinuria • Large granular lymphocytic leukemia

Treatment:

- Hematopoietic Stem Cell Transplant – **Best therapy***
- Immune suppression – with ATG (Antithymocyte Globulin)
- Androgens – Role unclear
- Hematopoietic Growth factors (Erythropoietin, G-CSF) – Role unclear.

Ans: (a) Bone marrow biopsy is the confirmatory test

Ref: *Harrison, 19th Edition, page 663*

19. Poor prognostic indicators of primary sclerosing cholangitis:

(a) Intractable pruritis (b) Hepatomegaly
(c) Low serum albumin (d) Splenomegaly

Explanation:

Primary sclerosing cholangitis (PBC)

- Autoimmune liver disease that generally affects middle-aged women
- The presence of **antimitochondrial antibodies (AMA)** in serum is highly characteristic of the disease
- PBC is characterized by:
  - **Progressive intrahepatic duct destruction**, which leads to cholestasis

- Complications and symptoms related to cholestasis
- Cirrhosis, and portal hypertension

- The typical patient with symptomatic disease is a middle-aged woman with a complaint of fatigue or pruritus. Clinical features include:
  - Hyperpigmentation
  - Hepatomegaly
  - Splenomegaly
  - Xanthelasma
  - Jaundice
  - Right upper quadrant pain
- Associated disorders include:
  - Sjögren's syndrome
  - Scleroderma
  - RA
  - Renal tubular acidosis
  - Thyroiditis
- The frequency of malignancy is increased in patients with PBC
- The diagnosis of PBC is established when 2 out of 3 of the following criteria are met:
  - Chronic cholestatic liver biochemical test elevation (typically with alkaline phosphatase ≥ 1.5 times)
  - Elevated serum ama (titer ≥ 1 : 4)
  - Liver biopsy consistent with PBC

Treatment:

- UDCA ,Obeticholic acid, Farnesoid X Receptor Agonist
- Pruritus is treated with antihistamines, Cholestyramine, naltrexone, rifampin

Poor prognostic factors:

- Jaundice
- High serum bilirubin level
- Low serum albumin
- Prolonged prothrombin time

Ans: (c) Low serum albumin

Ref: *Harrison's Principles of Internal Medicine, 20th Edition, page 2335*

20. Patient presents with history of recurrent falls. Examination revealed vertical gaze palsy. Most probable diagnosis?

(a) Idiopathic Parkinson disease
(b) Multiple system atrophy
(c) Progressive supranuclear palsy
(d) Shy Drager syndrome

Explanation:

History of falls + **Vertical gaze palsy** in an elderly patient suggests **Steel Richardson syndrome (Progressive Supranuclear Palsy)**

Progressive Supranuclear Palsy

- Elderly
- Early postural instability – Presents as frequent falls

- Vertical gaze palsy – Down > Up
- Apraxia of Eye opening
- Square wave jerks
- Surprised look
- Disease carries a poor prognosis and response to L-Dopa is poor
- Idiopathic Parkinson's disease does not present with early postural instability and also does not have Vertical gaze palsy
- Also Shy Drager syndrome would have predominant Autonomic features which is a distinguishing feature which this patient does not possess

Ans: (c) Progressive supranuclear palsy

Ref: *Harrison's 20th Edition, page 3116*

21. Bone scan of multiple myeloma shows:

(a) Diffuse increased uptake
(b) Diffuse decreased uptake
(c) Hot spot
(d) Cold spot

Explanation:

Bone scintigraphy

- **Scintigraphy with radioactive technetium** for finding bone lesions is dependent on
  - **Osteoblastic activity**
  - **Increased blood flow** to involved areas, which generally occur as a result of a reparative process in reaction to bone destruction.
- Bone scans show **hot spots** in case of **bony metastases** from
  - **Breast** carcinoma
  - **Prostatic** carcinoma
- **Hot spots**
  - Healing fracture
  - Bone cancer
  - Osteomyelitis
  - Arthritis
  - Paget's disease
- **Cold spots**
  - Multiple myeloma
  - Bone infarction

Bone scintigraphy in Multiple Myeloma

- **Bone scintigraphy** is much **less sensitive** than **radiography** in the diagnosis of **multiple myeloma**, which is usually an almost **purely osteoclastic** disease process, except when **fractures** occur
- Only exceptions where Bone scan is useful than conventional radiography are
  - **Osteoblastic response** to a **compression fracture** of a **vertebral body** or **pelvic insufficiency fracture.**
  - In evaluating areas not well demonstrated in plain radiography, such as **ribs and sternum**

Ans: (d) Cold spot

Ref: *South Med J 2000, 93(10), Radiology, Vol., 125, No. 1, pages 171-176, 1977*

SURGERY

1. A 24-year-old burns patient weighing 60 kg presents with involvement of face, neck, anterior chest wall and abdominal wall and both arms circumferential burns. Calculate the fluid to be given in the first 8 hours:

(a) 5.4 L (b) 6.5 L
(c) 7 L (d) 10.8 L

Explanation:

Let us start calculating based on the Parkland Formula:

Amount of Fluid needed = 4 × Weight in Kg × TBSA burns

So, our next step is to calculate the TBSA of Burns:

- Face and Neck - 9%
- Anterior Chest wall + Abdominal wall - 18%
- Both Arms - 9 + 9%
- TBSA = 45%

So as per formula:

- Amount of Fluid needed = 4 × 60 × 45 = 10800 ml
- Of this half the amount is given in 8 hours = 5400 ml as per Parkland Formula.

Ans: (a) 5.4 ml

Ref: *Sabiston, 20th Edition, page 514*

2. A 4-year-old child presented with burns. The burns seen in Head and neck fully, Right upper limb fully except palm and Right lower limb fully including foot. What is the percentage of Burns?

(a) 14 (b) 72
(c) 41 (d) 24

Explanation:

- Based on Berkow Formula, the burns percent is calculated for this case:
- Head and Neck–17+2%
- Upper Limb–7%
- Lower limb–15%

Berkow Formula to Estimate Burn Size (%) Based on Area of Burn in an Isolated Body Part						
Body Part	**0-1 year**	**1-4 years**	**5-9 years**	**10-14 years**	**15-18 years**	**Adult**
Head	19	17	13	11	9	7
Neck	2	2	2	2	2	2
Anerior trunk	13	13	13	13	13	13
Posterior trunk	13	13	13	13	13	13
Right buttock	2.5	2.5	2.5	2.5	2.5	2.5
Left buttock	2.5	2.5	2.5	2.5	2.5	2.5
Genitalia	1	1	1	1	1	1

Contd.

Contd.

Right upper arm	4	4	4	4	4	4
Left upper arm	4	4	4	4	4	4
Right lower arm	3	3	3	3	3	3
Left lower arm	3	3	3	3	3	3
Right hand	2.5	2.5	2.5	2.5	2.5	2.5
Left hand	2.5	2.5	2.5	2.5	2.5	2.5
Right thigh	5.5	6.5	8	8.5	9	9.5
Left thigh	5.5	6.5	8	8.5	9	9.5
Right leg	5	5	5.5	6	6.5	7
Left leg	5	5	5.5	6	6.5	7
Right foot	3.5	3.5	3.5	3.5	3.5	3.5
Left foot	3.5	3.5	3.5	3.5	3.5	3.5

Ans: (c) 41%

Ref: *Sabiston, 20th Edition, page 823*

3. Suture used for bile duct surgery:

(a) Vicryl (b) Catgut

(c) Polypropylene (d) Silk

Explanation:

Polyglactin (VICRYL) uses:

- Color–Violet color
- Bile duct anastomosis – 3'0 vicryl is used.
- Bowel anastomosis
- Subcuticular sutures monocryl (poliglecaprone) is better than Vicryl

Ans: (a) Vicryl

Ref: *Surgery Sixer, 4th Edition, page 44*

4. A patient admitted to emergency department with head injury. He opens eyes to painful stimulus, Localizes pain and produces Incomprehensible sounds. What would be his Glasgow coma scale?

(a) 13 (b) 9

(c) 7 (d) 6

Explanation:

Glassgow coma scale (EVM-456)

Eye opening	**Verbal**	**Motor**
• Spontaneous-4 • To loud voice-3 • To pain stimuli-2** • Do not open-1	• Normal Oriented-5 • Confused-4 • Inappropriate words-3 • Incomprehensile Sounds only-2** • No sounds-1	• Obeys commands-6 • Localizes to pain-5** • Withdrawal flexion-4 • Abnormal flexion-3 (decorticate) • Extension-2 (Decerebrate) • No motor response-1

Contd.

Contd.

Mnemonic:
- Verbal–One Confused Word Sounds Nowhere* (54321)
- Motor–Obey Localities With Flexion and Extension Now. (654321)
- Motor component–most predictive of future neurologic outcome
- Score represents the best performance elicited, *Example:* Flexion response to pain in left limb and localising pain in right limb-take into consideration the best which is in right limb-M5**

Classification of Head injury based on GCS:
- Minor: GCS 15 with no LOC
- Mild: GCS 14 or 15 with LOC
- Moderate: GCS 9-13
- Severe: GCS 3-8

Ans: (b) 9

Ref: *Surgery Sixer, 4th Edition, page 87*

5. According to ATLS guideline, in a patient with paraplegia 'Hard neck collar' is indicated in:

(a) All trauma patients
(b) Presence of Neck pain
(c) History of neck injury
(d) Neurological deficit present

Explanation:

- Patient's with Trauma – Airway management is first done alone with Cervical spine stabilisation.
- All trauma patients – Unless proved otherwise consider them as vertebral column is injured, and take appropriate precautions. Carefully apply a hard cervical collar and use LOG ROLL (rotating the patient as a whole while examining the spine)
- Rigid long boards with straps are helpful in transport of the patient from one place to other. Conscious and alert patient indirectly means they don't need Intubation and their airway is patent

Ans: (a) All trauma patients

Ref: *Surgery Sixer, page 124*

6. Long acting thyroid stimulator (LATS) is responsible for which of the following disease?

(a) Papillary Ca of Thyroid
(b) Hashimoto's
(c) Graves' disease
(d) MNG

Explanation:

- The long-acting thyroid stimulator (LATS) has been thought to be responsible for the hyperthyroidism of Graves' disease.

Long-acting thyroid stimulator (LATS)

- Found in the serum of some patients with Graves' disease.
- Although serum LATS levels correlate with several parameters of thyroid activity in thyrotoxicosis, the role of this abnormal stimulator in the pathogenesis of Graves' disease remains **uncertain**.
- High levels of LATS are frequently associated with **pretibial myxedema** but the relation of LATS to the ophthalmopathy of Graves' disease is less clear.
- Demonstration that LATS is an immunoglobulin G (IgG) and evidence that the distribution of thyroid-stimulating activity in the polypeptide chains of the IgG parallels antigen-binding activity in known antibodies has led to speculation that LATS is an **antibody** to **thyroid antigen(s)**.

- The evidence for and against this hypothesis is discussed in detail and it is concluded that present information is insufficient to confirm or disprove this postulate.
- Although both in vivo and in vitro studies indicate that LATS and TSH act on the same thyroidal site(s), the precise mechanism of action of these thyroid stimulators has not yet been determined.

Ans: (c) Graves' Disease

Ref: *Internet Sources*

7. A 36-year-old woman presents with thyroid swelling. Radio-iodine uptake scan showed diffuse uptake. Which intervention would benefit the patient best?

(a) Hemithyroidectomy
(b) Radioactive iodine
(c) No treatment
(d) Anti-thyroid drug

Explanation:

- Diffuse Radio-iodine uptake is seen in Graves' disease and the gold standard treatment for Graves' is RAI therapy with I-131.

Radioactive Iodine Uptake study:

- I^{123} and I^{131} are used to image thyroid gland.
- I^{123} has half-life of 12-14 hours* and emits low dose radiation hence used to detect Ectopic thyroids and Nodular goiter activities.
- I^{131} has long half-life of 8 days hence used to diagnose and treat differentiated thyroid cancers.
- Diagnostic dose–< 5 micro curie, Therapeutic doses may be given upto 200 micro curie in single sitting.
- Therapeutic uses–Graves' disease, Treat secondaries after surgery in Thyroid differentiated cancers.

Ans: (b) Radioactive iodine

Ref: *Surgery Sixer, 4th edition, page 225*

8. Cervical rib passes between:

(a) Scalenus anterior and medius
(b) Scalenus medius and posterior
(c) Clavicle and 1st rib
(d) Scalenus posterior and vertebra

Explanation:

Potential area of compression of Subclavian Artery

- **Interscalene space**: Anteriorly – Scalenus anterior, posteriorly – Scalenus medius, inferiorly – 1st rib
- **Intercostoclavicular space**: Between 1st rib and clavicle
- **In the axilla**: Between pectoralis minor tendon attaching to coracoid process

Cervical rib passes between Scalenus anterior and Medius and compresses the Subclavian artery and Lower trunk of brachial plexus

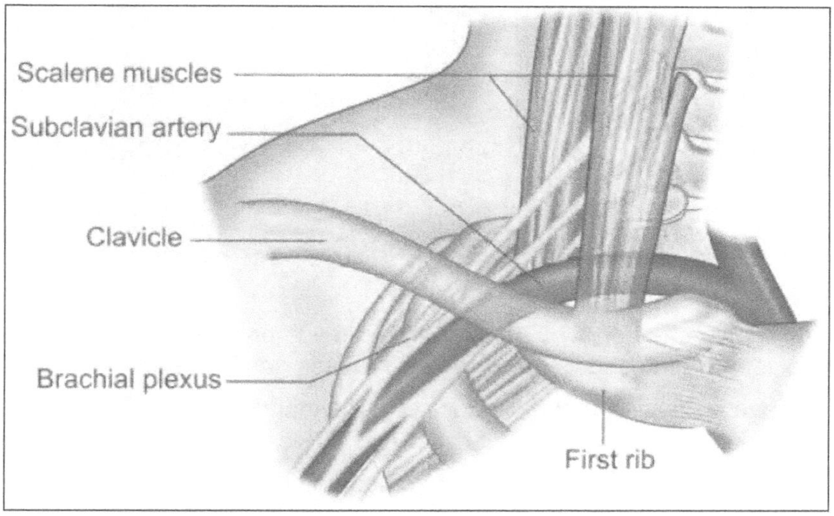

Ans. (a) Scalenus anterior and medius

Ref: *Surgery Sixer, 4th Edition, page 205*

9. A 12 weeks pregnant woman presents with Right lower quadrant pain, Leucocytosis, and inflamed appendix of 10 cm in USG. What is the next step in management? (JIPMER December 2019 Pattern)

(a) Immediate appendicectomy

(b) Conservative management with antibiotics and wait till 20 weeks for appendicectomy

(c) Conservative management with antibiotics and wait till delivery for appendicectomy

(d) Only Conservative management with antibiotics

Explanation:

Pregnancy and Appendicitis:

- Typical presentation seen in **50-60%** cases.
- Symptoms are nausea, vomiting and febrile response which can be seen in Normal pregnancy also.
- Appendix is pushed more **cephalad** by **gravid uterus**.
- Most common trimester of appendicitis-**2nd trimester**.
- Some lab values like Leucocytosis, CRP increase may be physiological also.
- High rate of negative appendectomy in pregnant is seen (25-50%) due to all the above reasons.
- Risk of preterm labour and fetal loss is seen in appendicitis cases and is less in uncomplicated appendicitis.
- IOC – **USG** done in Left posterior **Oblique or Left lateral Decubitus position**. (Sensitivity–78% and Specificity–83%)
- **MRI without Gadolinium** has excellent Sensitivity and specificity.
- In patients for whom MRI is normal needs no appendectomy and is shown to be cost effective.
- If MRI is not available–CT scan can be done, as by 2nd and 3rd trimester organogenesis has already happened.
- Laparoscopic Appendectomy is current recommendation, but Hasson Open technique is preferred for Primary port to avoid injury to gravid uterus.

Ans: (a) Immediate appendectomy

Ref: *Sabiston, 20th Edition, page 1306-1307*

10. Patient with history of CAD came with C/O Abdominal pain, Vomiting, diarrhea. On X-ray no gas is seen in small intestine but CT scan shows gas present in small intestine wall. What is true?

(a) Inferior mesenteric artery is commonly involved

(b) Thrombotic disease more common than non-thrombotic

(c) SMA is usually occluded by thrombosis commonly.

(d) Embolic occlusion of SMA

Explanation:

From the History, a known case of CAD, has risk of embolus and thrombus. Most common cause of SMA ischemia is – Embolus. CT scan shows bowel wall containing gas is a feature of bowel gangrene.

- Small bowel ischaemia usually presents as lack of wall enhancement, dilation and in more advanced cases, pneumatosis intestinalis and portal venous gas. The CT scan finding explained here is classical NOMI.

Mesenteric Ischemia is discussed under three broad headings:

- Acute mesenteric artery Ischemia
- Chronic mesenteric Ischemia
- Mesenteric Vein Thrombosis
- Non Occlusive Mesenteric Ischemia (NOMI)

Etiology:

1. Sudden occlusion of superior Mesenteric Artery [50%]
   - Atherosclerosis (Most common cause of Chronic Mesenteric Ischemia)
   - Embolism (Most common cause of Acute SMA ischemia 90% cases)**
   - Vasculitis (Poly arteritis nodosa)
   - Fibro muscular dysplasia
2. Mesenteric vein occlusion [25%]
   - Thrombosis due to OCP, Polycythemia, Neoplasm infiltrating
3. Non occlusive obstruction [25%]
   - Severe shock

Acute Mesenteric Ischemia:

Clinical features:

- Sudden severe abdominal pain, vomiting, abdominal distension
- Central abdominal pain with Symptoms out of Proportion to signs present* (Hall Mark feature**)
- Functional obstruction with absent bowel sounds
- Shock and peritonitis is rapid
- 100% mortality if untreated.
- In emboli cases the obstruction is in mid to distal SMA, distal to origin of Middle colic artery. In such cases some part of bowel is viable. (Figure)
- In thrombosis cases the obstruction is at origin of SMA. In such cases the bowel is gangrenous from DJ flexure to right Colon.
- Investigation to diagnose–Laparotomy**

Treatment

- Resection of non viable bowel with its mesentery

- Second look operation

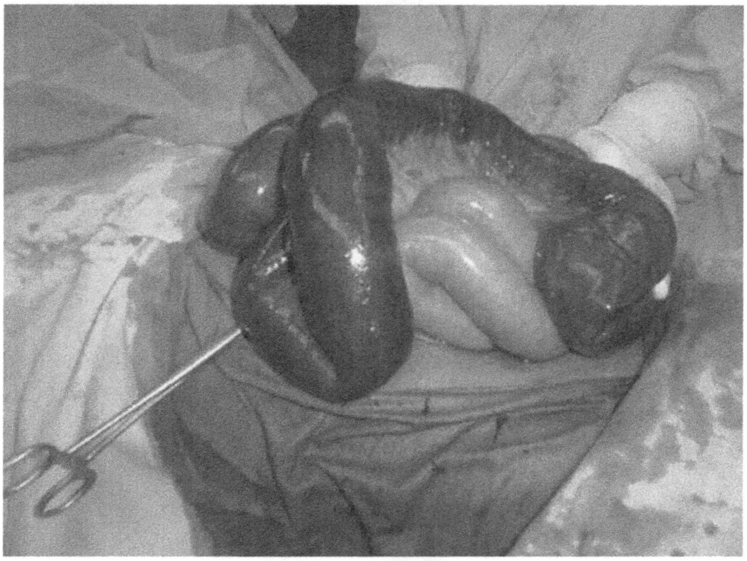

Figure: Acute SMA ischemia by Embolus

Chronic Mesenteric Ischemia:

- Presents with intestinal angina, weight loss, chronic diarrhoea
- Gold standard for chronic mesenteric ischemia–Mesenteric angiography.
- Atherosclerosis in main splanchnic artery (coeliac, IMA, SMA) is the most common cause of chronic mesenteric ischemia.

> **Recent Advances:**
> - SQUID–superconducting quantum interference device (SQUID) magnetometer to detect mesenteric ischemia noninvasively

Mesenteric Vein thrombosis:

- Mesenteric vein thrombosis is usually due to small peripheral vein thrombosis** [SMV OR IMV thrombosis is rare]
- Hence thrombectomy is not needed** (not indicated)
- Fluid resuscitation
- Heparin anticoagulation is sufficient
- If peritoneal signs are present-urgent laparotomy needed
- If peritoneal signs absent-Heparin [5 days], oral anticoagulation lifelong along with bowel rest and fluids is enough.

> **Extra Mile:**
> **Colonic Ischemia:**
> - Most common site of Ischemic Colitis–Splenic Flexure (Griffith Point)
> - Watershed area in colon–Splenic Flexure
> - Most common site of Ischemic Stricture–Sigmoid Colon (Sudeck's Point)

Ans: (d) Embolic Occlusion of SMA

Ref: *Surgery Sixer, 4th Edition, page 479*

11. Following total pancreatectomy on Day 4 Postoperative day, the drain fluid output is greater than 100 ml and patient is fully stable without any complaints. What is the next step in management?

(a) Remove drain and suture
(b) Amylase estimation of the drain fluid
(c) Perform drain fluid culture sensitivity
(d) Replace drain amount with IV Ringer's lactate

Explanation:

Pancreatic leak or pancreatic fistula, which has been defined by the International Study Group on Pancreatic Fistula as:

- "Output via an intraoperatively placed drain (or percutaneous drain) of any measurable volume on or after postoperative day 3, with amylase >3 times normal serum value"
- Incidence–5- 22%

Ans: (d) Replace drain amount with IV Ringers lactate

Ref: *Sabiston, 20th Edition, page 1548*

VERSION – 2

12. What to look for in the liver abscess wall on Pathological examination?

(a) Cyst
(b) Trophozoite
(c) Both
(d) Daughter cysts

Explanation:

- Cysts ingested in contaminated food reaches the stomach–intestine and in intestine, the cysts release trophozoites which enter and invade the colon.
- Trophozoites reach the liver via Portal vein. It does not invade via lymphatics.
- It causes necrosis of tissues in liver. The cavity will have acellular proteinaceous debris surrounded by a rim of Amoebic trophozoites in wall.
- Leucocytes will be there initially but later lysed by Trophozoites.

Ans: (b) Trophozoite

Ref: *Sabiston, 20th Edition, page 1451*

13. A patient suspected to have Pancreatitis. Which of the following intervention is the most beneficial according to the current level of Evidence?

(a) Early enteral feeds
(b) Prophylactic antibiotics
(c) PPI
(d) Octreotide

Explanation:

- In management of Acute pancreatitis, previously TPN was the treatment of choice. But TPN was associated with increased Bacterial Translocation in GUT and hence the enteral feeding is now supported if patient has sufficient BP.
- Enteral Feeding is suggested by Nasogastric tube and if patient has vomiting or unable to tolerate NG feeding we go with Nasojejunal tube.

Ans: (a) Early enteral feeds

Ref: *Bailey and Love, 27th Edition, page 1225*

14. 40 years female presents with severe right hypochondrial pain, she has Gall bladder stones with pericholecystic edema on USG. On examination she had Murphy's sign +, WBC count was 19000/mm3, Temperature 102 degree, Pulse rate 120/minute, Serum creatinine > 3mg/dl, PT elevated. What is the grading according to Tokyo guidelines?

(a) Mild (b) Moderate

(c) Severe (d) None

Explanation:

Tokyo Consensus Guidelines for Severity grading of Acute Cholecystitis:

Grade III (Severe) Acute Cholecystitis:

Associated with any one of the following organ dysfunction:

- CVS: Hypotension requiring Dopamine or Noradrenaline
- Neurological: Decreased consciousness level
- Respiratory: PaO_2/FiO_2 ratio <300
- Renal dysfunction: Oliguria: creatinine > 2 mg/dl
- Liver dysfunction: PT – INR elevated
- Hematological Dysfunction: Platelet count < 1 lakh/mm^3

Grade II (Moderate Cholecytitis)

- Elevated WBC count > 18000/mm^3
- Palpable Tender mass in Right Upper Quadrant.
- Duration of Complaints > 72 hours.
- Marked Local inflammation (Gangrene, Abscess, Biliary peritonitis, Emphysematous Cholecystitis)

Grade I (Mild Acute Cholecystitis)

- Grade 1 has none of the above features.
- Healthy person with mild inflammation only.
- Cholecystectomy is a safe and Low risk procedure.

In Grade III high-risk cases sometimes if patient is unfit for cholecystectomy a percutaneous Cholecystostomy can be performed by Radiologist.

Ans: (c) Severe

Ref: *Bailey and Love, 27th Edition, page 1200*

15. Examine the schematic diagram of hydrocele carefully. Which of the following types does this fit in?

(a) Congenital Hydrocele (b) Vaginal Hydrocele

(c) Infantile Hydrocele (d) Hydrocele of cord

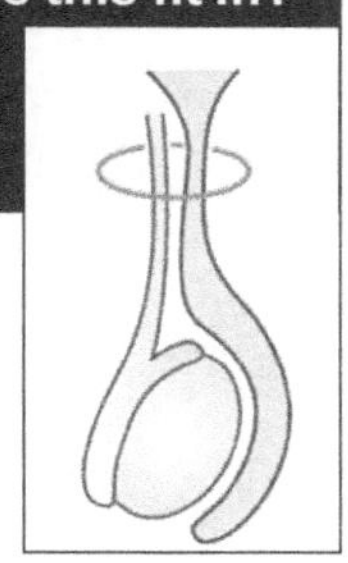

Explanation:

- The picture clearly shows the communication of the peritoneal cavity to the root of scrotum. Hence, the fluid collects in the entire sac.
- Typical Inverted ink Bottle Effect is seen in this case of hydrocele.

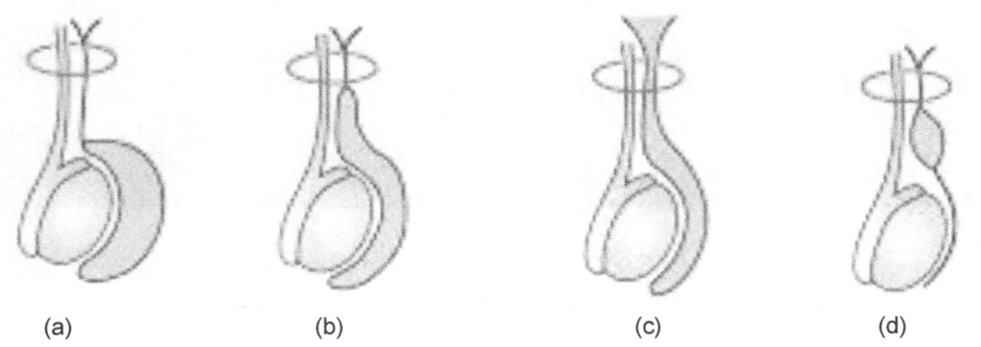

(a) Vaginal hydrocele (very common); (b) 'Infantile' hydrocele; (c) Congenital hydrocele; (d) Hydrocele of the cord

Ans: (a) Congenital Hydrocele

Ref: *Surgery Sixer, 4th edition, page 752*

16. A 28-year-old male presents with sudden detumescence, swelling and pain in penis following a loud pop sound during sexual intercourse. Which of the following is true?

(a) Tear of tunica vaginalis
(b) Rupture of Buck's fascia leads to bleeding limited only to penis (intrapenile hematoma)
(c) Immediate surgical exploration and repair
(d) Urethral injury is always associated

Explanation:

Penile Fractures:

- Traumatic Rupture of Tunica Albuginea during Sexual intercourse with female partner on top.
- The penile corporal bodies can rupture if sufficient force is exerted by partner's pubic symphysis or perineum.

Clinical feature:

- Immediate audible Pop heard by the man and rapid penile swelling.
- If Buck's fascia is disrupted patient may have Butterfly shaped hematoma (Butterfly sign) in perineum.
- Eggplant appearance of penis is seen.

Treatment:

- Exploration by a circumcising (degloving) incision and repair of the defect offers the best chance at avoiding permanent ED and penile deformity while also minimizing the risk of infection.
- A retrograde urethrogram should be performed to rule out urethral injury at the time of surgery, which may be seen sometimes.
- If present, the urethra should be repaired, taking care not to significantly narrow the lumen.
- A Foley catheter is left in place for several days after surgery

Ans: (c) Immediate surgical exploration and repair

Ref: *Schwartz, 10th Edition, page 1661*

17. False statement regarding Peyronie's disease:

(a) Immediate surgery during active stage gives best results

(b) Dorsal deviation is most common

(c) Associated with Dupuytren's contracture

(d) Nesbitt procedure is done

Explanation:

Peyronie's disease

- Peyronie's disease is characterized by- Penile deformity+ Palpable Penile Plaques+ Erectile dysfunction+ Pain on Erection.
- Etiology may be following microhemorrhages going for secondary fibrosis
- Results in Deformity more curvature dorsally (towards abdomen*)
- It is also called as penile fibromatosis
- Palmar fibromatosis (Dupuytren's contracture), plantar fibromatosis and penile fibromatosis (peyronie's disease) are components of the same pathological process called superficial fibromatosis

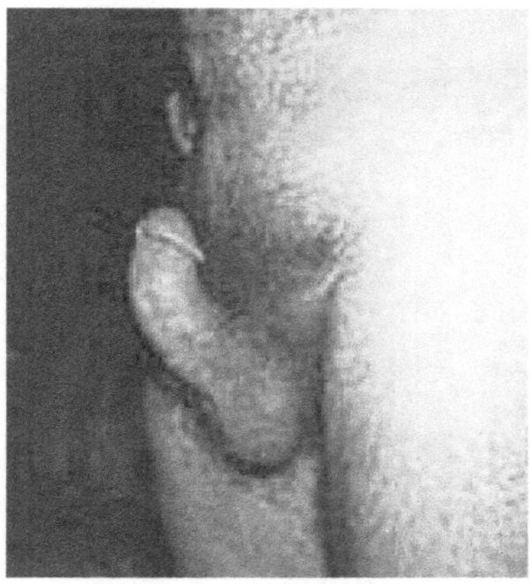

Figure: Peyronie's disease

- Treatment is difficult but some cases may show spontaneous regression
- In the penile deformity is distressing, Nesbitt's operation can be performed to straighten the penis.

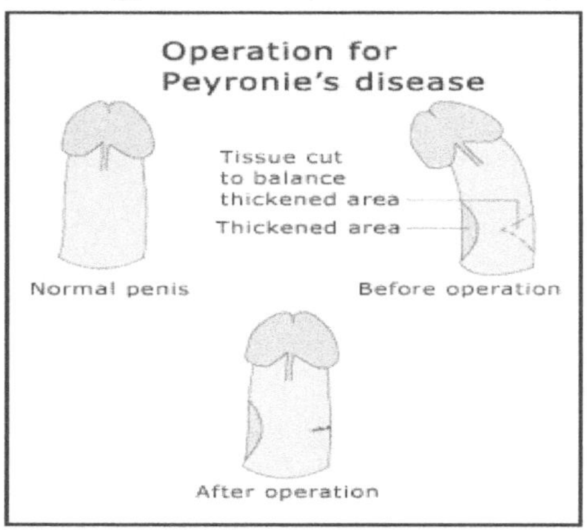

Nesbitt operation

Ans: (a) Immediate surgery during active stage gives best results

Ref: *Surgery Sixer, 4th Edition, page 749*

18. All are radio opaque stones *except*:

(a) Uric acid (b) Oxalate

(c) Cystine (d) Staghorn

Explanation:

Types of Renal Calculus

- **Calcium oxalate calculus (Most common*)**
  - They have hard, small and jagged surface.
- **Phosphate calculus**
  - Usually Calcium phosphate but sometimes is combined with ammonium and magnesium to form the triple phosphate calculus: ammonium magnesium phosphate
  - Also k/a struvite stone
  - Smooth, dirty white and solitary
  - Seen in alkaline urine especially with proteus infection which split urea to ammonia
  - This type of calculus may enlarge to fill all or most of renal collecting system forming a staghorn calculus*

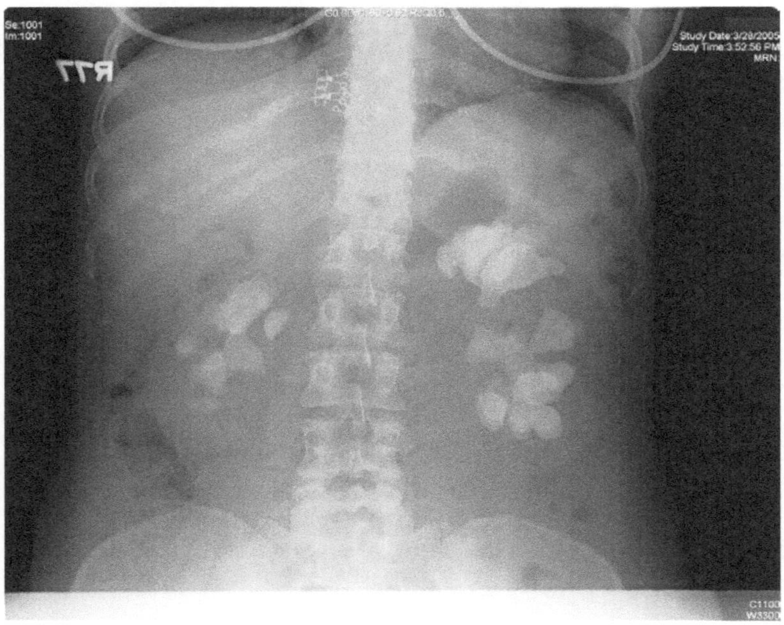

- **Uric acid and urate calculus**
  - These are **radiolucent**
- **Cystine stones**
  - Uncommon, seen in cystinuria
  - Appear only in acidic urine*
  - They are pink to yellow when first removed but they change colour to a greenish hue when exposed to air
- **Xanthine calculi**
  - Are **radiolucent**
  - Are secondary to a congenital deficiency of xanthine oxidase

- **Indinavir calculi**
  - Indinavir is protease inhibitor used in AIDS patients. It results in calculi in ~6% patients.
  - Indinavir calculi are **radiolucent****

Ans. (a) Uric acid

Ref: *Surgery Sixer, 4th Edition, page 695*

OBSTETRICS AND GYNAECOLOGY

1. In low risk delivery all of the following can be done *except:*

(a) Ambulation in I stage of labor
(b) Cut short II stage of labor
(c) Continuous monitoring of FHR in all cases
(d) Episiotomy

Explanation:

INTRAPARTUM CARE IN LOW RISK LABOR

First Stage of Labor

Latent Labor

- Encourage and help the woman to move and adopt **whatever positions she finds most comfortable throughout labor**
- Offer all nulliparous women **antenatal education** about the signs of labor
- Advise the woman and her birth companion(s) that **breathing exercises, immersion in water and massage may reduce pain** during the latent first stage of labor
- Record her pulse, blood pressure and temperature, and carry out urinalysis
- Palpate the woman's abdomen to determine the fundal height, the baby's lie, presentation, position, engagement of the presenting part, and frequency and duration of contractions

Active Phase

- **Offer cardiotocography if intermittent auscultation indicates possible fetal heart rate abnormalities**. If the trace is normal after 20 minutes, return to intermittent auscultation
- Inform the woman that she may drink fluids during established labour and that **isotonic drinks may be more beneficial than water**
- Inform the woman that she may eat a light diet in established labour
- If a woman is contemplating regional analgesia, talk with her about the **risks and benefits and the implications for her labour**
- **Do not offer cardiotocography to women at low risk of complications**
- Record the following observations during the first stage of labour:
  - Half-hourly documentation of frequency of contractions
  - Hourly pulse
  - 4-hourly temperature and blood pressure – Frequency of passing urine
  - Offer a vaginal examination 4-hourly

Second Stage of Labor

- Record all the following observations in the second stage of labour, on the partogram and assess whether transfer of care may be needed:
  - Half-hourly documentation of the frequency of contractions
  - Hourly blood pressure
  - Continued 4-hourly temperature
  - Frequency of passing urine
- Offer a **vaginal examination hourly in the active second stage**
- Perform **intermittent auscultation of the fetal heart rate immediately after a contraction for at least 1 minute, at least every 5 minutes**
- **Do not carry out a routine episiotomy** during spontaneous vaginal birth
- Perform an **episiotomy if there is a clinical need**, such as instrumental birth or suspected fetal compromise
- Think about offering **instrumental birth if there is concern about the baby's wellbeing or there is a prolonged second stage**

Third Stage of Labor

- **Active management of the third stage** involves a package of care comprising the following components:
  - **Routine use of uterotonic drugs**
  - Deferred clamping and cutting of the cord
  - **Controlled cord traction after signs of separation of the placenta**
- For **active management, administer 10 IU of oxytocin by intramuscular injection** with **the birth of the anterior shoulder or immediately after the birth of the** baby and before the cord is clamped and cut

Ans: (c) Continuous Monitoring of FHR

Ref: *NICE guidelines-intrapartum care 2020*

2. In a young woman with unilateral ovarian carcinoma Grade I confined to the ovary, management of choice is:

(a) Unilateral oophorectomy
(b) Unilateral oophorectomy with chemotherapy
(c) Bilateral oophorectomy
(d) Hysterectomy

Explanation:

MANAGEMENT OF OVARIAN CARCINOMA

Stage 1A and 1B, grade 1

Premenopausal patients

- After staging laparotomy, **unilateral oophorectomy** to preserve fertility
- **Follow up** with regular **pelvic examination** and **CA 125 levels**
- The **other ovary and uterus are removed** when **child bearing is completed**

Postmenopausal patients

- Should undergo **TAH and BSO and staging**

Stage 1A and 2B [grade 2 and 3]

- Treated **with TAH/BSO and staging followed by chemotherapy**

Stage 2,3,4

- Surgery–**cytoreductive surgery**
- Chemotherapy

Algorithm for management of ovarian cancer

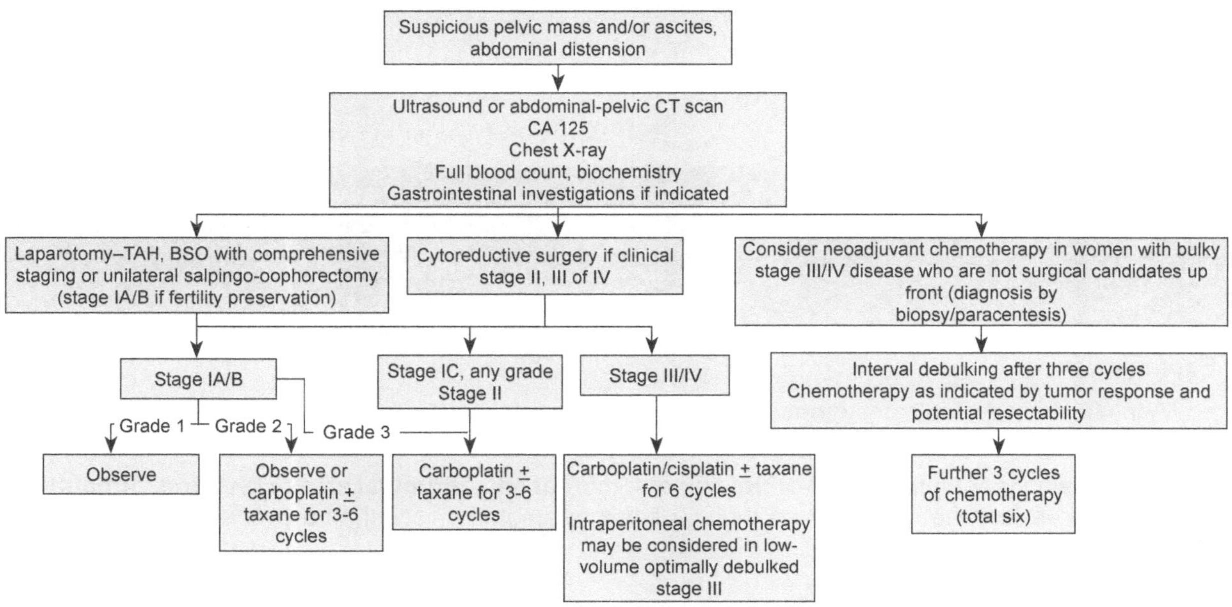

Figo Staging Criteria for Cancer of the Ovary, Fallopian Tube and Peritoneum	
Stage I	**Tumor limited to the ovaries or fallopian tubes**
IA	Tumor limited to one ovary (capsule intact) or fallopian tube No tumor on the external surface of the ovary or fallopian tube No malignant cells in ascites or peritoneal washings
IB	Tumor limited to both ovaries (capsules intact) or fallopian tubes No tumor on the external surface of the ovaries or fallopian tubes No malignant cells in ascites or peritoneal washings
IC	Tumor limited to one or both ovaries or fallopian tubes with any of the following: Stage IC1: Surgical spill Stage IC2: Capsule ruptured before surgery; or tumor on ovarian or fallopian tube surface Stage IC3: Malignant cells in the ascites or peritoneal washings
Stage II	**Tumor involves one or both ovaries or fallopian tubes with pelvic extension (below pelvic brim) or primary peritoneal cancer.**
IIA	Extension and/or implants on the uterus and/or ovaries and/or fallopian tubes
IIB	Extension to other pelvic intraperioneal tissues
Stage III	**Tumor involves one or both ovaries or fallopian tubes, or primary peritoneal cancer, with cytologically or histologically confirmed spread to the peritoneum outside the pelvis and/or metastasis to the retroperitoneal lymph nodes**
III A1	Positive (cytologically or histologically proven) retroperitoneal lymph nodes only Stage IIIA (i) Metastasis up to 10 mm in greatest dimension Stage IIIA(ii) Metastasis more than 10 mm in greatest dimension
III A2	Microscopic extrapelvic (above the pelvic brim) peritoneal involvement with or without positive retroperitoneal lymph nodes
III B	Macroscopic peritoneal metastasis beyond the pelvis up to 2 cm in greatest dimension, with or without metastasis to the retroperitoneal lymph nodes
III C	Macroscopic peritoneal metastasis beyond the pelvis more than 2 cm in greatest dimension, with or without metastasis to the retroperitoneal lymph nodes Stage IIIC includes extension of tumor to the capsule of liver and spleen without parenchymal involvement of either organ
Stage IV	**Distant metastasis, excluding peritoneal metastases**
IV A	Pleural effusion with positive cytology
IV B	Parenchymal metastases and metastases to extra-abdominal organs (including inguinal lymph nodes and lymph nodes outside of the abdominal cavity)

Ans: (a) Unilateral oophorectomy

Ref: *Berek and Novak's Gynecology, 16th Edition, page 2345*

3. An adnexal mass is palpable during bimanual examination in an asymptomatic woman. The next investigation to be done is:

(a) CA-125
(b) Transvaginal sonography
(c) CT- abdomen and pelvis
(d) All of the above

Explanation:

- Adnexal masses can have **gynecologic or nongynecologic etiologies**, ranging from normal luteal cysts to ovarian cancer to bowel abscesses
- Women who report **abdominal or pelvic pain, increased abdominal size or bloating, difficulty eating, or rapid satiety** that occurs more than 12 times per month in less than a year should be **evaluated for ovarian cancer**

- **Pelvic examination has low sensitivity for detecting an adnexal mass**; negative pelvic examination findings in a symptomatic woman should not deter further workup
- Ectopic pregnancy must be ruled out in women of reproductive age
- **Transvaginal ultrasonography (TVS)** is the **first choice for imaging of an adnexal mass**. **Large mass size, complexity, papillary projections, septation, irregularity, or bilaterality may indicate cancer**. If disease is suspected outside of the ovary, computed tomography may be indicated; magnetic resonance imaging may better show malignant characteristics in the ovary
- **A cancer antigen 125 (CA 125) test may assist in the evaluation of an adnexal mass** in appropriate patients. **However, CA 125 levels are elevated in conditions other than ovarian cancer**
- Due to substantial overlap in CA 125 levels between pre- and postmenopausal women may occur, CA **125 level alone is not recommended for differentiating between a benign and malignant adnexal mass**
- **Serial ultrasonography and periodic measurement of CA 125 levels may help in differentiating between benign or potentially malignant adnexal masses.** If an adnexal mass larger than 6 cm is found on ultrasonography, or if findings persist longer than 12 weeks, referral to a gynecologist or gynecologic oncologist is indicated

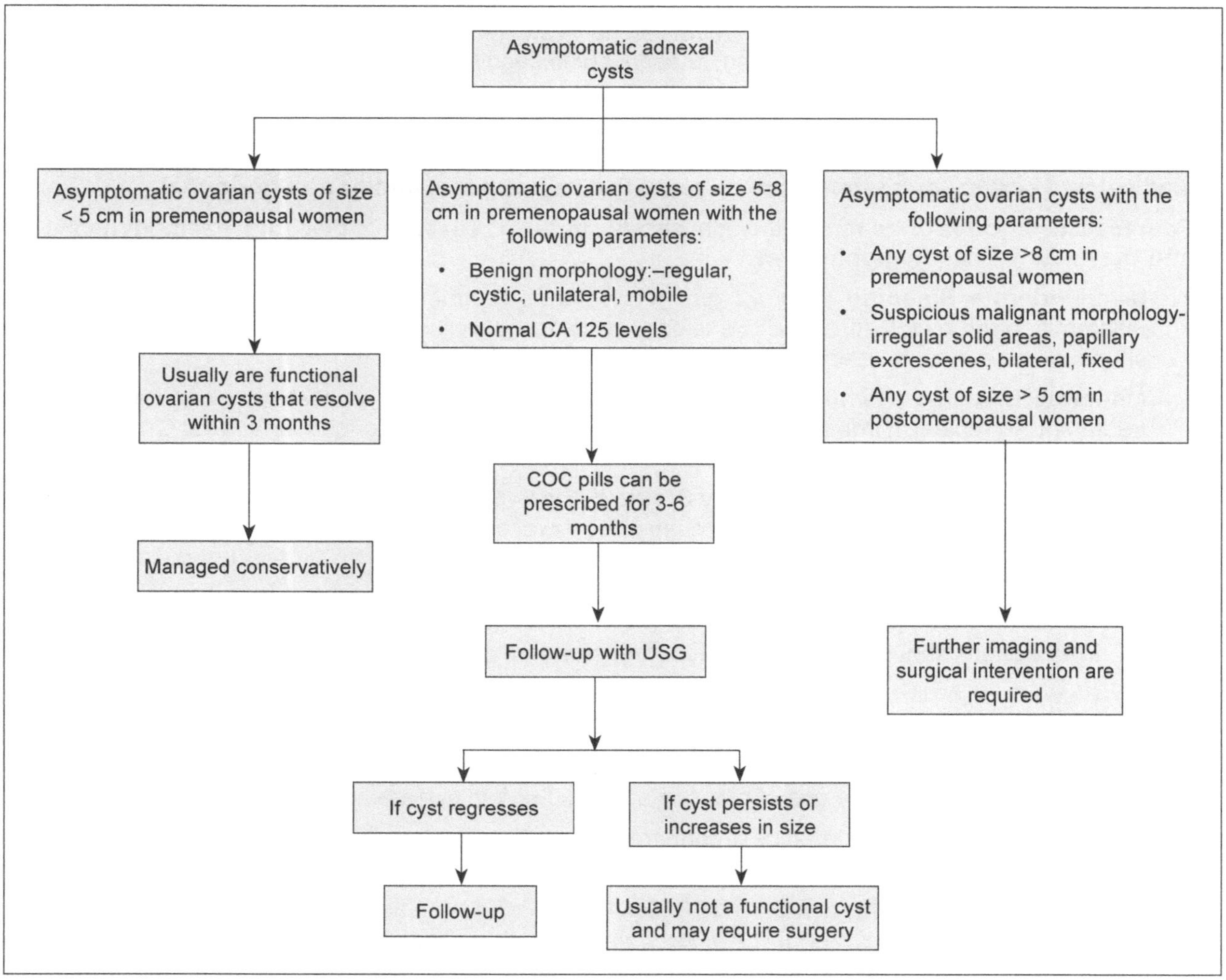

Flowchart: Management of asymptomatic adnexal cyst

Ans: (b) Transvaginal sonography

Ref: *Clinical Obstetrics and Gynecology by Sharmila Arun Babu, 1st Edition, 2019, page 356*

4. Which of the following is the first line management for abnormal uterine bleeding (AUB) in adolescent age group?

(a) Oral contraceptives
(b) Tranexamic acid
(c) Progesterone
(d) Progesterone IUCD

Explanation:

- Menstrual disorders and abnormal uterine bleeding (AUB) are among the most frequent gynecologic complaints in adolescents
- **Anovulatory uterine bleeding** is the primary cause of AUB in adolescents and generally resolves with maturation of the hypothalamic-pituitary-ovarian axis
- Additionally, endocrine disorders such as hypothyroidism, hyperprolactinemia and polycystic ovary syndrome are possible causes of AUB. Exclusion of bleeding disorders, especially of von Willebrand disease is important for diagnosis and treatment of HMB, particularly in cases with AUB, which has been present since menarche
- Management of HMB is based on the underlying etiology and severity of the bleeding. After other causes are excluded, anovulatory heavy bleeding can be treated successfully with combined oral contraceptives and iron supplementation either as an outpatient or in hospital depending on the clinical findings and level of anemia

Treatment

Medical and surgical treatments can be classified as hormonal and/or non-hormonal

Four main categories of treatment are administered based on **severity of bleeding, haemodynamic status and the patient's haemoglobin level**

- **Mild/Moderate Bleeding (Hb> 12 g/dL)**–Hormonal treatment is not considered. Non-steroid anti-inflammatory drugs (NSAIDs) can be used. The patient should be followed up at 3-month intervals and should be instructed to keep a menstrual-cycle diary
- **Moderate Bleeding (Hb 10–12 g/dL)**–Oral contraceptives or oral progesterone can be prescribed for treatment. To replenish iron stores, iron supplements should be prescribed for at least 6 months. NSAIDs can be added to the treatment
- **Severe Bleeding, Haemodynamically Stable (Hb = 8–10 g/dL)**–The use of OCPs, an approach that is similar to that for patients with moderate bleeding is recommended
- Severe Bleeding (Hb ≤7 g/dL) or Haemodynamically Unstable
  - The patient should be hospitalized and monitored.
  - Preparations should be made for blood transfusions, as they may be required.
  - Bleeding disorders must be eliminated before starting hormonal treatment.
  - The **first treatment of choice is to prescribe OCPs containing high doses of oestrogen (35-50** μg **ethinyloestradiol)** because OCPs promote rapid endometrial regrowth to cover denuded epithelial surfaces. The use of pills containing 50 μg ethinyloestradiol is usually considered.
  - Intravenous (IV) conjugated oestrogen treatment (25 mg at intervals of 4-6 hours) may be considered for patients who cannot tolerate high-dose oral oestrogen therapy.
  - Medroxyprogesterone acetate (MPA, 20-40 mg) or norethindrone acetate (NETA, 5-10 mg) are administered three times per day for 7 days. Another recommended treatment for acute HMB is depot-MPA (150 mg), administered intramuscularly and followed by MPA (20 mg) orally, every 8 hours for 9 doses
  - **The levonorgestrel-containing intrauterine system (LNG-IUS) is regarded as the most effective medical treatment option for patients with HMB**
  - **Other Hormonal Treatments**–Although danazol and GnRH analogues are quite effective in the treatment of severe bleeding, they are not the first choice due to their side effects

- **Non-hormonal Treatments**
    - **Tranexamic Acid**, a lysine derivative, is bound to lysine in its fibrinogen structure. Tranexamic acid prevents the destruction of fibrin and decreases bleeding by 30%-55%
    - **Mefenamic acid** -The recommended usage is 500 mg at intervals of 3-5 hours on the first day and a 250-500-mg dose, 3- 4 times per day thereafter
    - **Desmopressin** is a synthetic analogue of arginine-vasopressin. It is used to control and prevent bleeding episodes in patients with coagulation disorder
- **Surgical Treatment** More than 90% of the severe bleeding that occurs in adolescents is controlled with medical treatment. However, surgical treatment is required in the event of life-threatening bleeding, when medical treatment is unsuccessful and in situations where a histopathology evaluation is needed. Surgical treatment options include:
    - Dilatation and curettage
    - Uterine artery embolization
    - Endometrial ablation
    - Hysterectomy

Ans: (b) Tranexamic acid

Ref: *Berek and Novak's Gynecology, 16th Edition, page 1363*

5. Which one of the following is a second generation endometrial ablation technique?

(a) Roller ball endometrial ablation
(b) Transcervical resection of endometrium
(c) Nd: YAG laser endometrial ablation
(d) Thermal balloon endometrial ablation

Explanation:

Endometrial ablation (minimal invasive surgery)

Definition: Endometrial ablation involves destruction of the endometrium by resection or thermal energy

Minimal invasive surgery (MIS) is a safe and effective alternative to hysterectomy in women with DUB who do not respond to medical management

Indications

- Failed medical therapy in DUB
- Poor surgical candidates for hysterectomy
- Patients who do not want surgery
- Women with a desire to preserve the uterus

Endometrial ablation is especially beneficial in perimenopausal age group women who are not desirous of fertility or menstrual function

Contraindications

- Premalignant or malignant lesion of the cervix and endometrium
- Acute pelvic infection
- Previous upper segment uterine scar (chance of perforation)
- Uterine size >12 weeks
- Uterine malformations
- Desire for future fertility

Advantages of Endometrial ablation over hysterectomy

- Less morbid procedure
- Short recovery time

Preoperative preparation

Prior therapy with **GnRH analogues or danazol or MPA for 4–6 weeks reduces endometrial thickness** that facilitates the procedure (it is easier to resect a thin endometrium).

Various techniques

First-generation techniques: Resectoscopic endometrial ablation

- Transcervical resection of endometrium (TCRE)
- Rollerball endometrial ablation (REA)
- Laser endometrial ablation (LEA)—Nd:YAG laser commonly used

Second-generation endometrial ablation: Nonresectoscopic endometrial ablation

- Thermal balloon ablation
- Hydrothermal ablation
- Microwave endometrial ablation
- Radio-frequency–induced endometrial ablation
- Cryotherapy
- Photodynamic therapy

Second-generation endometrial ablation devices seem to be as effective as first-generation devices

Advantages of Second-generation endometrial ablation include:

- Reduces operating time
- Can be used more often with local anaesthesia
- Fewer complications
- More cost-effective than first-generation devices

Disadvantage: Endometrial tissue is not obtained for histopathology

Outcome

- Improvement in symptoms occurs (reduced rate of dysmenorrhea, blood loss) in 90% of cases
- Amenorrhea following the procedure occurs in 40–50% of cases
- Success is not absolute and symptoms may recur or persist—20% of cases may require surgery later

Complications of endometrial ablation

- Uterine perforation
- Hemorrhage

Ans: (d) Thermal balloon endometrial ablation

Ref: *Clinical Obstetrics and Gynecology by Sharmila Arun Babu, 1st Edition, 2019, page 318*

6. Which of the following is a feature of malignant ovarian tumor?

(a) Unilocular cyst
(b) Papillary growth
(c) Size > 5 cm
(d) Anechoic cyst

Explanation:

Features of Benign and Malignant Ovarian Tumors:

Clinical features differentiating a benign from a malignant ovarian mass		
Feature	**Benign ovarian mass**	**Malignant ovarian mass**
Age	Younger age group	Extremes of age (< 20 and > 50 years)
Duration of progression of illness	Slow	Rapid progression within a short period of few months
Cachetic symptoms (loss of weight and appetite)	Absent	Present
Palpation	Smooth surface, borders well defined, cystic consistency, mobile mass	Irregular surface, borders may be ill defined, variable consistency (due to presence of solid areas), restricted mobility or fixed mass
Site	Unilateral (80%)	Bilateral (70%)
Ascites	Absent	Present
POD deposits	Absent	May be present

Ultrasound features differentiating a benign ovarian tumor from a malignant ovarian tumor	
Benign ovarian tumor	**Malignant ovarian tumor**
Usually unilateral	Usually bilateral
Unilocular	Multilocular
Thin cyst wall	Thick cyst wall
Thin septations	Thick septae
Anechoic	Mixed echogenicity due to solid areas, papillary projections from inner wall of cyst may be present
No ascites, no lymphadenopathy	• Presence of ascites and pelvic and para-aortic lymphadenopathy suggest malignancy • Hepatosplenomegaly and omental thickening or caking may be present in advanced tumors
High-resistance flow pattern in Doppler	Doppler shows low-resistance flow pattern (increased vascularity)

Ans: (b) Papillary growth

Ref: *Clinical Obstetrics and Gynecology by Sharmila Arun Babu, 1st Edition, 2019, page 347*

7. In carcinoma cervix, which of the following lymph node involvement may indicate possibility of distant metastasis?

(a) Paracervical nodes

(b) Parametric nodes

(c) Obturator nodes

(d) Common iliac nodes

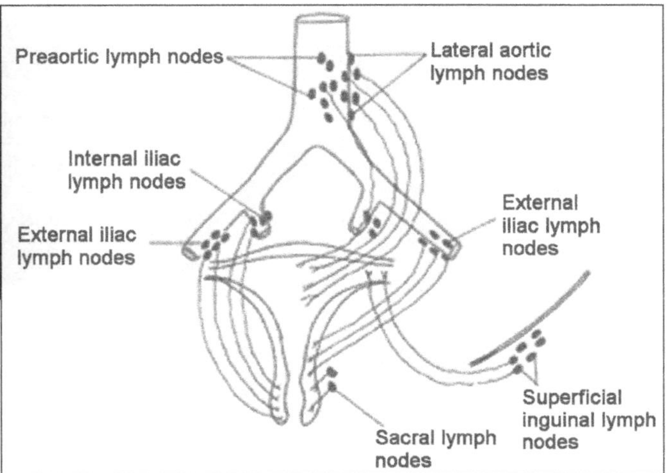

Explanation:

- Non-squamous cell carcinoma (non-SCC), common iliac lymph nodes metastasis (LNM) and bilateral pelvic LNM (PLNM) were identified as risk factors for distant metastasis

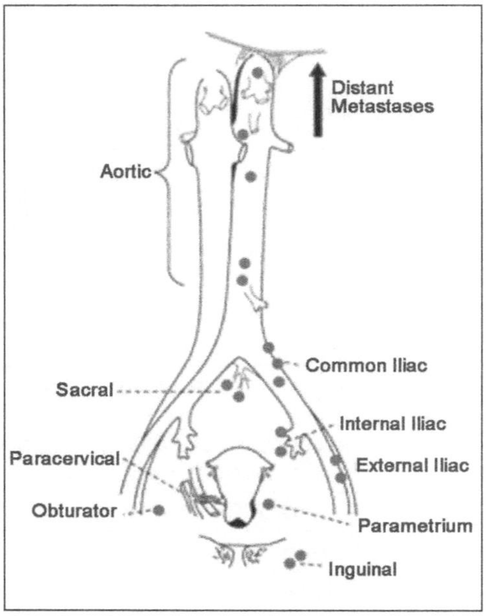

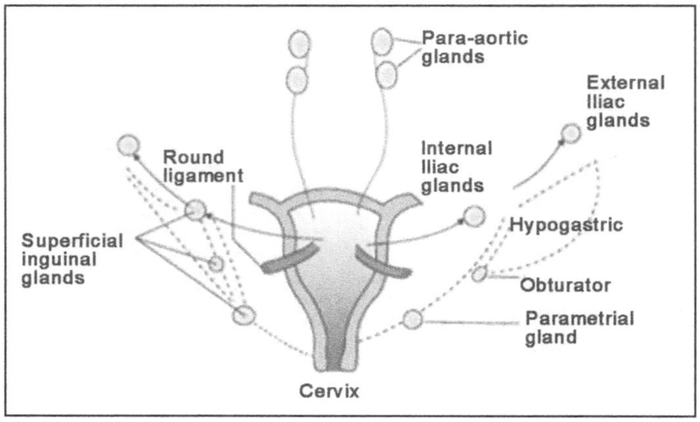

- Drains principally into the paracervical (parametrial, sacral and pre sacral lymph nodes→external iliac (obturator) and the internal iliac (hypogastric) lymph nodes
- The pelvic lymphatics drains into the common iliac and the para-aortic lymph nodes
- Fundus: Para-aortic lymph nodes, some part into inguinal nodes (along the found ligament) and common iliac lymph nodes

Ans: (d) Common iliac nodes

Ref: *Predictors of Distant Metastasis in Patients with Cervical Cancer Treated with Definitive Radiotherapy Xiaoliang Liu J Cancer 2019, 10(17): 3967-3974, doi:10.7150/jca.31538*

8. A K/C/O Rheumatic heart disease patient at 32 weeks of gestation, develops sudden dyspnea. Which of the following should not be done?

(a) Refer to cardiologist
(b) Hospitalize in ICU
(c) Reassure it is normal
(d) Rest in propped up position

Explanation:

- **Breathlessness, syncope, chest pain and nocturnal cough are warning symptoms of heart disease** of pregnancy. **Patient needs admission and early diagnosis of risk factors** and its management
- This patient comes under grade **4 NYHA classification. Hence needs admission and ICU care**

MANAGEMENT
New York Heart Association Functional Classfication (NYHA) of Heart Disease
• Class I → No signs or symptoms of cardiac decompensation
• Class II → No symptoms at rest but minor limitation of physical activity
• Class III → No symptoms at rest but marked limitation of physical activity
• Class IV → Symptoms present at rest increases discomfort with any kind of physical activity

Admission: Elective
• **Grade I:** At least two weeks prior to the expected date of delivery
• **Grade II:** At 28th week specially in case of unfavorable social surroundings
• **Grade III and IV:** As soon as pregnancy is diagnosed

Risks of Maternal Mortality with Heart Disease (NYHA, 1992)	
Cardiac Disease	**Mortality (%)**
Group 1 (Minimal Risk): ASD, VSD, PDA, Fallot tetralogy (corrected) Mitral stenosis (NYHA–Grade I and II), bioprosthetic valve	0–1
Group 2 (Moderate Risk): MS (NYHA–III and IV) AS, Marfan syndrome (Normal aorta), Fallot tetralogy (uncorrected), MS with atrial fibrillation, artificial valve	5–15
Group 3 (Major Risk): Pulmonary hypertension, Marfan syndrome (aortic involvement), aortic coarctation with valvular involvement	25–50

Ans: (c) Reassure it is normal

Ref: *DC Dutta, Textbook of Obstetrics, 9th Edition, page 258*

9. A 28-year-old woman was suspected to have genital tuberculosis. What is the percentage that fallopian tube would be involved in this case?

(a) 100% (b) 80%

(c) 60% (d) 50%

Explanation:

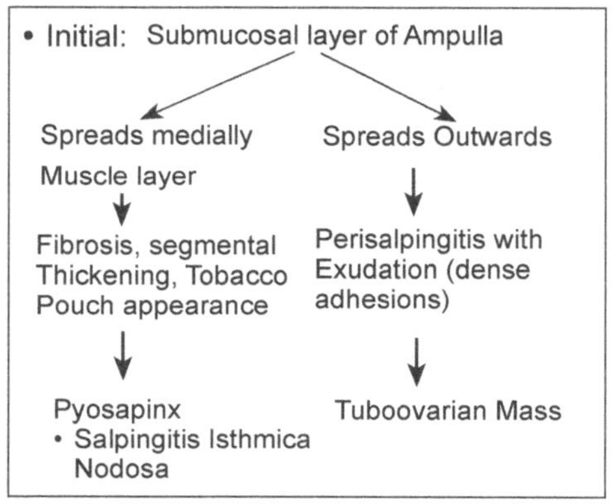

- **Fallopian tubes are involved** in 90-100% cases
- **Endometrium** is involved in **50-80% cases**
- Ovaries are involved in 20-30% cases
- Cervix is involved in 5-15% cases of genital TB.
- Tuberculosis of vagina and vulva is rare (1-2%)
- Genital TB is caused by mycobacterium tuberculosis
- In fallopian tubes it causes **salpingitis and pyosalpinx**
- In **HSG, moth eaten appearance, tobacco pouch appearance, beaded appearance, pipe stem appearance of fallopian tubes** are seen
- **Symptoms** include infertility, vaginal discharge, mass abdomen, fever, pain abdomen, abnormal uterine bleeding and amenorrhea
- **Investigations** include CBC, ESR, Manteaux test, chest X-ray, pelvic ultrasound, AFB staining of endometrial aspirate or curetting's
- **Treatment** – ATT

Ans: (a) 100%

Ref: *DC Dutta, Textbook of Gynecology, 7th Edition, page 113*

10. Which of the following types of HPV is least associated with cervical malignancy?

(a) Type 16 (b) Type 31

(c) Type 33 (d) Type 42

Explanation:

- **HPV-16 and 18 account for more than 70% of cervical cancers**
- **HPV-16 is most common HPV** seen in invasive CA and CIN 2/3 found in 50% cases
- **HPV-16 is not very specific** and is most common HPV type in women with normal cytology

- **HPV-18 is more specific** than HPV-16 for invasive tumors
- **After HPV, the six most common cervical cancer causing HPV types are 31, 33, 35, 45, 52 and 58**
- HPV is detected in more than 95% of cervical cancers and precancers
- It is also detected in 50% of vaginal cancers/precancers, over 50% of vulvar cancers/precancers, 50% of penile cancers, and over 70% of anal cancers

Clinical Association of Human Papillomavirus (HPV) Types			
HPV Type	**Most Common Clinical Lesion**	**Less Frequent Lesion**	**Potential Oncogenicity**
1	Deep plantar/palmar warts	Common warts	
2, 4, 27, 29	Common warts	Plantar, palmar and mosaic warts	
3, 10, 28, 49	Flat warts	Flat warts in EV	HPV-10 rare in cervical and vulvar carcinomas
7	Butcher's warts		
13, 32	Oral focal epithelial hyperplasia		
5, 8, 9, 12, 14, 15, 17, 19-26, 36, 47, 50	EV warts in immunosuppression	Normal skin (?)	HPV-5, –8, –9 isolated from SCCs
6, 11	Anogenital warts, cervical condylomata	Bowenoid papulosis, oral warts; respiratory papillomatosis	Buschke-Lowenstein tumor; rare in penile, vulvar, cervical and other urogenital tumors; "low risk"
16, 18, 31, 33-35, 39, 40, 51-60	Cervical condylomata; anogenital warts; bowenoid papulosis	Common warts	Genital and cervical dysplasias and carcinomas; rare in SCC of the digit, "high risk"

EV–epidermodysplasia verruciformia; SCC–squamous cell carcinoma

Pathogenesis of HPV Infection

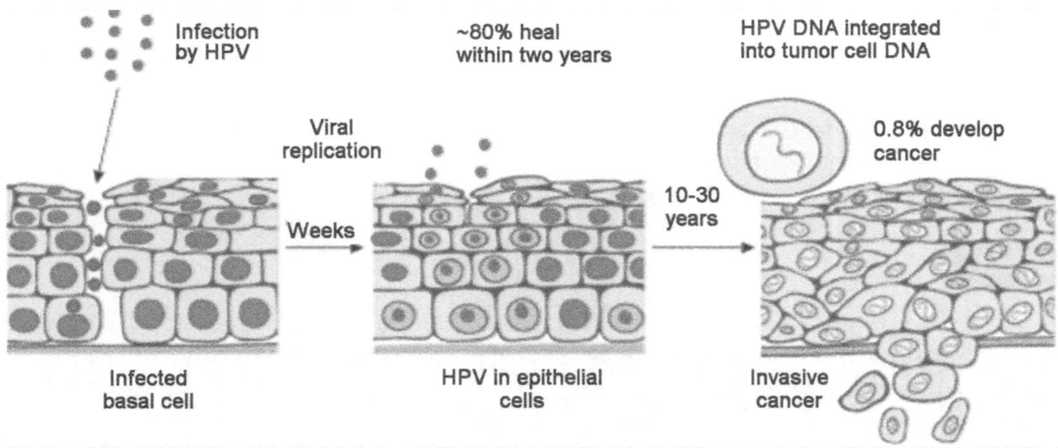

- **HSV-2 DNA and messenger RNA sequences** have been found in cervical cancer cells and may increase the likelihood of HPV infection.

Ans: (d) Type 42

Ref: *DC Dutta, Textbook of Gynecology, 7th Edition, page 265*

11. During instrumental vaginal delivery, there was extension of episiotomy downwards to involve the rectal sphincter but anal mucosa intact. Which grade of perineal tear does this belong to?

(a) I degree perineal tear
(b) II degree perineal tear
(c) III degree perineal tear
(d) IV degree perineal tear

Explanation:

Perineal tears are classified into four categories:

- **First-degree tear**: laceration is limited to the fourchette and superficial perineal skin or vaginal mucosa
- **Second-degree tear**: laceration extends beyond fourchette, perineal skin and vaginal mucosa to perineal muscles and fascia, but not the anal sphincter
- **Third-degree tear**: fourchette, perineal skin, vaginal mucosa, muscles, and anal sphincter are torn; third-degree tears may be further subdivided into three subcategories
  - **3a**: partial tear of the external anal sphincter involving less than 50% thickness
  - **3b**: greater than 50% tear of the external anal sphincter
  - **3c**: internal sphincter is torn
- **Fourth-degree tear**: fourchette, perineal skin, vaginal mucosa, muscles, anal sphincter, and rectal mucosa are torn
- **Button-hole tear**: the tear involves rectal mucosa with an intact anal sphincter complex

Ans: (c) III degree perineal tear

Ref: *DC Dutta, Textbook of Obstetrics, 9th Edition, page 397*

12. A pregnant woman at 32 weeks gestation presents with jaundice. Which of the following is unlikely to be a differential diagnosis?

(a) Acute hepatitis
(b) HELLP
(c) Cholestasis of pregnancy
(d) Thalassemia

Explanation:

- In Thalassemia, jaundice usually doesn't occur unless iron overload causes liver cirrhosis and failure. Anemia is seen in thalassemia

Causes of Jaundice in Pregnancy	
Unrelated to Pregnancy	**Pregnancy Specific**

Hepatic causes
• Acute viral hepatitis
• Drug induced hepatitis
• Chronic hepatitis
  – Viral (HBV, HCV)
  – Autoimmune hepatitis
• Wilson's disease
• Cirrhosis of liver
• Budd-Chiari syndrome
Pre-Hepatic Causes
• Hemolytic anemia
Post-Hepatic causes
• Common bileduct stone/strictures
• Biliary parasitosis
	• Hyperemesis gravidarum
	• Intrahepatic cholestasis of pregnancy
	• Pre-eclampsia/eclampsia
	• HELLP syndrome
	• Acute fatty liver of pregnancy

Ans: (d) Thalassemia

Ref: *DC Dutta, Textbook of Obstetrics, 9th Edition, page 269*

13. The oral contraceptive pill 'Mala N' contains which of the following type of progesterone component?

(a) Levonorgestrol (b) Etonorgestrel
(c) Desogestrel (d) Drosperinone

Explanation:

- MALA N (Govt of India) contains Levonorgestrel 0.15 mg + Ethinyl estradiol 30 mcg
- MALA-D contains Levonorgestrel 0.15 mg + Ethinyl estradiol 30 mcg

The composition of other common OCPs available in market are:

Brand Name	Estrogen component	Progesterone component
Novelon	Ethinylestradiol (30 µg)	Desogestrel (0.15 mg)
Femilon	Ethinylestradiol (20 µg)	Desogestrel (0.15 mg)
Loette	Ethinylestradiol (20 µg)	Levonorgestrel (0.1 mg)
Yasmin	Ethinylestradiol (30 µg)	Drospirenone (3 mg)

Ans: (a) Levonorgestrol

Ref: *DC Dutta, Textbook of Obstetrics, 9th Edition, page 503*

14. Which of the following is the most common cause of death in Carcinoma Cervix?

(a) Uremia (b) Metastasis
(c) Bleeding P/V (d) Sepsis

Explanation:

- **Uremia is the most common cause of death in cervical carcinoma**

Causes of Death in Carcinoma Cervix

- Uremia
- Hemorrhage
- Sepsis
- Cachexia
- Metastasis to lung, lymph nodes, bones and abdominal cavity

Ans: (a) Uremia

Ref: *DC Dutta, Textbook of Gynecology, 7th Edition, page 285*

15. Which of the following is not true regarding 'Diaphragm' barrier contraceptives?

(a) Diaphragm can be used with lubricant oil
(b) Should not be removed till 6 hours after last intercourse
(c) Spermicide is used with diaphragm
(d) Some local vaginal medicines may reduce the efficacy of barrier contraceptive

Explanation:

Diaphragm:

- A diaphragm is a shallow rubber dome with a flexible rim that covers the cervix on insertion
- It is **often used in combination with spermicidal jelly**

- It is available in various sizes. Diaphragm diameter varies from 5-10 cm
- Only water- or silicone-based **lubricants** can be used if the **diaphragm** is made of latex. Products made with **oil** cannot be used as **lubricants** because they damage latex
- It can be inserted up **to 3 hours before intercourse.** It should remain **in place for at least 6 hours** after the intercourse. However, it **must not be left inside the vagina for more than 24 hours**
- Following insertion, the anterior rim of the diaphragm rests behind the pubic symphysis and the dome of the diaphragm covers the cervix
- It can **be reused**. After usage, it is washed with soap and water, dried, and stored in a case

Disadvantages:

- It can cause irritation or allergic reaction
- Failure rate is high
- Not suitable in prolapse

Advantages

- Cheap
- Reduces STD/PID

Ans: (a) Diaphragm can be used with lubricant oil

Ref: *DC Dutta, Textbook of Obstetrics, 9th Edition, page 412*

16. Which of the following is not true regarding theory of endometriosis?

(a) Endometriosis lesions have aromatase

(b) Endometriosis patients have increased reactive oxygen species [ROS]

(c) Coelomic metaplasia

(d) Monocyte chemotactic protein [MCP-1] is found in peritoneal fluid of endometriosis

Explanation:

Theories of Endometriosis:

- **Retrograde menstruation (Sampson's theory)**–retrograde flow of menstrual blood through the tubes during menstruation. Endometrial tissue sheds at peritoneal surfaces, ovaries and uterosacral ligaments
- **Coelomic metaplasia (Meyer and Ivanoff)**–chronic irritation of pelvic peritoneum by the menstrual blood cause coelomic metaplasia which results in endometriosis
- **Direct implantation**–in abdominal scar, episiotomy scar, vagina or cervix
- **Lymphatic theory (Halban)**–normal endometrium can metastasise to pelvic lymph nodes
- **Vascular theory**–distant sites like lungs, arms and thighs
- **Genetic and immunological**–multifactorial inheritance, defect of local cellular immunity, subclinical peritoneal inflammation
- **Environmental**–somatic mutations of cells due to pollutants
- **Reactive oxygen species** and oxidative stress
- **Monocyte chemotactic protein [MCP-1]** is found in peritoneal fluid of endometriosis

Ans: (a) Endometriosis lesions have aromatase

Ref: *DC Dutta, Textbook of Gynecology, 7th Edition, page 251*

17. One of the following is True regarding prediction of risk of IUGR:

(a) Increased Sflt-1
(b) Increased PAPP-A in 1st trimester
(c) Decreased AFP
(d) Increased placental growth factor

Explanation:

Maternal Circulating Biochemical Markers in IUGR:

- **Decreased PAPP–**A in 1st and 2nd trimester
- **Decreased HCG** in 1st trimester and increased in 2nd trimester
- **Decreased UE3** in second trimester
- **Low Placental growth factor (PLGF)** in 1st and 2nd trimester
- **Low PP–13 and ADAM 12**
- **Increased AFP** in 2nd trimester
- **Increased inhibin A** in 2nd trimester
- **Increased or decreased Sflt 1** in 1st and 2nd trimester and increased in 3rd trimester
- **Increased SENG** in all trimesters

Ans: (a) Increased Sflt-1

Ref: *DC Dutta, Textbook of Obstetrics, 7th Edition, page 431*

18. A woman presents with history of recurrent abortion. Which of the following is not to be done?

(a) TSH
(b) APLA
(c) USG Scan
(d) Wait until next pregnancy

Explanation:

Etiology of Recurrent pregnancy loss (RPL)

Etiology	Causes	Incidence (%)
Genetic	Chromosomal abnormalities – Aneuploidy—trisomy, monosomy Parental chromosomal rearrangements—balanced reciprocal or Robertsonian translocation	3–5
Anatomical	Congenital causes: Mullerian anomalies (septate uterus, bicornuate uterus, cervical incompetence, etc.) Acquired causes: Uterine synechiae, fibroid, cervical incompetence	10–15
Endocrine	Corpus luteal insufficiency • Polycystic ovarian disease • Hypothyroidism • Uncontrolled diabetes mellitus	15–20
Immunological	Antiphospholipid antibody syndrome	20–30
Thrombotic factors	Inherited thrombophilias–factor V Leiden deficiency, protein C and protein S deficiency	
Infections	Chlamydial and *Mycoplasma* infections	5
Miscellaneous	Smoking, alcohol, drugs, radiation, subchorionic hematoma	10
Unexplained	Cause not known	50

- Abortions with normal karyotyping are associated with a higher recurrence rate than abortions with abnormal karyotyping. Hence, in the presence of normal karyotyping of the abortus, the cause of pregnancy loss has to be evaluated.

INVESTIGATIONS FOR RECURRENT PREGNANCY LOSS

Evaluation during pregnancy in a woman with RPL

- Complete hemogram with platelet count
- Blood grouping and typing
- Urine analysis
- Glucose tolerance test (GTT)
- VDRL
- APLA titers—ACA and LAC
- Thyroid function test in case of clinical feature suggestive of thyroid dysfunction (It is routinely done in clinical practice, although it is not indicated in the definitive tests for RPL)
- Cervical swab culture for *L. monocytogenes*, *M.hominis* and *Ureaplasma urealyticum*
- USG—for cervical length, uterine malformations, and fibroid uterus
- Karyotyping of both the partners

Evaluation for RPL that can be done only in the interconceptional period

- **HSG:** Uses of HSG in RPL include the following:
  - To diagnose cervical incompetence
  - To study the endometrial cavity—endometrialpolyps, submucous fibroid, and septate uterus
  - To diagnose uterine synechiae—Asherman syndrome
  - To check for tubal patency

However, HSG cannot differentiate a septate uterusfrom bicornuate uterus.

- **Hysterolaparoscopy:** Uses of hysterolaparoscopyin RPL include the following:
  - Detects uterine anomalies such as bicornuate/unicornuate/septate uterus
  - Differentiates a septate uterus (normal-lookinguterine fundus) from bicornuate uterus (depression between the two horns)
  - Helps in identifying non-communicating rudimentary horn of uterus
- **Luteal phase endometrial biopsy:** To identify LPD
- **Tests for diagnosis of cervical incompetence:** Passage of No. 8 Hegar's dilator without difficulty or HSG showing funnel-shaped cervical canal

Summary of evaluation and treatment of the causes of RPL

Category	Evaluation	Treatment
Genetic causes	Karyotyping of both parents Ovarian reserve test Genetic counseling	Donor gametes Preimplantation genetic diagnosis
Anatomic causes	Ultrasound examination Hysterosalpingogram Hysterolaparoscopy MRI	No surgery possible in unicornuate, didelphys, arcuate uterus Septate uterus—Jones and Tompkins' septoplasty, hysteroscopic resection of septum Bicornuate uterus—Strassman's metroplasty Cervical incompetence—cerclage Fibroid—myomectomy / hysteroscopic resection of submucous fibroid

Contd.

Contd.

Endocrine causes	Luteal phase defect—luteal phase endometrial biopsy PCOD—LH, FSH levels, USG DM—blood glucose, HbA1C TSH, Sr. prolactin	Progesterone supplementation Metformin, clomiphene citrate Insulin therapy Thyroxine therapy, dopamine agonists (for prolactinomas)
Immunological and thrombotic causes	APLA: LAC, ACA Thrombophilias: Factor V Leiden, protein C, protein S, antithrombin III deficiency	Heparin and aspirin
Infections	Endocervical culture: For *Chlamydia*, *Mycoplasma*, and *Ureaplasma*	Empirical antibiotics
Environmental causes	History	Behavioural modifications

Ans: (d) Wait till next pregnancy

Ref: *DC Dutta, Textbook of Obstetrics, 9th Edition, page 160*

19. A pregnant woman in 2nd trimester presents with groin pain. Patient symptomatically improves with Hot pad treatment. Which of the following is the probable diagnosis?

(a) Preterm labour (b) Spasm of round ligament
(c) Appendicitis (d) Renal calculus

Explanation:

- **Round ligament pain is** considered normal in pregnancy. It is a sudden sharp spasm in iliac fossa. It is usually relieved by mild exercises and hot pack

Non obstetrical causes of acute pain in pregnancy:

- Acute Appendicitis
- Gastric perforation
- Volvulus
- Cholecystitis
- Biliary colic
- Renal or ureteric calculi
- Torsion of ovarian cyst
- Red degeneration of fibroid
- Cystitis
- Hepatitis
- Acute fatty liver

Ans: (b) Spasm of round ligament

Ref: *DC Dutta, Textbook of Obstetrics, 9th Edition, page 286*

20. Which of the following reflects True statement regarding prevention of IUGR?

(a) High protein diet helps in prevention

(b) Aspirin and LMWH benefits fetal outcome in thrombophilic patients

(c) Aspirin reduces the risk of IUGR in low risk patients

(d) Aspirin and Clopidogrel reduces risk of IUGR in preeclamptic patients

Explanation:

Role of drug therapy in IUGR

- There are **no significant benefits with drug therapy in IUGR**
- There is **no concrete evidence to evaluate benefits and risks of nutrient therapy, nitric oxide donors, antioxidants, plasma volume expanders, and oxygen therapy** to the mother with IUGR fetus
- **Combined aspirin and heparin therapy may benefit fetal outcome in women with APLA**
- Maternal hyperalimentation by amino acids can improve fetal growth if it is due to maternal malnutrition only

Role of low-dose aspirin in IUGR

- **Low-dose aspirin** has been proved to be beneficial in women with **previous H/o IUGR and preeclampsia and in APLA syndrome, with history of thrombotic disease and recurrent FGR** if started early in gestation. It acts by inhibiting thromboxane A2 synthesis and thereby prevents vasoconstriction and platelet aggregation in uteroplacental circulation
- Fetal therapy by injecting amino acids into amniotic fluid or umbilical cord is under research.

Ans: (c) Aspirin reduces the risk of IUGR in low risk patients

Ref: *DC Dutta, Textbook of Obstetrics, 7th Edition, page 434*

21. A 32 year old female presents with hypotension 2 days after tubal ligation procedure. A Hematoma seen near anterior division of internal iliac artery on imaging. Which of the following is Likely to be injured?

(a) Uterine artery (b) Ovarian artery

(c) Superior vesical artery (d) Inferior vesical artery

Explanation:

- Uterine artery is a branch of anterior division of internal iliac artery which can be damaged during tubal sterilization and can cause broad ligament hematoma and cause hypotension

Branches of the Internal Iliac Artery

Anterior Division	Posterior Division
Uterine	Superior gluteal
Obliterated umbilical	Lateral sacral
Superior and inferior vesical	Iliolumbar
Obturator	
Internal pudendal	
Inferior gluteal	
Middle rectal	
Vaginal	

- Uterine artery is a branch of anterior division of internal iliac artery. In cases of severe hemorrhage when the internal iliac artery ligation is done, the anterior division should be ligated

Blood Supply

Organ	Arterial	Venous
Vagina	• Cervicovaginal branch of uterine • Vaginal • Middlerectal • Internal pudendal • Azygos (anterior, posterior)	Internal iliac and internal pudendal veins
Uterus	• Uterine artery • Ovarian and vaginal arteries	Uterine vein → internal iliac vein
Fallopian tube	• Uterine artery • Ovarian	Pampiniform plexus → ovarian veins
Ovary	Ovarian artery (branch of abdominal aorta)	Left ovarian vein → left renal vein Right ovarian vein → IVC

Ans: (a) Uterine artery

Ref: *DC Dutta, Textbook of Gynecology, 7th Edition, page 25*

ORTHOPEDICS

1. A 5-year-old Child presents with fever and diffuse thigh swelling. Most probable diagnosis:

(a) Scurvy (b) Osteomyelitis

(c) Suppurative Arthritis (d) Infantile hyperostosis

Explanation:

- Presence of fever points to an infective cause. Since there is a diffuse thigh swelling, the most probable cause would be osteomyelitis. In septic arthritis, swelling will be typically present around the joint.

Acute Osteomyelitis

- Acute osteomyelitis is infection of bone.
- **Etiology**
  - **Staphylococcus aureus** is the most common organism in all age groups
  - **Salmonella** is commonest organism in **sickle cell anaemia** patients
  - **Pseudomonas aeruginosa** is commonest organism in **Drug abusers**
  - Animal bite – Pasteurella multocida
  - Human bite – Eikenella corrodens
  - Diabetic ulcer and Fight bites – Anaerobes
  - Immunocompromised (HIV) – Staphylococcus aureus
  - Post-traumatic osteomyelitis/Post-surgical osteomyelitis – S. aureus
  - Open injuries – Staphylococcus
  - Foot injuries – Pseudomonas
- **Pathology**
  - Most common mode of infection is **hematogenous**
  - In children metaphysis of long bone (usually lower end femur upper end tibia) is earliest and most commonly involved site
  - In adults commonest site of infection is thoracolumbar spine
  - Starts in Metaphysis because of:
    - Defective phagocytosis in metaphysis (Inherently depleted Reticuloendothelial System)
    - Rich blood supply
    - Hair pin bend of metaphyseal vessels (leads to vascular stasis)
    - Metaphyseal hemorrhage due to repeated trauma (acts as culture media)
- **Pathophysiology**
  - ***Metaphyseal Abscess*** *is formed initially and* it spreads subperiosteally in children because periosteum is loosely attached to bone in children and in adults, pus spreads to Medullary cavity involving the Diaphysis
  - Infection rarely crosses growth plate because it has no blood vessels and periosteum is firmly attached to the plate at this level
  - Joint involvement can take place if - metaphysis is intracapsular (e.g. hip, shoulder, elbow)

- The pathological sequence is inflammation, suppuration, necrosis, reactive new bone formation and ultimately resolution and healing
- **Clinical Feature and Investigation**
  - Presenting complaints are Fever (>38.3°C), **swelling of the limb, pain, systemic symptoms, toxic look, and increased levels of Total leucocyte counts, ESR and CRP**
  - Systemic signs are absent in immunocompromised and neonates
  - Absent movements of a limb after ruling out trauma in pediatric population is osteomyelitis till proved otherwise
  - **X-rays in <24 hours is normal**
  - 1st change on X-rays is **loss of soft tissue planes***
  - 1st bony change is **Periosteal reaction** seen on day **7–10** (2nd week or day 10) Solid Periosteal Reaction
  - Later features of **bone destruction** appear
  - **MRI** is considered the best radiological investigation for bone infections because it can identify **marrow edema** (seen **within 6 hours**) and soft tissue extension in bone infections
  - **Tc99-MDP, Ga-67-citrate or Indium 111** labelled leucocytes (Best out of 3) are the 2nd best radiological investigation
  - **Gold standard** is always **tissue diagnosis** (from the lesion) hence growth of organism on **culture media** is the best investigation for infections
  - **Blood Culture** is positive in **60% cases**

Ans: (b) Osteomyelitis

Ref: *Fundamentals of Orthopedics by Mohindra and Jain, 2nd Edition, Jaypee Brothers, Publishers, page 282*

2. Most common type of fibrodysplasia:

(a) Monostotic
(b) Polyostotic
(c) Mc Cune-Albirght
(d) Osteofibrous dysplasia

Explanation:

- **Monostotic** form **is 6 times** more common than **polyostotic** form in **Fibrous dysplasia**
- **Osteofibrous dysplasia** (**ossifying fibroma of long bones**, also known as **Campanacci disease**) is also relatively less common and usually affects patients in their **first two decades** of life
- The **diaphysis of the tibia** followed by **fibula** is the most frequently affected location
- Tibia is often bowed anterolaterally and the radiographs show **eccentric, intracortical osteolysis with the expansion of the cortex**
- Management primarily involves **observation** as some lesions regress spontaneously

Ans: (a) Monostotic

Ref: *Fundamentals of Orthopedics by Mohindra and Jain, 2nd Edition, Jaypee Publishers, page 313*

3. 65 years old patient, chronic smoker, chronic alcoholic, who has lost 6 kg over 3 months. Comes with back pain and lytic lesions on X-ray pelvis with hematuria. No limitation of movement. Diagnosis?

(a) Chondroblastoma
(b) Mets from prostate adenocarcinoma
(c) Adenocarcinoma lung
(d) Multiple Myeloma

Explanation:

- **Chronic smoker** and **osteolytic lesions** point towards the possibility of **secondary's** from **carcinoma lung**

Metastatic Bone Disease

- Most common primary is Breast > Prostate overall
- **Most common sites of primary for bone metastasis**
  - In males – Prostate > Lung
  - In Female – Breast > Lung
  - In Children – Neuroblastoma
- **Skeletal sites most frequently involved**
  - Spine (Dorsal)
- **Lytic expansile metastasis seen in**
  - Renal Cancer
  - Thyroid carcinomas
- **Purely Osteoblastic secondaries**
  - Prostate/Carcinoid/Medulloblastoma
- **Metastasis distal to knee and elbow is rare and usually arises**
- **From primary tumors of the**
  - Bronchus, Bladder and Colon

Extra Edge

METASTASIS TO BONE

- Osteoblastic lesions–Prostate, Seminoma, Carcinoids, Medulloblastoma
- Osteolytic lesions–Kidney, Thyroid, Lung
- Mixed–Breast (more commonly Lytic)

Ans: (c) Adenocarcinoma lung

Ref: *Fundamentals of Orthopedics by Mohindra and Jain, 2nd Edition, Jaypee Publishers, page 334*

4. Examine the schematic picture of epiphyseal fracture. What is the grade according to Salter Harris classification?

(a) Type 2
(b) Type 3
(c) Type 4
(d) Type 5

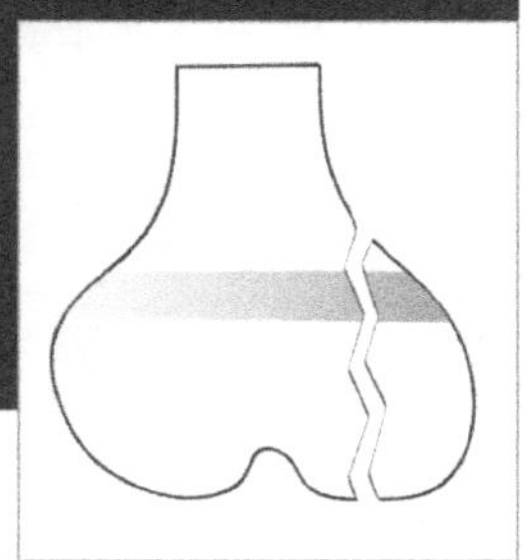

Explanation:

- **Since there is a fracture within the epiphysis, it is Type IV injury.**

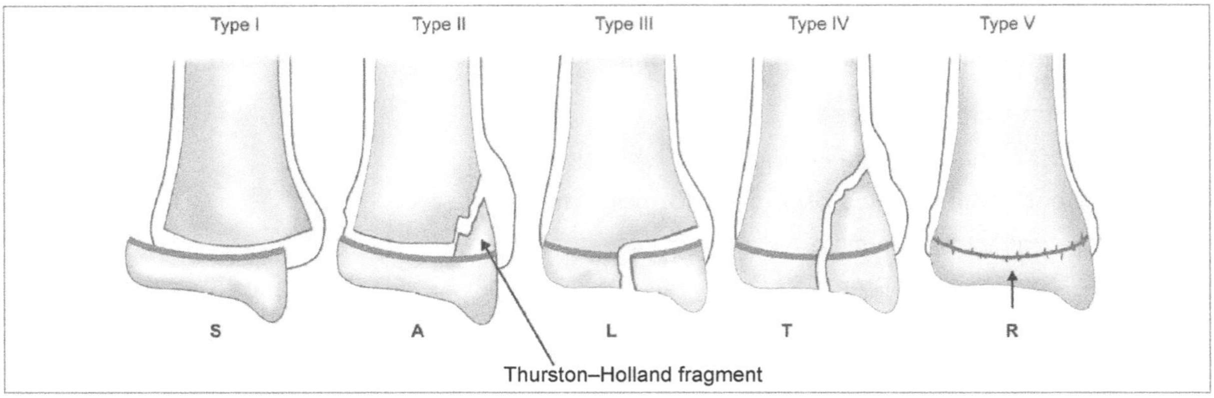

Figure: Salter Harris Classification

Mnemonic for Salter-Harris Classification–"SALTR"				
Type I	**Type II**	**Type III**	**Type IV**	**Type V**
Slipped (Slippage of epiphysis)	Above (fracture passes up in the metaphysis)	Lower or below (fracture passes below in epiphysis)	Through (fracture passes through all; epiphysis, physis and metaphysis)	Rammed or crushed physis

Ans: (c) Type 4

Ref: *Fundamentals of Orthopedics by Mohindra and Jain, 2nd Edition, Jaypee Publishers, page 334*

5. A polytrauma patient presents with fracture wound >10 cm, high energy, extensive soft-tissue damage which is contaminated. What is the grading according to Gustilo Anderson classification?

(a) II
(b) III A
(c) III B
(d) III C

Explanation:

Gustilo Anderson classification is used to classify open fractures.

Gustilo-Anderson classification of compound fractures*	
Type/Grade	**Features**
I	Fracture wound <1 cm with minimal soft tissue injury and fracture comminution. Usually, it is low energy trauma with clean wound
II	Fracture wound >1 cm without extensive soft tissue damage and fracture comminution. There is mild-to-moderate soft tissue injury and mild-to-moderate wound contamination
IIIA	Fracture wound > 10 cm with extensive soft tissue injury and wound contamination, but with adequate soft tissue coverage (at least periosteum over bone is intact)
IIIB	Fracture wound > 10 cm with extensive soft tissue damage and contamination. Soft tissue coverage is inadequate (periosteal stripping occurs and bone may be exposed) and require skin or flap grafting
IIIC	Any size of open wound with major vascular injury requiring repair
*Gunshot wounds with fractures and open segmental fractures are classified as type IIIA Gustilo-Anderson injuries	

Ans: (c) III B

Ref: *Fundamentals of Orthopedics by Mohindra and Jain, 2nd Edition, Jaypee Publishers, page 334*

6. A patient presents with joint swelling. Joint effusion aspirate with cloudy appearance, high WBC and normal glucose. Probable diagnosis:

(a) Osteoarthritis (b) Septic arthritis
(c) Tubercular arthritis (d) Rheumatoid arthritis

Explanation:

- **Normal glucose** rules out possibility of infectious arthritis. **Cloudy appearance** and high WBC but normal glucose point more towards **RA**

Synovial fluild analysis in various types of arthritis						
		Degenerative	**Inflammatory**		**Infectious**	
Parameters	**Normal**	**Osteoarthritis**	**Gout**	**Rheumatoid arthritis**	**Pyogenic arthritis**	**Tuberculous arthritis**
Appearance	Straw or clear yellow	Clear yellow	Yellow to turbid milky	Yellow, cloudy	Purulent	Yellow, turbid
Viscosity	Normal	Normal	Decreased	Decreased	Decreased	Decreased
Total white blood cell (WBC) count	≤ 200	≤ 2,000	2,000-50,000	2,000-50,000	> 50,000	10,000-20,000
Polymorphonuclear leukocytes	<20%	<20%	60-70%	50-60%	90%	60%
Crystals	Negative	Negative	Urate crystals	Negative	Negative	Negative
Glucose level	A bit lower than plasma level	↓	↓	↓	↓↓	↓↓

Ans: (d) Rheumatoid arthritis

Ref: *Fundamentals of Orthopedics by Mohindra and Jain, 2nd Edition, Jaypee Publishers, page 418*

7. A 7-year-old boy presents with painless limp, limitation of abduction and internal rotation. Probable diagnosis:

(a) TB hip (b) Perthes' disease
(c) SCFE (d) Aseptic chondrolysis

Explanation:

- Age, painless limp and limited abduction and internal rotation are classical of **Perthes' disease** in the above question. Limp in **TB hip** and **SCFE** is generally **painful**

Idiopathic chondrolysis of hip (ICH)

- Rare condition and is more commonly seen in **females**
- The condition presents with loss of articular cartilage (joint space on X-ray <3 mm) that occurs without obvious reason
- Condition is postulated to be autoimmune but exact etiology is unknown

Differential Diagnosis of Limping Child

Painless Limp	Painful Limp
• **1–3 years age group:** – DDH (Developmental dysplasia of hip) – Cerebral palsy – Muscular dystrophy – Infantile coxa vara • **4–10 years age:** – Limb length discrepancy, Poliomyelitis	• Legg calves Perthes' disease (**NOTE:** Classically Perthes' is described as painless limp) • Slipped capital femoral epiphysis • Osteochondritis dissecans (knee) (Lateral surface of medial femoral condyle) • Arthritis/Synovitis/Osteomyelitis

- Order of investigation in Limping child X-ray followed by **ultrasound** followed by **MRI**

Ans: (b) Perthes' disease

Ref: *Fundamentals of Orthopedics by Mohindra and Jain, 2nd Edition, Jaypee Publishers, page 368*

8. A patient has a suspected Tumor in distal femur involving Epiphyseal-metaphyseal junction, ill-defined with reactive bone formation. Probable Diagnosis:

(a) Fibrous dysplasia
(b) Ewing sarcoma
(c) Osteosarcoma
(d) Giant cell tumor

Explanation:

- **Site** (distal femur), **location** (metaphyseal-epiphyseal junction), **ill-defined borders** and **reactive bone formation** (Codman's triangle/sunray appearance) point to diagnosis of **Osteosarcoma**

Characteristic histologic finding of osteosarcoma

- **Bone forming tumor** (osteo = bone)
- Presence of **osteoid**

Characteristic radiologic features of osteosarcoma

- **Codman's** triangle
- **Sunburst** appearance

Ans: (c) Osteosarcoma

Ref: *Fundamentals of Orthopedics by Mohindra and Jain, 2nd Edition, Jaypee Publishers, page 325*

9. Light bulb sign is seen in:

(a) Anterior dislocation of shoulder
(b) Posterior dislocation of shoulder
(c) Posterior dislocation of hip
(d) Anterior dislocation of hip

Explanation:

- **"Light Bulb Sign"** is seen in Posterior dislocation of shoulder.

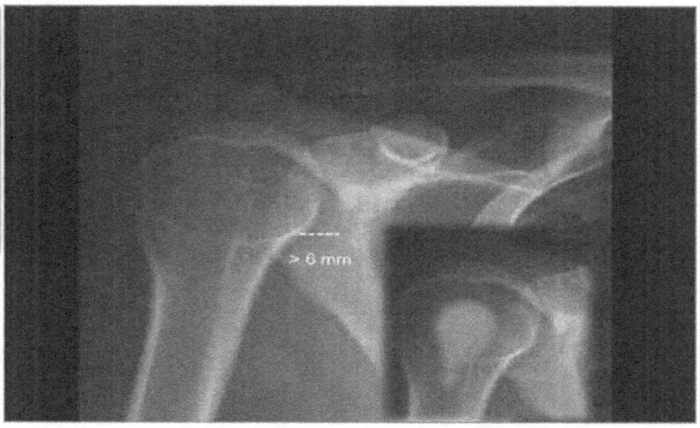

Figure: Light bulb sign and Rim Sign seen in posterior dislocation of shoulder (note the head is appearing in a reduced position though the same is dislocated posteriorly)

SHOULDER DISLOCATION

- **Shoulder** – Most common joint to undergo **recurrent dislocation** (2nd most common—fpatella)
- **Shoulder** – Most common joint to undergo **non recurrent (traumatic) dislocation**
- **Anterior (Antero-inferior) dislocation** is the **commonest type** of shoulder **dislocation (97%)**
- **Sub coracoid** is the most common sub type of **anterior dislocation**.
- Most common early complication of anterior dislocation of shoulder: **Nerve injury (circumflex branch of Axillary nerve)**
- **Mode of injury:**
  - **Recurrent anterior dislocation**: Abduction and external rotation force
  - **Posterior dislocation**: Indirect force producing marked internal rotation and adduction
  - **Inferior dislocation**: Severe hyper abduction force

Anterior Dislocation

- **Lesions**
  - **Bankart's lesion**: avulsion of glenoidal labrum from neck of scapula
  - **Hill Sach's lesion**: compression fracture of postero lateral humeral head
  - Humeral avulsion of Glenohumeral ligaments (HAGL)
  - Concurrent rotator cuff or superior labrum anterior to posterior (**SLAP**) tear
  - **Bony Bankart** (associated glenoid rim fracture) can lead to recurrent instability
- **Clinical features:**
  - Hand is kept at **abduction, external rotation and extension**
  - **Dugas test**: patient is unable to touch the opposite shoulder
  - **Callaway's test**: increased vertical circumference of shoulder
  - **Bryant's test**: anterior axillary fold is at a lower level
  - **Hamilton ruler test:** a straight ruler can touch if placed between acromion process and lateral epicondyle of humerus
  - **Regiment badge sign:** area of anesthesia around the deltoid due to injury to axillary nerve

- **Management**
  - ***Kocher's method*** *(preferred)*
  - ***Stimson's gravity method***
  - ***Hippocratic method***
  - ***Hippocrates and Milch maneuver***

Recurrent Shoulder Dislocation

- ***Tests for recurrent dislocation:***
  - Shift and load test
  - Sulcus test
  - Apprehension test
  - Lachman test
  - Relocation test
- ***Causes of recurrence***:
  - Inadequate immobilization

- High velocity initial injury
- Larger defect
- Younger age

Treatment options:

- **TUBS** – Trauma -> Unidirectional -> Bankart's lesion -> Surgery
- **AMBRI** – Atraumatic ->Multidirectional, Bilateral -> Rehabilitation, If surgery, Inferior capsular shift

Surgical Procedures

- **Bankart's repair** – detached anterior structures attached to glenoid rim by sutures
- **Putti platt** – double breasting subscapularis muscle
- **Bristow procedure** – transplantation of coracoid process to anterior rim of the glenoid cavity

Posterior Dislocation

- **Causes:**
  - *Direct blow from front*
  - *Epileptics*
  - *Electroconvulsive therapy*
- **Signs**
  - **Vacant glenoid sign** (6 mm)
  - **Light bulb sign**
  - Trough line or reverse Hill-sach lesion
  - Void superior and inferior glenoid fossa
  - Loss of profile of neck of Humerus.

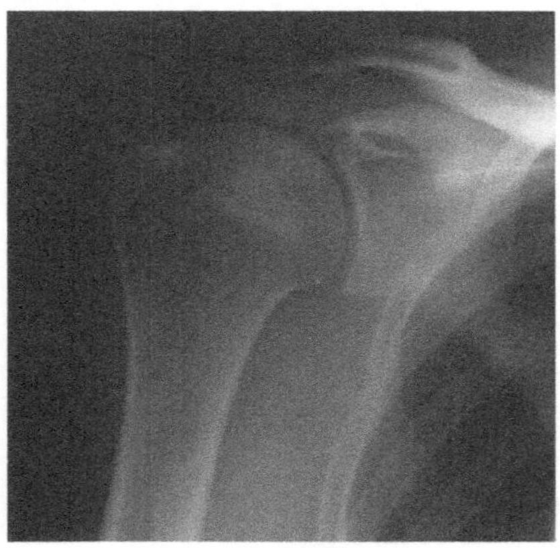

- Normal appearance of shoulder in X-ray.

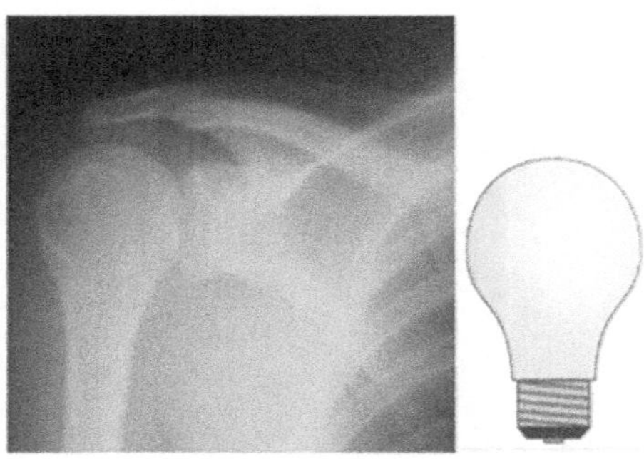

- **Light bulb appearance** of humeral head in X-ray due to **internal rotation of the humeral head** in **posterior dislocation**

Inferior dislocation

- **Rare injury** caused by **severe hyper abduction** force.
- Called **luxatio erecta**
- The humeral head is **subluxated** (dislocated inferiorly and shaft points upwards (erected)
- **Arm locked in almost full abduction / elevation** is the **common symptom**.
- The patient comes with his arm fixed almost by the side of his head.
- Axillary nerve is commonly injured

Position of arm in shoulder dislocation

- **Anterior Dislocation (Preglenoid, Subcoracoid, Subclavicular type)**
  - By the **side of body** in slight abduction
  - Locked in **external rotation** and **internal rotation is restricted**.
- **Posterior Dislocation**
  - Difficult to diagnose because the patient may have normal contour of shoulder
  - Holds injured shoulder in internal rotation and examiner cannot externally rotate it.
- **Inferior Dislocation (Luxatio erecta / Subglenoid)**
  - Locked in full abduction / elevation, fixed almost by the **side of head**

FINDINGS IN INSPECTION

- **Anterior dislocation:**
  - **Squaring of the shoulder** secondary to a relative prominence of the acromion anteriorly
  - A **palpable mass** (the humeral head) anteriorly
  - A hollow beneath the acromion posteriorly
- **Posterior dislocation:**
  - A **flattening** of the **shoulder anteriorly**
  - A **palpable mass** (the humeral head) posteriorly
  - A **prominent coracoid** anteriorly
  - Mechanical block to external rotation
- **Inferior dislocations:**
  - Humeral head is palpable on the lateral chest wall and axilla.
  - Do not confuse this dislocation with a step-off between the distal clavicle and the acromion in a shoulder separation.
- **Superior dislocations:**
  - The humeral head rides above the level of the acromion.
  - The arm is shortened compared with the contralateral side.
  - Shoulder movement is restricted.

	Anterior dislocation (95%)	Posterior dislocation (5%)
Mechanism of injury	• **Direct force**—blow from the posterior aspect of the shoulder • **Indirect force**—due to **Abduction** + **External rotation** + **Extension injury** (**common**)	• **Direct force**—blow from the anterior aspect of the shoulder • **Indirect force**—due to **Internal rotation + Adduction + Flexion** injury (**common**)
Clinical features	• Severe pain • Arm is held in **abduction and external** rotation • Adduction is restricted • Normal contour of shoulder is lost • Anterior shoulder fullness	• Severe pain • Arm is in position of **adduction and internal rotation (Classical 'sling' position)** • Abduction is restricted • Normal contour of shoulder is lost • Posterior shoulder fullness
Clinical test	• Posterior aspect is flat • Coracoid process is not identified • **Axillary nerve injury** may be present	• Anterior aspect is flat • Coracoid process is more prominent
X-ray	• **Bankart's lesions** (Lateral defect anterior) • **Hill-Sachs lesion** (posterolateral defect in the head of the humerus seen in 100% of cases). • **Erosions of rim of glenoid**	• Anterolateral defect • **Vacant glenoid sign** • **Daylight sign** (complete gap) • **The trough line.** Similar to Hill - Sachs lesion and is found on the anteromedial aspect of the head of the humerus
Transthroracic lateral X-ray	• C- shaped rolling line	• V-shaped rolling line
Techniques of reduction	• **Closed reduction:** Three methods – **Hippocrates's** method – **Stimson's** gravity method – **Kocher's** method: Most effective and commonly followed method. • **Open reduction**: Indicated in – Failed closed reduction – Soft tissue interposition – Greater tuberosity fracture displaced > 1 cm after reduction – Large glenoid rim fractures	• Reduction under general anesthesia • Distal traction on the injured limb with • Lateral rotation on the upper arm
Complications	• Recurrent dislocation • Unreduced dislocation • Traumatic osteoarthritis • Secondary osteoarthritis • Axillary nerve damage	• Recurrent dislocation • Unreduced dislocation • Traumatic osteoarthritis

Ans: (b) Posterior dislocation of shoulder

Ref: *Fundamentals of Orthopedics by Mohindra and Jain, 2nd Edition, Jaypee Publishers, page 68*

PEDIATRICS

1. A 2-year-old boy was brought with 2nd degree burns involving 20% Body Surface Area (BSA). At initial assessment his airway was stable, breathing was normal and he is normotensive. What is the volume of crystalloid fluid you would like to start?

(a) 1 ml/kg/day/% BSA burned
(b) 2 ml/kg/day/% BSA burned
(c) 3 ml/kg/day/% BSA burned
(d) 4 ml/kg/day/% BSA burned

Explanation:

- This question is based the PARKLAND FORMULA for calculation of resuscitation fluid in burns

Classification of burns:

1. Based on depth of involvement:

Superficial (1st degree)	Superficial partial thickness (2nd degree)
• Epidermis involved • ***Dry***, red and ***painful*** (***sun burn, scalds***) • ***No need to estimate the BSA*** (Burned Surface Area) • ***Do not require Intra venous fluids*** • ***Heals without scarring in a week***	• Epidermis and partial dermis involved • ***Moist (blisters),*** cherry-red skin and very painful • Nails, hair, sebaceous glands, nerves - intact • Can progress further • ***Heals in 2–3 weeks***
Deep partial thickness (3rd degree)	**Full thickness (4th degree)**
• Epidermis and dermis completely involved • ***Dry and white, usually painless*** • ***Nails, hair, sebaceous glands–involved*** • Heals with scarring • Skin grafting usually required	• All layers of skin involved • ***Charred black color ± dry or white*** • Pain ± depending on nerve ending involvement • Heals with scarring • Skin grafting usually required

2. Based on the Total Body Surface Area (TBSA) burned: Burn Assessment chart (number in percentage)

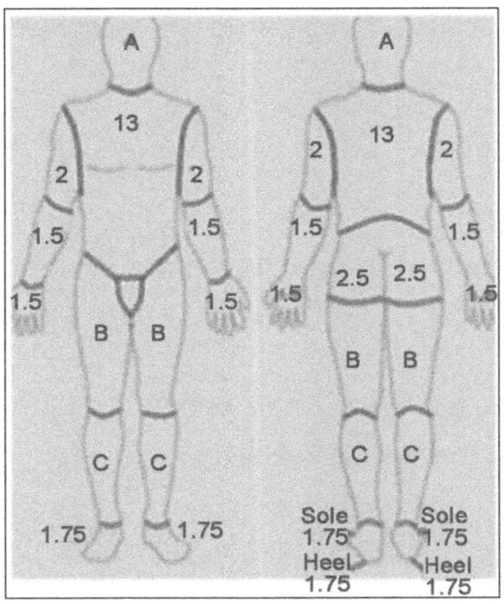

	Area	<1 year	1 year	5 years	10 years	15 years
A	HEAD (Front and Back)	9.5	8.5	6.5	5.5	4.5
B	THIGH (Front and Back)	2.75	3.25	4	4.25	4.5
C	LEG (Front and Back)	2.5	2.2	2.75	3	3.25

Indication of inpatient management

- TBSA > 10%
- Full thickness burns
- Circumferential burns
- Electrical / chemical / inhalational injuries
- Critical anatomical areas like face, hand, perineum and joints
- Suspicion of abuse

Fluid management of life threatening burns (crystalloid like lactated Ringer solution)

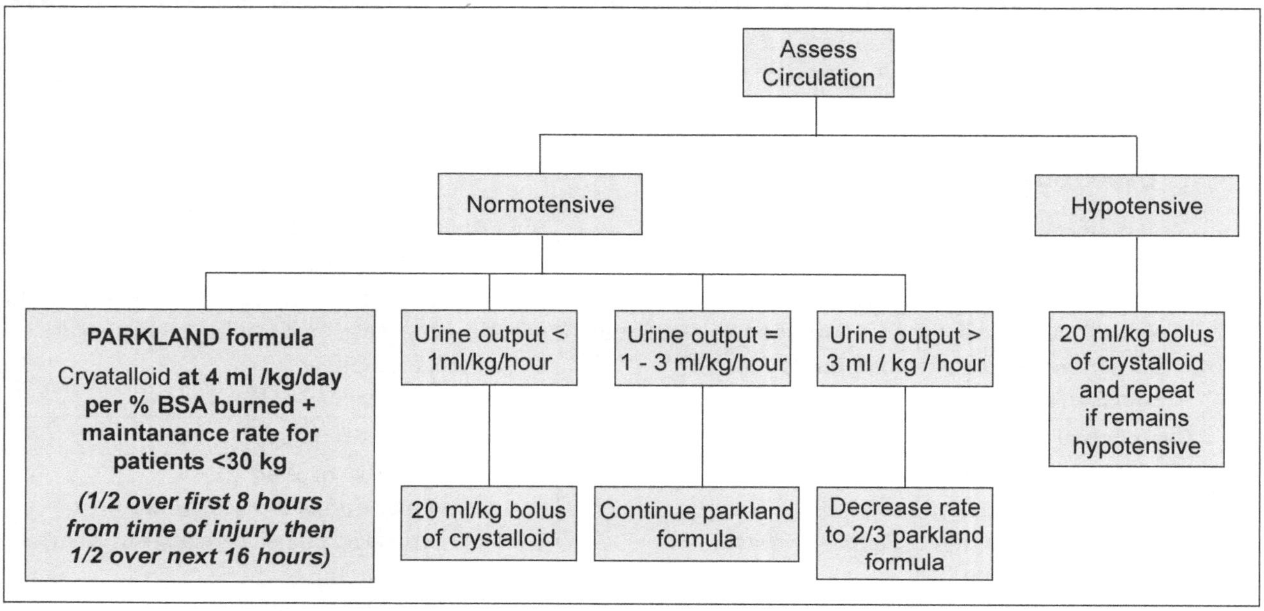

- Central venous access for burns ***25% BSA***
- Use the Parkland formula as a guideline to estimate fluid needed
- Consider adding colloid after 18 to 24 hours (albumin, 1 g/kg/day) to maintain serum albumin 2 g/dL
- ***Withhold potassium generally for the first 48 hours*** because of a release of potassium from damaged tissues

Outpatient management:

- Clean with warm saline and water
- Debride open wounds and necrotic tissue
- Topical antibacterial agent (***oral antibiotic not necessary***) and cover with non-adherent dressing
- Daily cleaning and dressing
- Follow up after 1 week

Burn prevention – Install smoke detectors and keep water heater temperature ***<49°C***

Exclude other option – The question had a direct answer (mutually exclusive)

Extra Edge:

- ***Upper airway obstruction*** progresses rapidly with thermal or chemical burns to the face / oropharynx
- Administer humidified 100% O_2 through a non rebreather mask until carboxyhemoglobin (COHb) level <10%
- Elimination half-life of COHb is dependent on PaO_2 (use ***hyperbaric*** $\boldsymbol{O_2}$ if pH <7.4 and COHb elevated)

- Make decisions based on ***PaO_2 rather than pulse oximetry***
- Risk of rhabdomyolysis and hyperkalemia from ***succinylcholine*** following burns for many months

Ans: (d) 4 ml/kg/day/% BSA burned

Ref: *The Harriet Lane Handbook, 12th Edition, page 78-82*

2. Which of the following epileptic syndromes will not present during infancy?

(a) Ohtahara syndrome (b) West syndrome

(c) Lennox-Gastaut syndrome (d) Dravet Syndrome

Explanation:

Clinical characteristics of Common Epileptic Syndromes:

Specific syndromes	Age of onset	Age at remission	Prognosis	Drug of choice	Role of surgery
Benign neonatal seizures	Newborn	Newborn	Good	LEV, PB	No
Early myoclonic encephalopathy and Ohtahara syndrome	Newborn / infant	Ohtahara syndrome evolves into West syndrome	Ominous	PB, steroids, VGB	No
West syndrome	Infant	Variable	Variable	ACTH, steroids, VGB	Lesionectomy ± cortical resection
Dravet syndrome (severe myoclonic epilepsy in infancy)	Infant	No remission	Severe	CLB, stiripentol, TPM, VPA	No
Benign myoclonic epilepsy in infancy	3 mo-3 years	3-5 years	Variable	LEV, TPM, VPA	No
Febrile seizures	3-5 years	3-5 years	Good	PB or VPA if repeated and prolonged	No
Landau-Kleffner syndrome	3-6 years	8-12 years	Guarded	LEV, nocturnal DZP, steroids, VPA	Multiple subpial transections, rarely lesionectomy
Lennox-Gastaut syndrome	3-10 years	No remission	Severe	CLB, LTG, RFD, TPM, VPA	Callosotomy
Benign childhood epilepsy with centrotemporal spikes	3-13 years	16 years	Good	CBZ, LEV, OXC, VPA	No
Childhood absence epilepsy	5-6 years	10-12 years	Good	ESM, LTG, VPA	No
Juvenile absence epilepsy	10-12 years	Usually lifelong	Good	ESM, LTG, VPA	No
Juvenile myoclonic epilepsy	12-18 years	Usually lifelong	Good	LEV, TPM, VPA	No
Epilepsy with generalized tonic-clonic seizures only	12-18 years	Usually lifelong	Good	LEV, LTG, TPM, VPA	No

(PB – Phenobarbitone, PHT – Phenytoin, CBZ – Carbamazepine, VPA – Sodium Valproate, CLB – Clobazam, CZP – Clonazepam, ESM – Ethosuximide, OXC – Oxcarbazepine, LTG – Lamotrigine, TPM – Topiramate, LEV – Levetiracetam, VGB – Vigabatrin)

Lennox-Gastaut syndrome (LGS)

- Starts between the ages of **2 and 10 years**
- **Consists of a triad of**
  - ***Developmental delay***
  - ***Multiple seizure types*** – rule include atypical absences, myoclonic, astatic, and tonic seizures (either in wakefulness (***causing falls and injuries***) or also, typically, in sleep)
  - ***EEG findings*** – 1-2 Hz spike–and– slow waves, polyspike bursts in sleep, and a slow background in wakefulness
- **Difficult to control** (long-term cognitive impairment and intractable seizures despite multiple therapies)

Few start with Ohtahara syndrome → West syndrome → Then progress to LGS

Myoclonic astatic epilepsy (Doose syndrome)

- Is a (mild) syndrome similar to LGS (***does not*** have tonic seizures or polyspike bursts in sleep)
- Prognosis is more favorable than LGS

Nodding syndrome (etiology is unknown)

- Characterized by atonic seizures–head nodding as well as tonic, clonic and stimulus sensitive seizures
- Epidemic type of epilepsy seen in some African countries and
- Associated with encephalopathy, stunted growth, and variable degrees of cognitive deficits

Treatment: (difficult-to-treat epilepsy syndrome) According to the preponderant seizure type

- **For drop attacks** (tonic, atonic, or myoclonic astatic seizures)
  - Valproate, lamotrigine, topiramate, clobazam, felbamate, and rufinamide are effective
  - ***Felbamate*** – is used as a last resort medication because of its potential toxicity
- **Preponderance of atypical absence seizures**
  - Lamotrigine or ethosuximide , valproate
  - Clonazepam is as a rescue medication (significant sedation, hyperactivity, and drooling, and often tolerance to its antiepileptic effects develops in a few months)
- **Resistant cases**
  - Zonisamide, levetiracetam, acetazolamide, methsuximide, corticosteroids, ketogenic diet, or IVIG can be used
- **Surgery – corpus callosotomy** is used for drop attacks

Prolonged period of seizure freedom on treatment is often warranted before AEDs are withdrawn (if attempted)

Exclude other options:

(a) Ohtahara syndrome
(b) West syndrome
(c) Dravet Syndrome

} Age of onset during the **Infancy**

Extra Edge:

Change in seizure type classification from 1981 to **2017 (ILAE – International League against Epilepsy)**

- The term ***partial*** was changed to ***focal***
- ***Awareness*** is used as a classifier of focal seizures

- *Eliminated terms* like–dyscognitive, simple partial, complex partial, psychic and secondary generalized
- *New generalized seizure types* – include absence with eyelid myotonia, myoclonic absence, myoclonic – tonic – clonic, myoclonic – atonic and epileptic spasms.

Ans: (c) Lennox-Gastaut syndrome

Ref: *Nelson Textbook of Pediatrics, 20th Edition, page 2826-2848*

3. Highest risk of development of epilepsy in case of febrile seizures is with:

(a) Complex seizure (b) Neurodevelopmental abnormalities

(c) Family history of epilepsy (d) Recurrent febrile seizures

Explanation:

Febrile Seizures:

- Occurs between the age of ***6 and 60 months*** with a temperature of 38°C (100.4°F) or higher
- That are not the result of central nervous system infection or any metabolic imbalance
- Occur in the absence of a history of prior afebrile seizures

A. Simple febrile seizure–

- ***Criteria for diagnosis***
  - Primary generalized, usually tonic–clonic
  - Attack associated with fever
  - Lasting for a maximum of 15 minutes
  - Not recurrent within a 24 hours period.
- Do not have an increased risk of mortality

B. Complex febrile seizure–prolonged *(>15 min), is focal, and/or reoccurs within 24 hours*, fold long-term increase in mortality

C. Febrile status epilepticus is a febrile seizure lasting longer than *30 minutes*

D. Simple febrile seizure plus for those with recurrent febrile seizures within 24 hours

Recurrence:

- **30%** of those experiencing a first episode
- **50%** after 2 or more episodes, and
- **50%** of infants younger than 1 year old at febrile seizure onset.
- **2-7%** of children who experience febrile seizures proceed to develop epilepsy later in life

Risk factor for recurrence

Major	Minor	Recurrence Risk
• Age <1 year • Duration of fever <24 hours • Fever 38-39°C (100.4-102.2°F)	• Family history of febrile seizures • Family history of epilepsy • Complex febrile seizure • Daycare • Male gender • Lower Serum sodium at time of presentation	• With Nil risk factor – **12%** • With 1 risk factor – **25 – 50%** • With 2 risk factor – **50 – 59%** • With >3 risk factor – **73 – 100%**

Dravet syndrome (Severe Myoclonic Epilepsy in infancy)

- Phenotypic spectrum of febrile seizure-associated epilepsies
- Caused by a de novo mutation, located on 2q24-31 and encodes for ***SCN1A***
- The onset in infancy, characterized by ***febrile and afebrile unilateral clonic seizures*** recurring every 1 month
- Differ from the usual febrile convulsions
  - Have more prolonged, more frequent, focal and clusters of seizures
  - Seizures subsequently start to occur with lower fevers and then without fever
- In 2nd year of life – myoclonus, atypical absences, and partial seizures occur frequently with developmental delay
- ***Only small patients have abnormality in neuroimaging like–cortical dysplasia, hippocampal sclerosis and focal brain atrophy***
- Treated with ***valproate and benzodiazepines such as clobazam*** or clonazepam
- Lamotrigine, carbamazepine, and phenytoin are reported to exacerbate seizures
- They do not attain remission and have poor prognosis

Generalized Epilepsy with Febrile Seizures Plus (GEFS+)

- Autosomal dominant, variable phenotype
- Onset – early childhood and remission is usually in mid-childhood
- Multiple febrile seizures and afebrile generalized seizures with variable degrees of severity
- A focal febrile seizures plus epilepsy variant – in which the seizures are focal rather than generalized

Indication for lumbar puncture	Indication for Electro Encephalogram
• All infants ***younger than 6 months*** of age who present with fever and seizure • If the child is ill appearing or at any age if there are clinical signs or symptoms of concern. • Option in a child 6-12 months of age whose Haemophilus influenzae type b and Streptococcus pneumonia ***immunization status is unknown*** • A lumbar puncture is an option in children who have been ***pretreated with antibiotic***	• ***Do not predict the future recurrence*** of febrile seizures or epilepsy even if the result is abnormal • ***Performed within 2 weeks of*** a febrile seizure often have nonspecific slowing, usually posteriorly • Children with febrile status epilepticus

CT or MRI is not recommended in evaluating the child after a first simple febrile seizure

Treatment:

- Seizure lasts for longer than 5 min, acute treatment with diazepam, lorazepam, or midazolam is needed
- Parents are very anxious concerning their child's seizures, ***intermittent oral diazepam (0.33 mg/kg every 8 hours during fever) / clonazepam (0.1 mg/kg/day)***
- ***Antipyretics*** can decrease the discomfort of the child but do not reduce the risk of having a recurrent febrile seizure
- Future epilepsy does not change with or without antiepileptic therapy
- Iron deficiency is associated with an increased risk of febrile seizures

Prognosis:

Simple febrile seizures

- No long-term adverse effects of having 1 or more

- Do not have any increase in the incidence of abnormalities of behavior, scholastic performance, neurocognitive function, or attention

Complex febrile seizures

- May have an approximately 2-fold long-term increase in mortality

Future epilepsy

- Only 2-7% of children who experience febrile seizures proceed to develop epilepsy later in life.

Exclude other options: Risk factor for subsequent Epilepsy after a febrile seizure

Risk Factor	Risk for future Epilepsy (%)
Simple febrile seizure	1
Recurrent febrile seizures	**4**
Complex febrile seizures	**6**
Fever <1 hour before febrile seizure	11
Family history of epilepsy	**18**
Complex febrile seizures (focal)	29
Neurodevelopmental abnormalities	**33**

Extra Edge:

- **HHV-6B** (more frequently) and **HHV-7** infections - one-third of the febrile seizure cases
- Only the function of **FEB 2** (chromosome. 19p13.3) is known: it is a sodium channel gene, SCN1A
- **SCN1A**-related seizure disorders - inherited in an autosomal dominant pattern with variable expressivity
- Inherited from an affected parent or it can occur brand new (de novo) in an affected child
- If parent also has the disorder, the risk of having a child with an SCN1A-related seizure disorder is 50% with each pregnancy
- If a parent does not have the condition, the risk of other siblings being affected is very low
- SCN1A cause a spectrum of mild to severe epilepsy–**Dravet Syndrome** and the mild familial epilepsy syndrome of Genetic/**Generalized Epilepsy with Febrile Seizures Plus (GEFS+)**

Ans: (b) Neurodevelopmental abnormalities

Ref: *Nelson Textbook of Pedaitrics, 20th Edition, page 2829-2831*

4. A 1 year old child was brought with sudden spasm; on examination he had shagreen patch and 4 hypomelanotic macules on extremities. What is the drug of choice for the seizures?

(a) Carbamazepine (b) Phenytoin

(c) Vigabatrin (d) Steroids

Explanation:

- The scenario was consistent with infantile spasm and other findings suggests Tuberous Sclerosis as per the criteria (2 major) and vigabatrin is the drug of choice for infantile spasms secondary Tuberous Sclerosis.

Tuberous Sclerosis Complex (TSC): Extremely heterogeneous disease with a wide clinical spectrum

- ***Autosomal dominant***, prevalence of 1 in 6,000 newborns
- Spontaneous genetic mutations – 65%
- Molecular genetic studies 2 foci for TSC: (TSC 1 and 2 - tumor-suppressor genes)
  - The **TSC1 gene is on chromosome 9q34 (encodes a protein called hamartin)**
  - The **TSC2 gene is on chromosome 16p13 (encodes the protein tuberin)**

- Loss of either protein – leads to formation of numerous benign tumors (hamartomas)

Clinical Features:

Hallmark of TSC – ***CNS involvement (Cortical tuber)***, identified best by ***MRI*** brain

Diagnostic criteria (Atleast 2 Major or 1 Major + 2 minor)

Major features of tuberous sclerosis complex	Minor features of tuberous sclerosis complex
Cortical tuber	Cerebral white matter migration lines
Subependymal nodule	Multiple dental pits
Subependymal giant cell astrocytoma (SEGA)	Gingival fibromas
Facial angiofibroma or forehead plaque	Bone cysts
Ungula or **periungual fibroma (Koenen tumor)**	Retinal achromatic patch
Hypomelanotic macules (>3)	Confetti skin lesions
Shagreen patch	Non-renal hamartomas
Multiple **retinal hamartomas***	Multiple renal cysts
Cardiac **rhabdomyoma***	Hamartomatous rectal polyps
Renal **angiomyolipoma***	
Pulmonary lymphangioleiomyomatosis	

May present during infancy with infantile spasms and a hypsarrhythmic EEG pattern

- **Later may develop into myoclonic epilepsy**

Retinal, brain and other lesions

Retinal lesions	• Mulberry tumors and hamartomas or depigmented areas
Brain lesion	• Most common neurologic manifestations of TS consist of **seizures**, **cognitive impairment, and behavioral abnormalities including autism** • The characteristic brain lesion is a **cortical tuber** • Located in the convolutions of the cerebral hemispheres and subependymal region • **Undergo calcification and project into the ventricular cavity, producing a** candle-dripping appearance **(10% risk of developing *Subependymal Giant cell Astrocytoma)* SEGA** • The greater the number of tubers, the more neurologically impaired is the patient
Rhabdomyomas of the heart	• Seen in 50% of children with TS • Located at the apex of the left ventricle • Can cause congestive heart failure and arrhythmias • Tend to slowly resolve spontaneously
Angiomyolipomas of kidney	• Benign tumors • Single or multiple renal cysts are also commonly present in TS • Nephrectomy should be avoided
Lymphangiomyomatosis	• Is the classical pulmonary lesion in TS • Most common in the female patient

Skin lesions

- **Ash leaf macules**
  - On the trunk and extremities–Hypomelanotic macules in 90% cases
  - Visualization by the use of a wood ultraviolet lamp
  - At least three hypomelanotic macules must be present
- **Sebaceous adenomas**
  - Also known as Facial angiofibroma, Pringle nodules, adenoma sebaceum
  - Tiny red nodules over the nose and cheeks

- **Shagreen patch**
  - Roughened, raised lesion with an orange peel consistency
  - Located primarily in the lumbosacral region
- **Confetti lesions**
  - Variant of leukoderma spots
- **Subungual or periungual fibromas (Koenen tumor)**
  - Arise from the stratum lucidum of the finger and toe
  - During adolescence

Management and follow up:

- **Brain MRI** confirms the diagnosis in most cases
- Genetic testing for TSC1 and TSC2 mutations – **prenatal testing**
- **DOC for infantile spasms** associated with TS—**vigabatrin (ACTH if vigabatrin fails)**
- **FDA** approved drug —mTOR inhibitor—**Everolimus*** (Reduce the size of SEGA / renal angiomyolipoma / facial angiofibroma)
- **Neurosurgical emergency – increased ICP due to obstruction of foramen of Monro by SEGA**
- MRI brain / Renal imaging – every 1–3 year for development of astrocytoma

Excluding other option:

- Both carbamazepine and Phenytoin were not used in TSC.
- Adrenocorticotropic hormone (ACTH) was tried when vigbatrin fails.

Extra edge:

- Loss of peripheral vision and ***retinal toxicity*** were the serious side effect of vigabatrin.
- **Drug of choice for (infantile spasm) west syndrome is** Adrenocorticotropic hormone

Ans: (c) Vigabatrin

Ref: *Nelson Textbook of Pedaitrics, 20th Edition, page 2877-2879*

5. Which of the following primary immunodeficiency present during the neonatal period?

(a) Hyper-IgE syndrome
(b) Chronic granulomatous disease
(c) Leukocyte adhesion defect
(d) Ataxia-telangiectasia

Explanation:

Common clinical features of Immunodeficiency:

Occurrence	Common clinical features
Usually present	• Recurrent Upper respiratory infections • Severe bacterial infections • Persistent infections with incomplete or no response to therapy • Paucity of lymph nodes and tonsils
Often present	• Persistent sinusitis or mastoiditis / bronchitis or pneumonia • Failure to thrive or growth retardation for infants or children; weight loss for adults • Intermittent fever (Infection with unusual organisms)

Contd.

Contd.

	• Skin lesions: rash, seborrhea, pyoderma, necrotic abscesses, alopecia, eczema, telangiectasia / Recalcitrant thrush • Diarrhea and malabsorption • Hearing loss caused by chronic otitis / Chronic conjunctivitis / Arthralgia or arthritis • Bronchiectasis • Evidence of autoimmunity, especially autoimmune thrombocytopenia or hemolytic anemia • Hematologic abnormalities: aplastic anemia, hemolytic anemia, neutropenia, thrombocytopenia

Clinical patterns of primary immunodeficiency:

Clinical features	Diagnosis
Age of presentation < 6 months	
Hypocalcemia, unusual facies and ears, heart disease	**DiGeorge anomaly**
Delayed umbilical cord detachment, leukocytosis, recurrent infections	**Leukocyte adhesion defect**
Persistent thrush, failure to thrive, pneumonia, diarrhea	**Severe combined immunodeficiency**
Bloody stools, draining ears, atopic eczema	**Wiskott-Aldrich syndrome**
Age of presentation 6 months to 5 years	
Severe progressive infectious mononucleosis	**X-linked lymphoproliferative syndrome**
Recurrent staphylococcal abscesses, staphylococcal pneumonia with pneumatocele formation, coarse facial features, pruritic dermatitis	**Hyper-IgE syndrome**
Oculocutaneous albinism, recurrent infection	**Chédiak-Higashi syndrome**
Abscesses, suppurative lymphadenopathy, antral outlet obstruction, pneumonia, osteomyelitis	**Chronic granulomatous disease**
Age of presentation > 5 years	
Progressive dermatomyositis with chronic enterovirus encephalitis	**X-linked agammaglobulinemia**
Sinopulmonary infections, neurologic deterioration, telangiectasia	**Ataxia-telangiectasia**
Sinopulmonary infections, splenomegaly, autoimmunity, malabsorption	**Common variable immunodeficiency**

Initial immunological screening test for suspected Immunodeficiency:

<table>
<tr><td colspan="4">Complete blood count, Manual differential and Erythrocyte Sedimentation Rate
• Absolute lymphocyte count (normal result rules against T-cell defect)
• Absolute neutrophil count (normal result rules against congenital or acquired neutropenia and leukocyte adhesion deficiency)
• Platelet count (normal result excludes Wiskott-Aldrich syndrome)
• Howell-Jolly bodies (absence rules against asplenia)
• Erythrocyte sedimentation rate (normal result indicates chronic bacterial or fungal infection unlikely)</td></tr>
<tr><td colspan="4">Screening Tests</td></tr>
<tr><td>B-Cell Defects</td><td>T-Cell Defects</td><td>Phagocytic Cell Defects</td><td>Complement Deficiency</td></tr>
<tr><td>• Immunoglobulin (Ig) A measurement
• If abnormal, IgG and IgM measurement</td><td>• Absolute lymphocyte count (normal result indicates T-cell defect unlikely)</td><td>• Absolute neutrophil count</td><td>• CH50</td></tr>
</table>

Contd.

Contd.

• Isohemagglutinins • Antibody titers to blood group substances, tetanus, diphtheria, Haemophilus influenzae, and pneumococcus	• Flow cytometry to examine for the presence of naïve T cells (CD3+CD45RA+ cells)	• Respiratory burst assay	

Exclude other options:

(a) Hyper-IgE syndrome - Age of presentation 6 months to 5 years

(b) Chronic granulomatous Disease - Age of presentation 6 months to 5 years

(c) Ataxia-telangiectasia - Age of presentation > 5 years

Ans: (c) Leukocyte adhesion defect

Ref: *Nelson Textbook of Pedaitrics, 20th Edition, page 999–1006*

6. All of the following are true for selective IgA deficiency except:

(a) Can occur due to phenytoin administration
(b) Intestinal giardiasis is rare
(c) IgG2 subclass deficiency
(d) Treated with intravenous immunoglobulin

Explanation:

Selective IgA Deficiency

- Autosomal dominant inheritance with variable expressivity
- Isolated absence or near absence ***(<10 mg/dL)*** of serum and secretory IgA with normal blood B cells
- Commonly in pedigrees containing individuals with CVID and ***IgA deficiency may evolve into CVID***
- Susceptibility gene common to these 2 conditions may reside in the MHC region on chromosome 6
- IgA deficiency and CVID seen in patients receiving (***phenytoin***, d-***penicillamine, gold and sulfasalazine***)
- IgA deficiency ***remits spontaneously*** or after discontinuation of phenytoin therapy

Clinical Manifestations

- Infections – respiratory, gastrointestinal, and urogenital tracts.
- ***Intestinal giardiasis is common***.
- Serum concentrations of other immunoglobulins are usually normal
  - ***Although IgG2 (and other) subclass deficiency*** has been reported, and
  - ***IgM (usually elevated***) may be monomeric
- Associated with a ***celiac-like syndrome***, which may or may not respond to a gluten-free diet
- The incidence of autoantibodies, autoimmune diseases, and malignancy is increased
- 44% have serum antibodies to IgA (these antibodies are of the IgE isotype)
  - Cause ***severe or fatal anaphylactic reactions*** after intravenous administration of blood products containing IgA
  - 5-times washed (in 200-mL volumes) normal donor erythrocytes or blood products from other IgA-deficient individuals, should be administered
- Many intravenous immunoglobulin (IVIG) preparations contain sufficient IgA to cause anaphylactic reactions
- Administration of IVIG, which is >99% IgG, is not indicated (these ***IgG antibodies normal***)

Treatment:

- ***Antibiotics + regular administration of IVIG*** are the only effective treatments
- Replacement therapy are either intravenous or subcutaneous immunoglobulin (IVIG or SCIG)
  - Provide missing antibodies, not to raise the serum IgG or IgG subclass level
  - IVIG or SCIG at a dose of 400 mg/kg per month achieves trough IgG levels close to the normal range
- Anaphylactic reactions caused by a patient's IgE antibodies to IgA in the IVIG occur in patients with CVID or IgA deficiency

Exclude other options:

(a) Can occur due to phenytoin administration – True
(b) ***Intestinal giardiasis is rare*** ***– False***
(c) IgG2 subclass deficiency – True
(d) Treated with intravenous immunoglobulin – True

Extra Edge:

- Maternal (Fetal therapy) intravenous immunoglobulin is used as a treatment for:
  - Autoimmune / Isoimmue thrombocytopenia (ITP) in neonate
  - Neonatal iron storage disease (alloimmune)

Ans: (b) Intestinal giardiasis is rare

Ref: *Nelson Textbook of Pedaitrics, 20th Edition, page 2221-22*

7. Fat content of breast milk:

(a) 2.4 percent (b) 3.4 percent
(c) 4.4 percent (d) 5.4 percent

Explanation:

Comparison of components of Human milk and cow's milk (per 100 ml):

Component	Human Milk	Cow's Milk
Non protein Nitrogen	0.2 g	0.03 g
Protein	***1.1 g***	***3.0 g***
Caesin: Whey	40:60 lactalbumin and lactoferrin	80:20 Lactoglobulin
Lactose	***7g***	***4.5g***
Fat	***3.8 g***	***3.7g***
Essential Fatty Acid	13%	2%
Calcium: phosphorus	>2	<2
Sodium	0.7 mEq	2.2 mEq
Potassium	55 mg	137 mg
Calcium	***33 mg***	***125 mg***
Phosphorus	15 mg	96 mg
Iron	***0.05 – 0.15 mg***	***0.1 mg***
Iodine	7 mg	21 mg
Vitamin A	53 ug	34 ug

Contd.

Contd.

Vitamin D	***0.4 – 10 IU***	***0.3 – 0.4 IU***
Vitamin E	2 mg	0.4 mg
Vitamin K	15 ug	60 ug
Vitamin C	4.3 mg	1.8 mg
Polyunsaturated fatty acid		
Osmolarity	***7.9 mOsm***	***22.1 mOsm***
Energy: protein ratio	70:1	25:1
Calories	***67 Kcal***	***67 Kcal***

Exclude other options: Since it's a direct question other options were mutually exclusive

Extra Edge:

- **Lipids**–major sources (**44%** of the total energy provided by human milk)
- **Triacylglycerols** represents **98%** of human **milk fat**
- **Milk lipids** (constituted by 35-40% of saturated fatty acids, 45- 50% of monounsaturated and 15% of polyunsaturated fatty acids)
- **Palmitic acid** provides the majority of saturated fatty acids.

Ans: (b) 3.4 percent

Ref: *Nutrition and Child Development, 4th Edition, Page 7–20 and Mosca F, Giannì ML (2017), Human Milk: Composition and Health Benefits, La Pediatria Medica E Chirurgica, 39(2),155*

8. Amount of iron in milk:

(a) 0.1 to 0.2 gm / L
(b) 0.1 to 0.2 mg / 100 ml
(c) 1000 to 2000 ug / L
(d) 1 to 2 µmol/L

Explanation:

Refer to previous question's explanation

Extra Edge:

- **Breast milk iron** concentration gradually decreased as **lactation progressed**
- Iron content of **preterm breast** milk is **higher** than term breast milk
- Iron content in breast milk is **bound** to **proteins**–preventing its use by harmful bacteria like (E.coli)

Ans: (b) 0.1 to 0.2 mg

Ref: *Nutrition and Child Development, 4th Edition, page 7-20*

9. Breastfeeding contraindicated in:

(a) MDR Tuberculosis
(b) Zika virus infection
(c) Hepatitis B infection
(d) Mastitis with abscess

Explanation:

- **Among the given options, option (a) can be considered as best option, though breast milk is not contraindicated as such but only direct breast feeding to be avoided**

BREASTFEEDING IN SPECIAL SITUATIONS:

Mother with Tuberculosis:

- Breastfeeding should be continued with cough hygiene
- Isolation with feeding with expressed breast milk is recommended if mother is
  - Sick
  - Infectious (less than 2 week of treatment)
  - MDR TB or non-adherent to treatment

Mother with Zika virus infection:

- Zika virus transmission through breast milk has not been confirmed
- CDC recommends continuation of breastfeeding even if the mother is infected, live, or travelled to an area with the risk of Zika.

Mother infected with hepatitis B virus:

- Breastfeeding do not increase the risk of transmission to the baby
- Breastfeeding can be continued provided the baby received immunoprophylaxis

Mother with HIV infection:

- Exclusive breastfeeding is the recommended infant feeding choice in the first 6 months, irrespective (mother is on ART or infant ART prophylaxis for 6 weeks)
- No Mixed Feeding is to be done during the first 6 months
- Infants are HIV uninfected or of unknown HIV status–breastfeeding should be continued for the first 12 months of life
- Infants are HIV infected – breastfeeding should be continued for 24 months of life

Mother with COVID-19 infection:

- The COVID-19 virus has not, to date, been detected in the breast milk of any mother with confirmed/ suspected COVID-19
- There is no reason to avoid or stop breastfeeding
- Immediate and continued skin-to-skin care, including kangaroo mother care and early initiation of breastfeeding
- While breastfeeding, a mother should still implement appropriate **hygiene measures**
  - Hygiene measures
  - Wash hands frequently with soap and water
  - Wear a medical mask while feeding
  - Sneeze or cough into a tissue, immediately dispose of it
  - Regularly clean and disinfect surfaces

Mastitis with breast abscess:

- Its is safe to continue breastfeeding from the affected breast

Extra Edge:

Definite Contraindication of breastfeeding:

- Congenital lactose intolerance
- Galactosemia
- Mother on

- Anti neoplastic drugs
- Anti thyroid drugs
- Lithium (anti psychotic drugs)

- Maternal intake of Radioactive Iodine

Ans: (a) MDR Tuberculosis

Ref: *1. Mittal H, Das S and Faridi M M (2014), Management of Newborn Infant Born to Mother Suffering from Tuberculosis: Current Recommendations and Gaps in Knowledge. The Indian Journal of Medical Research 140(1), 32-39*
2. https://www.cdc.gov/pregnancy/zika/testing-follow-up/zika-in-infants-children.html
3. https://www.indianpediatrics.net/aug2016/703.pdf
4. https://www.who.int/docs/default-source/maternal-health/faqs-breastfeeding-and-covid-19.pdf?sfvrsn=d839e6c0_1
5. Nutrition and Child Development, 4th Edition, KE Elizabeth, page 9

10. Ebstein anomaly all *except:*

(a) PDA dependent in neonate
(b) VSD associated
(c) ECG: Tall broad p waves
(d) Cyanosis at birth

Explanation:

Ebstein anomaly of tricuspid valve:

- Downward displacement of an abnormal tricuspid valve into the right ventricle (RV)

Pathophysiology:

- Failure of separation of the tricuspid valve (TV) from the right ventricular myocardium during embryogenesis
- Anterior cusp of the valve attached to the valve ring (but the other leaflets are adherent to right ventricle)
- The right ventricle divided into 2 parts by this abnormal tricuspid valve:
  - ***Thin-walled "atrialized" portion***, is continuous with the cavity of the right atrium
  - ***Second, often smaller portion*** consists of normal ventricular myocardium
- Tricuspid valve regurgitation (TVR) leads to right atrium is enlarged
- Right heart output decreased by combination of the
  - Poorly functioning small RV +
  - Tricuspid valve regurgitation and
  - Obstruction of the right ventricular outflow tract (by the sail-like, anterior TV leaflet).

In neonate – cyanosis due to shunting of blood from dilated right atrium to left atrium

Clinical manifestation:

- Severity of symptoms and the degree of ***cyanosis*** depends on:
  - The displacement of the tricuspid valve and
  - The severity of right ventricular outflow tract obstruction
- Jugular venous pulsations - ***increased*** in those with tricuspid insufficiency
- On palpation, the precordium is quiet
- A ***holosystolic murmur***–tricuspid regurgitation (anterior left side of the chest)
- A gallop rhythm with multiple clicks and scratchy diastolic murmur at the lower left sternal border
- Newborns–***marked cyanosis, massive cardiomegaly and long holosystolic murmurs***

- Neonates die of cardiac failure, hypoxemia, and associated pulmonary hypoplasia
- Spontaneous improvement may occur–as pulmonary vascular resistance falls
- The majority are ***dependent on a PDA, and thus on a prostaglandin infusion***, for pulmonary blood flow

Diagnosis:

- ECG–a right bundle-branch block, tall and ***broad P waves with normal or prolonged P-R interval***
- Features of supraventricular tachycardia if associated with Wolff-Parkinson- White syndrome
- Chest X-ray–***box shaped cardiomegaly*** (enlarged right atrium)
- Echocardiography is diagnostic:
  - Shows the degree of displacement of the tricuspid valve leaflets,
  - A dilated right atrium, and
  - Right ventricular outflow tract obstruction
- Pulsed and color Doppler–Degree of tricuspid regurgitation

Treatment:

- ***Prostaglandin infusion*** if ductal dependent then single ventricle repair using the ***Fontan procedure***
- Persisting regurgitation–Glenn shunt is performed to reduce the volume load on the right ventricle
- Prognosis is guarded for neonates or infants with intractable symptoms and cyanosis

Exclude other options:

(a) PDA dependent in neonate – True
(b) ***VSD associated*** – ***False***
(c) ECG: Tall broad p waves – True
(d) Cyanosis at birth – True

Extra Edge:

Ductal dependent congenital cardiac conditions:

Ductal dependent pulmonary circulation	Ductal dependent systemic circulation
Pulmonary stenosis / Pulmonary atresia	Critical coarctation of Aorta
Tetralogy of fallot with severe Pulmonary stenosis	Interrupted Aortic Arch
Tricuspid atresia with Pulmonary stenosis	Critical Aortic Stenosis
Severe Ebstein Anomaly	

Ans: (b) VSD associated

Ref : *Nelson Textbook of Pediatrics, 20th Edition, page 2221-2223*

11. Most sensitive test for thyroid dysfunction in newborn:

(a) Total T3 (b) Total T4
(c) TSH (d) Free T3

Explanation:

Congenital Hypothyroidism:

- Prevalence: 1 in 1757, female-to-male ratio is 2:1
- Associated with Trisomy 21, congenital heart disease, gastrointestinal anomalies, and cleft palate

Causes of congenital hypothyroidism:

Permanent Congenital Hypothyroidism	Transient Congenital Hypothyroidism
Most common **Thyroid dysgenesis (>85% of cases)** • Includes aplasia, hypoplasia, and dysplasia, ectopy • Always sporadic with no increased risk to subsequent siblings. • Infants - have no goiter, low total and free T4 levels, elevated TSH, and normal TBG. • Ultrasound and thyroid radioactive iodine scan - absent or ectopic thyroid gland.	**Intrauterine exposure anti thyroid drugs** • Resolves within 1 week and does not require treatment. **Exposure to excess iodine during neonatal period** **Large liver hemangiomas**
Thyroid dyshormonogenesis (10 – 15%) • 25% recurrence risk in subsequent siblings • Most common - ***abnormal thyroid peroxidase activity*** • ***Pendred syndrome*** - goiter (mild organification defect) + sensorineural deafness • Total and free T4 levels are low, TSH is • Devated, and TBG is normal	**Transient hypothyroxinemia of prematurity** Infants born at <31 weeks' gestation Immature hypothalamic-pituitary axis

Clinical features:

- Birth weight and length – normal
- Head circumference – may be increased
- Prolonged jaundice (immaturity of hepatic glucuronyl transferase), poor feeding
- Constipation, hypothermia, poor tone, mottled skin (cutis marmoratus), umblical hernia
- Large tongue, open posterior fontanel, wide anterior fontanel

Diagnosis:

- 95% of newborns with CH are ***asymptomatic at birth***
- Best method – ***concomitant screening with both FreeT4 and TSH*** (thyroid Stimulating Hormone), after 72 hours of life
- Low FreeT4 and increased TSH suggest Congenital Hypothyroidism
- If birth weight < 1,500 g, repeat testing at 2, 6, and 10 weeks of age (delayed TSH elevation)
- ***TSH estimation (>20 mU/L) is more sensitive (98%) and specific (92%) test***
- Measurement of Thyroglobulin level and thyroid ultrasound / Radio Active Iodine scan can differentiate dysplasia from other hormone dysgenesis
- **ECHO–Pericardial effusion***
- **EEG–Low voltage QRS complexes**
- **Age > 2 years–Serum cholesterol** usually **elevated**

X-ray femur and vertebra	X-ray skull
• Epiphyseal dysgenesis (Multiple foci of ossification)	• **Wide fontanelle** and suture
• Absent **distal femoral epiphysis**	• Intrasutural **Wormian bones**
• **Deformity (beaking**) of the **12th thoracic or 1st or 2nd lumbar vertebra**	• **Enlarged and round sella turcica**—may be erosive and thinning

Approach to a child with hypothyroidism

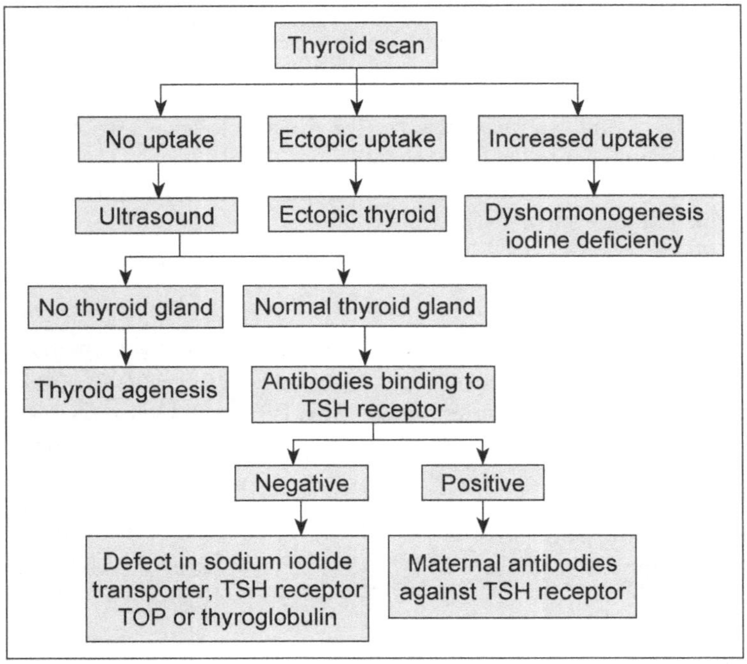

Treatment:

- Early diagnosis and immediate exogenous replacement of thyroid hormone are the basic principles of therapy
- Irrespective of the etiology, all cases of confirmed hypothyroidism should promptly receive thyroid hormone supplementation
- Thyroxine tablets should be crushed and fed directly to the infant or mixed in a small amount of **juice, water or breast milk**
  - **Infants–10–15 µg/kg***
  - Children–**4 µg/kg/24 hours**
  - Adults–**2 µg/kg/24 hours**
- Repeat T4 and TSH measurements should be performed
  - 1 week after starting therapy
  - 2 weeks after any dose change
  - Every 1 to 2 months in the first year of life
- Better IQ scores - If Diagnosis should be preferably made before **10–13 days** and euthyroid state should be achieved **by 3 weeks** of life
- **Overtreatment** can lead to
  - Premature fusion of cranial sutures (**Craniosynostosis**)
  - Acceleration of skeletal maturation
  - Neurobehavioral and psychological problems

Extra Edge:

- **Kocher–Debre–Semelaigne syndrome: Muscular pseudo hypertrophy particularly in the calf muscle in hypothyroidism**
- **TBG deficiency has X-linked dominant inheritance and needs no treatment as Free T4 levels are normal**

- **Quebec score** – Clinical scoring for congenital hypothyroidism
- **Bamforth – Lazarus Syndrome** – Autosomal Recessive condition
  - Loss-of-function missense mutations in the ***FOXE1 gene*** (9q22), encoding Thyroid Transcription Factor 2 (TTF-2)
  - Present at birth with thyroid dysgenesis
  - All of them have **cleft palate and spiky hair** (choanal atresia and bifid epiglottis rarely seen)

Ans: (c) TSH

Ref: *Cloherty–Manual Neonatal Care, 7th Edition, page 28-37*

12. Amount of iron in 1 unit of packed red cell:

(a) 500 milli gram (b) 500 gram

(c) 200 milli gram (d) 200 micro gram

Explanation:

The question is based on the Packed RBC transfusion and iron overload as in thalassemia receiving frequent transfusion.

Guidelines for RBC transfusions in children and adolescents:

Condition	Infants ≤ 4 months	Children and Adolescent
Maintain stable status in acute blood loss	> 75% of circulating blood volume	
Symptomatic anemia	Maintain Hb > 7 g/dL	Maintain Hb > 7 g/dL
Preoperatively and during major surgery	Maintain Hb > 10 g/dL	Maintain Hb > 7 g/dL
Severe cardiac/pulmonary disease	Maintain Hb > 12 g/dL	Maintain Hb > 12 g/dL
Moderate cardiac/pulmonary disease	Maintain Hb > 10 g/dL	Maintain Hb > 10 g/dL

- In chronic anemia - decision to transfuse RBCs (***not be based on blood hemoglobin levels***) as children compensate well even at Hb of 5 gm%.

RBC product of choice to transfuse

- Typed and cross-matched blood product is preferred (O-negative if transfusion cannot be delayed)
- Suspended in an anticoagulant/preservative storage solution at a ***hematocrit value of (55 – 70 %)***

Type of PRBCs:

- ***Prestorage leukocyte-reduced RBCs*** – to prevent ***CMV infection*** and non hemolytic febrile transfusion reaction or
- ***Washed RBC*** – for children with complete ***IgA deficiency*** / history of urticarial transfusion reactions or
- ***Irradiated (1500 cGy irradiation)*** – ***for prevention of GVHD***

Volume – 10-15 mL/kg, over 2 – 4 hours of fresh RBCs (no faster than 2–3 mL/kg/hr) (<7 days of storage)

Rule of thumb in severe compensated anemia:

Give an X mL/kg aliquot, where X = patient Hb (g/dL);
for example, if Hb = 5 g/dL, transfuse 5 mL/kg over 4 hours

To calculate the volume of PRBC to achieve a desired HCT, use the following equation:

$$\text{Volume of PRBCs (mL)} = \frac{\text{Estimated Blood Volume (mL/kg)} \times (\text{desired HCT} - \text{actual HCT})}{\text{HCT of PRBCs (55\%–70\%)}}$$

Autologous RBC transfusions (alternative to donor allogeneic RBC)–blood collections from the patient occur up to ***6 weeks before the surgery and replaced with saline***

1 unit of PRBS contains 200 mg of iron (vs daily iron intake is 1-2 mg vs normal total body iron 3-5 gm)

Changes during PRBC storage:

- The ***pH decreases*** from 7.55 to pH 6.5
- Potassium is released from the RBC
- 2,3-diphosphoglycerol (2,3-DPG) levels drop rapidly during the first 2 weeks of storage (increases the affinity of the hemoglobin for oxygen and decreases its efficiency in delivering oxygen to tissue)

Neonatal Anemia: Physiologic anemia of infancy:

- **In utero** – the ***fetal aortic oxygen saturation is 45%*** (thus ***erythropoietin levels are high*** and RBC production is rapid)
  - The ***fetal liver is the major site*** of erythropoietin production
- **After birth** – the ***oxygen saturation is 95***%, and the ***erythropoietin is undetectable*** and the hemoglobin level falls
- **8 to 12 weeks** – hemoglobin levels reach their nadir, oxygen delivery to the tissues is impaired, renal erythropoietin production is stimulated, and RBC production increases

Maturity of neonate	Hemoglobin nadir	Time of nadir (weeks)
Term	9.5 – 11	6 -12
Preterm babies (1200 – 2500 gm)	8 – 10	5 -10
Small preterm babies (<1200 gm)	6.5 – 9	4 -8

Transfusion guidelines for premature infants:

• Asymptomatic infants with Hct <21% and reticulocytes <100,000/UL (2%)
• Infants with Hct <31% and hood O_2 <36% or mean airway pressure <6 cm H20 by CPAP or IMV • >9 apneic and bradycardic episodes per 12 h or 2/24 h requiring bag-and-mask ventilation while on adequate methylxanthine therapy • HR > 180/min or RR >80/min sustained for 24 h or weight gain of <10 g/d for 4 don 100 Kcal/kg/d or having surgery
• Infants with Hct <36% and requiring >35% 0 2 or mean airway pressure of 6--8 em H_2O by CPAP or IMV

- Treatment of anemia of prematurity: Treatment with EPO and iron effectively stimulate neonatal erythropoiesis

Transfusional iron overload:

- Depends on the average number of units transfused
- Not influenced by – type of PRBC (CPD/washed)
- Serial serum ferritin levels – screening technique
- Standard method – Quantitative measurement of liver iron (MRI technology) and cardiac iron (T2* MRI cardiac software).
- Complication – Cardiac iron overload (failure/arrhythmias), Growth hormone deficiency, diabetes mellitus, hypothyroidism/parathyroidism and liver fibrosis

Iron Chelation:

1. Goal - prevent hemosiderosis-induced tissue injury and avoid chelation toxicity
2. ***Serum ferritin >1,000 ng/mL*** and/or a ***liver iron concentration of >2,500 μg/g dry weight***
3. 3 available iron chelators (deferoxamine, deferasirox and deferiprone)

4. Combination preferred – Deferoxamine, in combination with deferiprone
5. Iron stores in heart respond slowly than liver stores

Chelator	Deferoxamine	Deferiprone	Deferasirox
Half life	20 minutes	2 – 3 hours	8 – 16 hours
Route of administration	Subcutaneous	Per oral	Per oral
Frequency	5 – 7 days / week	3 times daily	Once daily
Iron excretion	Urine / stool	Urine	Urine

Ans: (c) 200 milli gram

Ref: *Nelson Textbook of Pediatrics, 20th Edition, page 2372-75*
The Harriet Lane Handbook, 12th Edition, page 329-31
Cloherty – Manual Neonatal Care, 7th Edition, page 529-31

13. A mother of 5-year-old boy feel that he is too tall for his age brought him to hospital for evaluation. On examination his height was 108 cm, arm span of 105 cm, upper segment to lower segment ratio 1.2 : 1.

What would be your advice to the mother?

(a) Order for karyotyping
(b) Reassure parents
(c) Echocardiography to rule out marfans syndrome
(d) Ophthalmogical examination and order for homocysteine levels

Explanation:

In this case scenario, the 1st step is to interpret the anthropometric measurement and common causes of tall stature.

Interpretation: Age : 5 years old boy

Present measurement	Expected measurement	Impression
Height **110 cm**	**Weech's formula** Expected height (cm) = (age in years × 6) + 77 So, height = (5 × 6) + 77 = **107 cm**	Height – Normal for age
Arm span **105 cm**	Armspan is **2 cm less than the height** in 5 year old children	Normal arm span
Upper segment to lower segment ratio **1.2: 1**	Upper segment to lower segment ratio : • At birth – 1.7:1 • 1 year 1.5:1 • **5 years 1.2:1**	Normal ratio

Impression: The measured anthropometric measurement were normal for age.

Definition of tall stature:

Crown – heel length > 97th percentile (>2 SD above the mean) for normal population of same age and sex.

Causes of tall stature:

Familial (constitutional)	Most common cause of tall stature in childhood
Nutritional	Exogenous obesity
Endocrine	Precocious puberty (early stage) Pituitary gigantism

Contd.

Contd.

	McCune-Albright syndrome Thyrotoxicosis Testicular feminization Adrenocorticotropic hormone (ACTH)/cortisol deficiency
Chromosomal	Klinefelter syndrome (XXY) Fragile X syndrome
Collagen vascular	Marfan syndrome
Metabolic	Homocystinuria
Fetal overgrowth syndromes	Maternal diabetes mellitus Cerebral gigantism (Sotos syndrome) Beckwith-Wiedemann syndrome

Approach to tall stature:

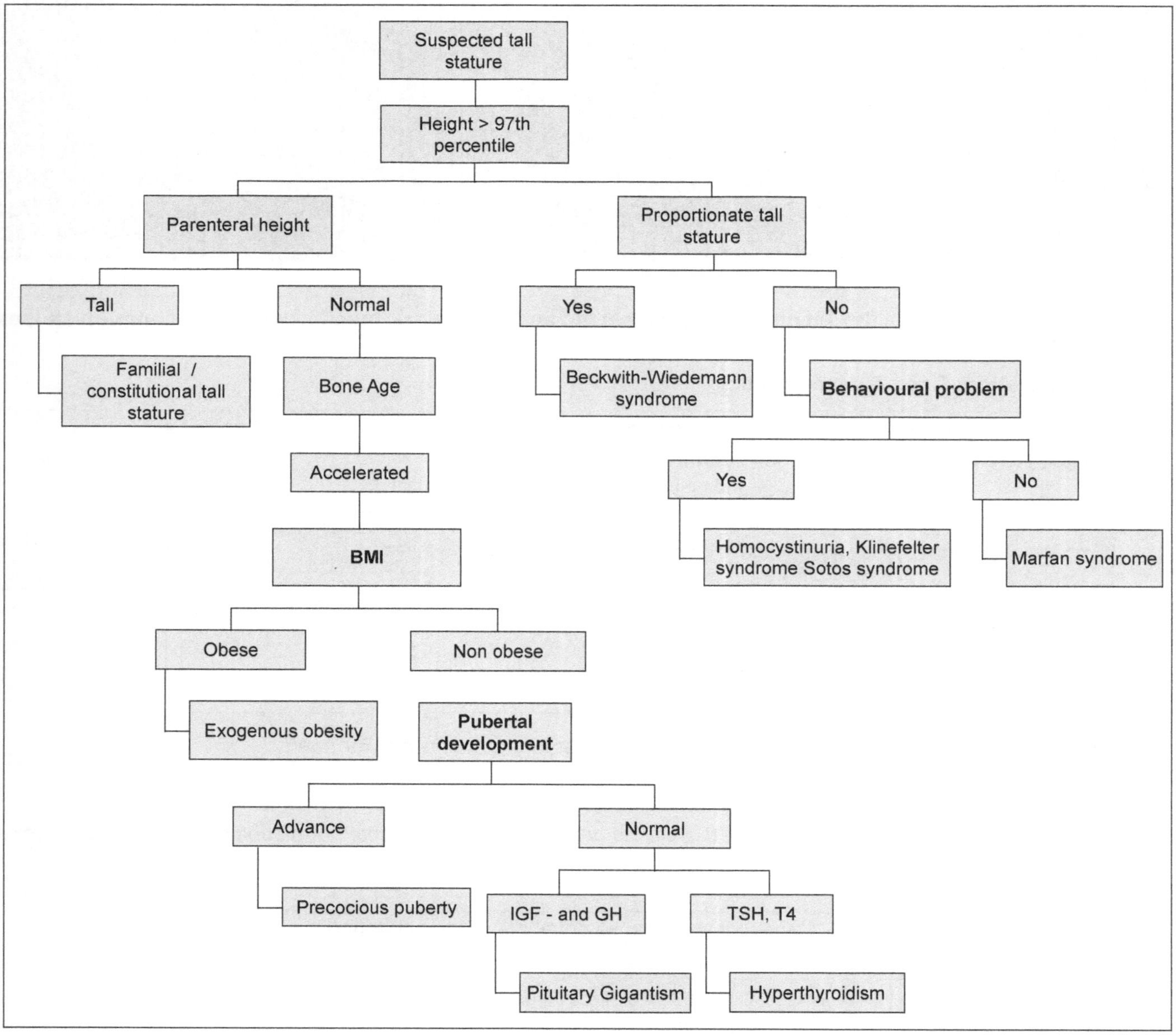

Investigations:

Suspected cause	Investigation
Beckwith-Wiedemann	Glucose, insulin, renal ultrasonography
Hyperthyroidism	T3, T4 and TSH levels
Homocystinuria	***Homocysteine, methionine***
Klinefelter syndrome	LH, FSH and testosterone levels; ***karyotyping***
Marfan syndrome	***Clinical diagnosis, Echocardiography, fibrillin-1 gene mutation***
Precocious puberty	Bone age

Extra Edge:

Characteristics	Homocystinuria	Marfan Syndrome
Inheritance	Autosomal recessive	Autosomal dominant
Intelligence Quotient	Low	Normal
Ectopia lentis	Displaced down and in	Displaced down and out
Joint mobility	Limited	Hyper flexibility
Aortic root	Normal	Dilated
Thromboembolic features	Present	Absent

Ans: (b) Reassure parents

Ref: *Nelson Textbook of Pediatrics, 20th Edition, page 2649*

14. The following were true about risk of delivering a Intra Uterine Growth Restriction (IUGR) baby *except:*

(a) High protein diet reduces risk of IUGR
(b) Antiplatelet intake reduces the risk of IUGR
(c) Antioxidants intake prevent IUGR
(d) Caffeine intake increases the risk of IUGR

Explanation: Intra Uterine Growth Restriction (IUGR):

- Fetuses weighing less than the 10th percentile for gestational age
- Major cause of IUGR in singleton pregnancies is abnormal placental vascular development

Risk factors for IUGR:

Maternal	Fetal	Placental
• Extremes of age • Fertility treatment • Insufficient energy and nutrient intake • Obesity and overweight • Substance use – smoking, illicit drugs, caffeine, alcohol • Medical conditions: e.g. malaria, diabetes, hypertension • History of previous growth restricted baby	• Genetic/chromosomal • Malformations • Infection • Multiple pregnancy	• Small size • Bleeding in pregnancy • Mosaicism • Vascular/cord abnormalities • Fetal arterial thrombosis • Placental tumors

Diagnosis:

- Ultrasonography improves the sensitivity and specificity to over 80%
- Fetal weight < 10th percentile + evidence of compromised intrauterine environment like
  - Oligohydramnios
  - Elevated head-abdomen ratio, or

   - Abnormal Doppler velocimetry in the umbilical cord
- Absent or reversed end diastolic flow of fetal umbilical artery/middle cerebral artery Doppler – poor prognosis

Prevention:

- Balanced energy/protein supplementation is associated:
   - Increase in birth weight and
   - 30% reduction in the incidence of SGA.
- In chronically undernourished women, high-energy supplementation – reduces IUGR
- High-protein supplementation is not beneficial in reducing IUGR
- Multiple-micronutrient supplementation in pregnancy results in less IUGR babies
- Smoking reduces birth weight by an average of 200 g, with a dose–response effect on birth weight
- Caffeine intake throughout pregnancy was associated with an increased risk of growth restriction
- Renal impairment and autoimmune disease in pregnancy are associated with abnormal fetal growth in pregnancy
- Antiplatelet agents are associated with a 10% reduction in the risk of an IUGR baby
- Antioxidants (vitamin C and E) – there was no reduction in the risk of the baby being IUGR
- Beta blocker agents (for treating hypertension in pregnancy) are used; there is an increase in IUGR

Ans: (c) Antioxidants intake prevent IUGR

Ref : *Grivell R, Dodd J, Robinson J, The Prevention and Treatment of Intrauterine Growth Restriction, Best Pract Res Clin Obstet Gynaecol 2009, 23:795-807 and Cloherty-Manual Neonatal Care, 7th Edition, page 86-88*

15. A screening test for mitochondrial myopathies:

(a) Creatinine Phospho Kinase (b) Growth differentiation factor 11 (GDF 11)

(c) Serum lactate (d) LDH

Explanation:

- **Lactic acidosis** is a primary component of Mitochondrial encephalomyopathies (like MELAS)

Mitochondrial encephalomyopathies:

- Caused by genetic lesions impairing energy production through oxidative phosphorylation
- Most common mutation - MELAS 3243 mutation on tRNA gene of mtDNA

Inheritance of mutations present on mtDNA

- Nonmendelian and complex.
- Transmitted by maternal inheritance
- Her daughters can pass it on to their children

Mitochondiral (mt) DNA containing mutations can be distributed unequally between cells in specific tissues

- Normal / Wild type Homoplasmy - cells receive few or no mutant genomes
- **Heteroplasmy -** others receive a mixed population of **mutant** and **wild-type** mtDNAs
- **Mutant homoplasmy -** still others receive primarily or exclusively **mutant** genomes

Signs of brain and muscle dysfunction:

- Seizures, ptosis, external ophthalmoplegia, psychomotor regression, hearing loss, movement disorders and ataxia

WITH

- Lactic acidosis (prominent features of mitochondrial disorders)

Types:

- Mitochondrial encephalomyopathy with lactic acidosis and stroke-like episodes (***MELAS***)
  - Present with developmental delay, weakness, and headaches, as well as focal signs that suggest a stroke
- Myoclonic epilepsy with ragged red fibers (MERRF)
  - Present with myoclonus and myoclonic seizures as well as intermittent muscle weakness.
- NARP syndrome (neuropathy, ataxia, and retinitis pigmentosa)
- Kearns-Sayre syndrome (KSS; ptosis, ophthalmoplegia, heart block)
- Leigh disease (subacute necrotizing encephalomyelopathy), and
- Leber hereditary optic neuropathy (LHON)

MELAS

Normal for several years, then display delayed motor, cognitive development, short stature.

Characterized by:

(1) Recurrent stroke-like episodes of hemiparesis or other focal neurologic signs

(2) Lactic acidosis, ragged red fibers (RRF), or both; AND

(3) At least 2 of the following:

- Focal or generalized seizures
- Dementia
- Recurrent migraine headaches, and
- Vomiting

- Single-photon emission CT studies – Regional cerebral hypoperfusion
- Lactic acidosis in the brain – MR spectroscopy
- Muscle biopsy – shows ragged red fibers (RRF)

Treatment tried – corticosteroids, nicotinamide, carnitine, creatine, riboflavin

Prognosis – poor

Extra Edge:

Difference between MELAS and Kearns-Sayre syndrome

Symptoms	MELAS	Kearns-Sayre syndrome
Ataxia	+	+
Cortical Blindness	+	–
Deafness	+	–
Hemi paresis	+	–
Myoclonus	+	–
Movement disorder	+	–
Seizures	+	–
Regression	+	+

Exclude other options:

(a) Creatinine Phospho Kinase
- Used in muscular dystrophy (Duchenne Muscular Dystrophy)

(b) Growth differentiation factor 11(GDF 11)
- GDF 15 is a new biomarker for screening mitochondrial myopathies

(c) LDH
- Used for screening myocardial injury (particularly LDH-1)

Ans: (c) Serum lactate

Ref: *Nelson Textbook of Pediatrics, 20th Edition, page 2900-92*

16. A neonate born as IUGR, with microcephaly, ptosis, epicanthic fold, toe syndactyly, cleft palate and ambiguous genitalia (micro penis, hypospadias and bilateral inguinal swelling) brought with feeding difficulty. On evaluation the mullerian structures were absent and the karyotyping was 46, XY. What will the next investigation you would like to order?

(a) 7 dehydrocholesterol
(b) 17 hydroxy progesterone
(c) Androstenedione/ testosterone ratio
(d) Testosterone/DHT ratio

Explanation:

The clinical and laboratory features suggests of Smith-Lemli-Opitz syndrome in which 7 dehydrocholesterol levels elevated

Smith-Lemli-Opitz syndrome:

- Multiple congenital anomalies and developmental delay caused by **low plasma cholesterol** and **accumulated precursors** (**7-dehydrocholesterol**)
- Autosomal recessive disorder
- Mutations in the sterol **Δ7-reductase gene** located on chromosome 11q12-q13
- **Deficiency of the microsomal enzyme DHCR7** (necessary to complete the final step in cholesterol synthesis)
  - 70% are male (with genital ambiguity)
  - Partial sex reversal or complete sex reversal with female external genitals
  - But müllerian duct derivatives were absent
  - Prenatal and postnatal growth retardation, retromicrognathia, Midline cleft palate
  - Low-set ears, microcephaly, ptosis, anteverted nares, broad alveolar ridges
  - Syndactyly of the 2nd-3rd toes, and cognitive impairment

Associated malformations:

CNS	CVS
• Frontal lobe hypoplasia • Agenesis of corpus callosum • Holoprosencephaly	• Atrioventricular canal • Secundum atrial septal defect • Patent ductus arteriosus • Membranous ventricular septal defect

Urinary Tract	Gastrointestinal	Pulmonary	Endocrine
• Renal hypoplasia • Renal cortical cysts • Hydronephrosis • Ureteral duplication	• Hirschsprung disease • Pyloric stenosis • progressive liver disease	• Pulmonary hypoplasia	• Adrenal insufficiency

- Type I – classical form (acrodysgenital syndrome) – lethal within 1 year and associated with Pyloric stenosis
- Type – II (extremely abnormal external genitalia) – associated with Hirschsprung disease

- Low plasma cholesterol (<20 mg/dL - lethal) with elevated 7-dehydrocholesterol seen in both type I and II.
- Maternal apolipoprotein E values do seem to correlate with severity.
- Treatment – Supplemental dietary cholesterol (egg yolk) and
  – HMG-CoA reductase inhibition (prevent the synthesis of toxic precursors)

Congenital adrenal hyperplasia (CAH)

Etiology

Group of **autosomal recessively** inherited disorders of **adrenal corticosteroid biosynthesis** due to deficiency of 1 of 5 enzymes in the cholesterol to cortisol biosynthesis pathway:

- ***21-hydroxylase—most common****
- *11 beta hydroxylase*
- *3 beta hydroxysteroid dehydrogenase*
- *17 alpha hydroxylase*
- *Cholesterol desmolase*

Enzymes involved in the **adrenal androgen (and gonadal**) biosynthetic pathway include

- 17,20 desmolase
- 17 beta hydroxysteroid dehydrogenase
- 5 alpha reductase

Pathophysiology

- Loss of feedback inhibition on ACTH due to **deficient cortisol**
- This causes excess ACTH secretion leading on to **hyperpigmentation*** and **hyperplasia of adrenal cortex***

Prenatal androgen excess	Postnatal androgen excess
Females • Masculinized **external** genitals • Internal genital organs are normal • Brain exposure leads to sexually dimorphic behaviours later **Males** • Males normal at birth • Signs of adrenaline insufficiency	**Common features:** • Rapid somatic growth • Accelerated skeletal maturation • Tall during childhood, but early fusion of epiphysis leading on to short stature during adulthood • Excessive muscle development • Pubic and axillary hair appear **In males** • Penis, scrotum, and prostate enlarged • Testes is pre-pubertal **In females** • **Breast development and menstruation does not occur**

21 Hydroxylase deficiency

- Most common type of CAH*
- Two genes encoding **CYP21B** (active) and **CYP21A** (inactive) mapped to the short arm of **chromosome 6**

Clinical features

- **Masculinization** of karyotype **female** results in ambiguous **external genitalia** recognized at birth
- Severe cases infant is thought to be a **male** but
  - Internal female structures include **ovaries, fallopian tubes and uterus**
  - Variable **labio scrotal fold** associated with **urogenital sinus**

  - Genital **hyperpigmentation** and **clitromegaly**
- **Males normal** at **birth** but present with
  - Penile enlargement
  - Rapid growth—tall stature
  - **Advanced skeletal maturation*** (leading to eventually **short stature**)
- Classical **salt wasting**
- Neonatal presentation (In both sexes)
  - Severe renal wasting of **sodium**
  - Vomiting, dehydration
  - Ambiguous genitalia

21 hydroxylase deficiency—classic form*

Features	Lab findings	Treatment
Due to glucocorticoid deficiency: • **Hypoglycemia** • **Hyperpigmentation** of **areola** and **scrotum** in males • **Hyperpigmentation** of **genital creases** in females	Cortisol - decreased ACTH - increased Baseline and ACTH stimulated **17-hydroxy progesterone** (17 OHP) - increased	• Glucocorticoid replacement (hydrocortisone)
Due to mineralocorticoid deficiency: • **Salt-wasting crisis***	Hyponatremia Hyperkalemia Renin levels - increased	• Mineralocorticoid replacement (Fludrocortisone) • Sodium chloride supplementation
Due to androgen excess: • **In females**: Virilization: Ambiguous genitalia and **pseudohermaphrodite** • **In males:** Phenotypically **normal** at birth and **precocious puberty**	Androgen levels - increased	• **In females:** Vaginoplasty and clitoris reduction • **In males**: Suppression with glucocorticoids

21 hydroxylase deficiency—Non-classical form (mild, late onset)

- Suspected in **women** presenting with **hirsutism** and **infertility**
- **Premature pubarche and adrenarche**
- Rapid growth (but reduced final height)
- **Acne, male type baldness** in **female**
- Delayed **menarche** or **secondary amenorrhea**
- Association with **PCOD**

Laboratory diagnosis:

- **Neonatal screening: 17 OHP** measurements at birth and at 2 weeks.
- **Plasma ACTH, androstenedione and urinary pregnanetriol levels** are raised
- Salt wasting form:
  - Urinary sodium loss (hyponatremia)
  - Aldosterone levels are low for the high renin levels

Management:

- Surgery for ambiguous genitalia (Virilized females surgery between 2 and 6 months of age)
- Prenatal treatment—**Dexamethasone** 20 μg/kg (crosses the placenta, reduces virilization in females)

- **Chorionic villous biopsy** is then performed to determine the sex and the genotype of the fetus, therapy is continued only if the fetus is an affected female

Glucocorticoid replacement	Mineralocorticoid replacement
• **Hydrocortisone**—15–20 mg/m^2/24 hours TDS lifelong • Double or triple doses—stress (infection/surgery) • Suppresses androgens from adrenal cortex thereby reducing excessive growth, skeletal maturation and virilization • Under treatment—when crossing higher height centiles instead of maintaining desirable linear growth along percentile lines • Over treatment—excessive weight gain • Monitoring pubertal development, evaluating skeletal maturation	• **Fludrocortisone:** 0.1–0.3 mg daily in 2 divided doses with sodium supplementation (8 mmol/kg) • Monitoring of vital signs (tachycardia and hypertension—overtreatment) • Serum electrolytes measured frequently • **Plasma renin**—adequacy of therapy • **Additional approaches** – Antiandrogen—Flutamide – Aromatase inhibitor—anastrazole – Growth hormone with or without LHRH agonist

Approach to diagnose CAH

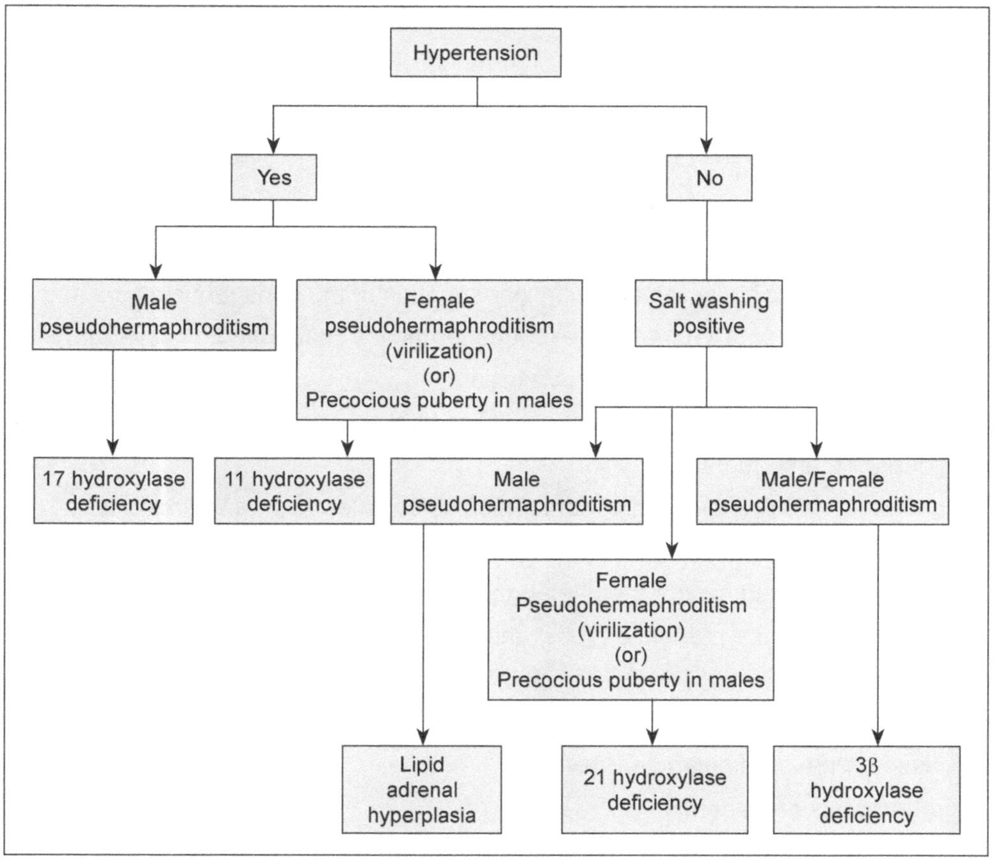

Exclude other options:

(a) 17 hydroxy progesterone – used to screen, **21-hydroxylase deficiency CAH (salt loosing type with virilisation)**

(b) Androstenedione/ testosterone ratio – used in the diagnosis of 17 beta-hydroxysteroid dehydrogenase 3 deficiency (feminized genitalia in newborns due to the low testosterone levels)

(c) Testosterone/DHT ratio – ratio is increased in 5alpha–reductase deficiency

Extra Edge:

- Types with **hypertension starts** with **1: 11** and 17 hydroxylase def
- Types with **virilization ends** with **1: 21** and 11hydroxylase def
- 17 has male pseudo herma PD and 11 has female pseudoherma PD – 17 >11; M comes later than F

Ans: (a) 7 dehydrocholesterol

Ref: *Nelson Textbook of Pediatrics, 20th Edition, page 700-01*

17. A 3-month-old infant brought with the complaints of not moving the upper limb with fever and irritability. On examination the upper limb was swollen with woody induration but without other signs of inflammation (like warmth and redness). The investigation showed anemia, thrombocytosis with increased ESR and serum alkaline phosphatase. X-ray of the upper limb revealed soft-tissue swelling and calcification and cortical hyperostosis. What could be the possible diagnosis?

(a) Inflammatory arthritis of shoulder (b) Infantile hyperostosis

(c) Garre's sclerosing osteomyelitis (d) Scurvy

Explanation:

- The clinical scenario (age of 3 months, sudden onset symptom limb swelling with minimal signs of inflammation. The laboratory tests of increased ESR and alkaline phosphatase. The X-ray clinches the diagnosis of **Infantile Cortical Hyperostosis**

Infantile Cortical Hyperostosis: (Caffey Disease)

- Etiology – unknown
- Characterized by cortical hyperostosis with inflammation of the contiguous fascia and muscle
- Reported mutations of the COL1A1 gene (codes for the α1 chain of type I collagen)
- Prenatal disease (high mortality) is characterized:
  - Typical bone lesions, polyhydramnios, hydrops fetalis, severe respiratory distress, prematurity
- Onset – younger than 6 months
- Manifestations – Irritability, swelling of contiguous soft tissue, fever, and anorexia
- Painful swelling with wood-like induration (minimal warmth or redness) and suppuration is absent
- All bones may be affected except the phalanges or vertebral bodies
- Most common bones – the mandible (75%), the clavicle, and the ulna

  Laboratory features
  - Erythrocyte sedimentation rate and serum alkaline phosphatase – elevated
  - Increased serum prostaglandin E levels
  - Thrombocytosis and anemia

  Radiographic features
  - Soft-tissue swelling and calcification and cortical hyperostosis

Differential Diagnosis: As for hyperostosis

- Chronic vitamin A intoxication
- Prolonged prostaglandin E infusion
- Primary bone tumors, and
- Scurvy

Complications:

- Pseudoparalysis with limb or scapula involvement
- Pleural effusions (rib)
- Torticollis (clavicle)
- Mandibular asymmetry
- Bone fusion (ribs or ulna and radius), and
- Bone angulation deformities (common with severe prenatal onset).

Treatment – Indomethacin and prednisone

Exclude other options:

(a) Inflammatory arthritis of shoulder

Swelling will be restricted to shoulder and signs of inflammation will be present

(b) Garre's sclerosing osteomyelitis

Specific type of chronic osteomyelitis (young adults) of the mandible / non tender

(c) Scurvy

Can produce pseudo paralysis and joint swelling (hemarthrosis), but fever and acute phase reactants will be absent. The X-ray would have shown subperiosteal hemorrhage with Pelken's spur, Wimberger's ring, trummerfeld zone, pencil thin cortex and white line of frankel.

Ans: (b) Infantile hyperostosis

Ref: *Nelson Textbook of Pediatrics, 20th Edition, page 3379*

DERMATOLOGY

1. Which of the following is true regarding Kerion?
(a) Often seen in Kashmir
(b) Causative agent is Trichophyton schoenleinii
(c) Painful boggy swelling in scalp with follicular pustules
(d) Yellow scutula

Explanation:

- The history of boggy inflammatory swelling of scalp in a child is suggestive of the diagnosis of inflammatory type of tinea capitis called as **Kerion.** The other inflammatory types of **tinea capitis** are **favus** and **agminate folliculitis**. The non-inflammatory types of tinea capitis are **black-dot tinea capitis**, **grey-patch tinea capitis** and **seborrheic dermatitis-like tinea capitis**.

Tinea capitis

- Endothrix and Ectothrix
- Most common – **Trichophyton violaceum***

***Varieties*:**

- **Non inflammatory**
  - Gray patch
  - Black dot
  - Seborrheic dermatitis
- **Inflammatory**
  - Favus
  - Kerion, agminate folliculitis

Black dot/Grey patch

- Breakage of hair gives rise to 'black dots'
- Patchy alopecia, often circular, numerous broken-off hairs, dull grey
- Wood's lamp examination: green fluorescence (occasional non-fluorescent cases)

Tinea capitis: Kerion, agminate folliculitis

- Inflammatory variety
- **Microsporum, Trichophyton verrucosum, Trichophyton mentagrophytes**
- Painful, inflammatory boggy swelling with purulent discharge.
- Hairs may be matted, easily pluckable
- Lymphadenopathy
- Co-infection with bacteria is common
- May heal with scarring alopecia

Tinea capitis: Favus

- Inflammatory variety

- Seen commonly in **Kashmir**
- **Trichophyton schoenleinii**
- Yellowish, cup-shaped crusts develop around a hair with the hair projecting centrally.
- Extensive patchy hair loss with cicatricial alopecia

Ans: (c) Painful boggy swelling in scalp with follicular pustules

Ref: *Rook, 8th edition, page 20, 26, 27, 36*

2. An adult with leprosy took overdose of dapsone and presented after 8 hours with cyanosis. What is the next step?

(a) Do ABG analysis (b) ECG
(c) Check for carboxy hemoglobin (d) Echo Heart

Explanation:

Dapsone induced Methemoglobinemia

- Life-threatening condition that can be difficult to diagnose
- Dapsone is particularly potent because of its pro-oxidant metabolite hydroxylamine which has a very long half-life (catalyzed by a variety of hepatic enzymes or via myeloperoxidase present in white blood cells).
- When administered in standard doses of 100 mg/day, it can induce significant **methemoglobinemia** in biochemically normal patients.
- It accelerates with coexistent anemia, fever, and coadministration of immunoglobulin.
- Thromboxane and prostaglandin synthesis in response to infection increases oxidative stress on erythrocytes.
- In a healthy and biochemically normal individual, cyanosis develops when levels reach **15%–20%** and symptoms ensue with levels of **25%–50%.**
- While **headache, dyspnea, lightheadedness, weakness and confusion** are reported in mild methemoglobinemia, individuals with more severe disease are at risk of **cardiac arrhythmias, seizures,** and coma.
- Diagnosis in patients with acquired methemoglobinemia requires high index of clinical suspicion and a thorough drug history.
- First, direct observation may reveal an **arterial sample** that is **chocolate-brown** in appearance.
- Second, the presence of **cyanosis** in an individual with a **normal PaO_2** level may suggest the **diagnosis**.
- The only reliable method of measuring methemoglobin concentration and confirming a diagnosis of methemoglobinemia is **CO-oximetry***
- **CO-oximetry** thus allows both identification and **quantitation** of all hemoglobin species, including **methemoglobin**. CO-oximetry also allows calculation of oxygen saturation; this is a more reliable method of assessing oxygen saturation in patients with methemoglobin than either pulse oximetry or blood gas analysis

Treatment

- Treatment depends on the clinical severity.
- In asymptomatic patients (with a methemoglobin level of <20%), simple measures such as discontinuing the offending agent may be all that is required.
- In symptomatic patients (or where the methemoglobin level exceeds 20%), administration of supplemental oxygen and methylene blue may be indicated.

Ans: (a) Do ABG analysis

Ref: *Indian J Dermatol 2015; 60:108*

3. Pterygium of nail is characteristically seen in:

(a) Lichen planus (b) Psoriasis

(c) Tinea unguium (d) Alopecia areata

Explanation:

LICHEN PLANUS

- It is a pruritic, inflammatory papulosquamous disorder affecting the skin, mucous membranes, nails and hair follicles.
- **Etiology** – Unknown
  - Genetic predisposition: **HLA B8- oral LP; HLA-Bw 35-cutaneous LP**
  - Exogenous: **Primary biliary cirrhosis, alcoholic cirrhosis, hepatitis B, hepatitis C**
  - Drugs cause lichenoid drug eruptions
  - Metals like **mercury** (dental amalgams), **palladium**, **gold** – oral lichenoid eruptions
- **Clinical Features:**
  - 30-60 years; children-4% of cases, childhood LP more common in India
  - ***Skin:***
    - Intensely **pruritic, flat topped, shiny, polygonal, violaceous papules** and plaques
    - Predominantly **flexor distribution**–flexor of wrist, forearm, legs, trunk, glans penis (cf-psoriasis another papulosquamous disorder has predominant extensor distribution)
    - **Wickham's striae**–network of greyish white streaks on papules seen on pressing with glass slide after application of oil–corresponds to wedge shaped hypergranulosis seen on histopathology
    - **Koebner/ isomorphic phenomenon** common
    - Annular LP–Glans penis
    - Hypertrophic LP–shins
    - Actinic LP–sun exposed areas
  - ***Oral:***
    - Classical type is reticulate pattern–white/violaceous **lacy reticular network** of coalesent papules in buccal mucosa and tongue; usually asymptomatic
    - Most common pattern–ulcerative/erosive LP
  - ***Nail:***
    - 5-10% cases
    - Thinning of nail plate (cf psoriasis–thickening of nail plate), longitudinal ridging, roughening of nail plate (**trachyonychia**) and nail dystrophy involving all 20 nails called 20 nail dystrophy (also seen in **alopecia areata**)
    - Classical/characteristic nail finding (but not common finding)–**pterygium** formation (proximal nail fold fuses with nail bed)
    - **Longitudinal furrows** alternating with portion of normal nail plate that appear as ridges
    - Uniform thinning of the nail plate (**Angel Wing deformity**)
    - Total nail area atrophy

    - **Pup tent sign**–Discrete red or violaceous papules in the nail bed may lift and split the overlying nail plate longitudinally, and the split lateral edges angle forward to give a pup tent appearance
    - Violaceous lines in nail plate
    - **Subungual hyperkeratosis**
  - Hair follicles: lichen planopilaris–scarring alopecia

- **Histopathology:**
  - Hyperkeratosis
  - Wedge shaped hypergranulosis (psoriasis–hypogranulosis)
  - Irregular acanthosis (psoriasis–regular acanthosis)
  - **Saw tooth rete ridges** (psoriasis–**elephant foot/camel foot like/club shaped rete ridges**)
  - Basal layer vacuolar degeneration
  - Band like dermal lymphocytic infiltrate hugging epidermis
  - **Max Joseph spaces**–subepidermal clear zone (subepidermal clear zone in lepromatous leprosy is called Grenz zone)
  - Melanin incontinence
- **Treatment**–steroids (topical/intralesionsal/systemic), retinoids, cyclosporine, PUVA photochemotherapy, dapsone, methotrexate
- **"8 P's of Lichen planus"**
  - Papulosquamous disorder
  - Pruritic
  - Plane topped
  - Polygonal/polyangular
  - Purple coloured
  - Papules
  - Plaques
  - Pigmentation after healing
  - Pterygium formation in nails

Ans: (a) Lichen planus

Ref: *Papulosquamous Disorders, In: Thappa DM, editor, Essentials in Dermatology, 2nd edition, New Delhi: Jaypee Brothers Medical Publishers (P) Ltd 2009, page 82-98*

4. Which of the following is true about HPV vaccine?

(a) Protects only from cervical cancer

(b) Live vaccine

(c) Cannot be taken with other vaccine

(d) Protects from cervical vaginal, anal, penile and nasopharyngeal cancer

Explanation:

HPV vaccines

- Three HPV vaccines are now being marketed in many countries throughout the world – a bivalent, a quadrivalent, and a nonavalent vaccine.

- All three vaccines are highly efficacious in preventing infection with virus types **16 and 18**, which are together responsible for approximately 70% of cervical cancer cases globally.
- The vaccines are also highly efficacious in preventing precancerous **cervical lesions** caused by these virus types.
- The quadrivalent vaccine is also highly efficacious in preventing **anogenital warts**, a **common genital** disease which is virtually always caused by infection with **HPV types 6 and 11.**
- The nonavalent provides additional protection against HPV types **31, 33, 45, 52 and 58.**

Ans: (d) Protects from cervical, vaginal, anal, penile and nasopharyngeal cancer

Ref: *https://www.who.int/immunization/diseases/hpv/en/*

5. Which is false regarding Behcet syndrome?

(a) Recurrent oral ulcers
(b) Recurrent ulcer on glans penis
(c) Erythema nodosum
(d) Superficial thrombosis

Explanation:

Behçet disease (BD)

- Primary variable vessel vasculitis
- Associated with **HLA-B5101**
- **Recurrent oral aphthous ulcerations** are sine qua non for the diagnosis
  - Ulcers are usually painful shallow or deep with a central yellowish necrotic base, appear singly or in crops.
  - Small ulcers <10 mm in diameter, seen in >85% patients
- **Genital ulcers**
  - Less common but more specific
  - Produce scrotal and vulvar ulcers leading to scars
  - Do not affect the glans penis or urethra
- **Skin involvement**
  - Folliculitis
  - Erythema nodosum
  - Acne like exanthema
  - Vasculitis
  - Sweet's syndrome
  - Pyoderma gangrenosum
- **Superficial and deep vein thrombosis in 30% patients**

Behçet's disease diagnostic criteria*
Major criteria
1. Recurrent oral and genital ulcerations 2. Eye lesions 3. Skin lesions (erythema nodosum-like or folliculitis) 4. Positive pathergy test (non infected pustules in the site of trauma)

Contd.

Contd.

Minor criteria
1. Arthritis or arthralgia 2. Deep venous thrombosis 3. Subcutaneous thrombophlebitis 4. Epididimitis 5. Family history 6. Gastrointestinal lesions 7. CNS symptoms 8. Vascular lesions
* International Study Group for Behçet's disease

Ans: (b) Recurrent ulcer on glans penis

Ref: *Harrison's Principles of Internal Medicine, 20th edition*

6. A 50-year-old female presents with violaceous lesions over knuckles and heliotrope rash. Most probable diagnosis is:

(a) SLE
(b) Dermatomyositis
(c) Behçet's syndrome
(d) CREST syndrome

Explanation:

Dermatomyositis

- **Connective tissue disorder characterized by:**
  - **Inflammatory myositis**
  - **Proximal muscle weakness**
  - **Cutaneous manifestations**

Pathognomonic features:

- **Gottron's papules**
  - Violaceous flat topped papules on **IP joints** and **knuckles**
  - Also seen in **knee, elbow, medial malleoli**
- **Gottron's sign**–Violaceous erythematous macules with or without edema at the above mentioned sites

Characteristic Features:

- **Heliotrope rash**
  - Periorbital violaceous erythema with edema
  - Oedema of the eyelids and periorbital tissues
- **Shawl sign**–Erythema and scaling with or without poikiloderma over shoulder region
- **Periungual telangiectasia and dystrophic cuticles**
- **Mechanic's hands**–Hyperkeratosis, scaling, fissuring and hyperpigmentation over fingertips, sides of thumbs and fingers
- **Oedema of the hands and arms**, and sometimes of much of the body
- Rash of dermatomyositis on the dorsa of the hands occurs as linear streaking over the extensor tendon sheaths
- **Other compatible features:**
  - Calcinosis cutis
  - Poikiloderma trophicans vasculare

Other options

- In **Behcet's syndrome** – Classically associated with triad of:
  - **Recurrent Aphthous Stomatis**
  - **Genital ulceration**
  - **Eye disease** (especially iridocyclitis and retinal vasculitis)
- In SLE there is:
  - **Malar rash** (cutaneous erythema on the sun-exposed area)
  - Discoid rash
  - Oral ulcer
  - Photosensitivity
- **CREST Syndrome**
  - Limited form of systemic scleroderma
  - Anti centromere antibody

C–Calcinosis cutis
R–Raynaud's phenomenon
E–Esophageal dysmotility
S–Sclerodactyly
T–Telangiectasia

- **Progressive systemic sclerosis–cutaneous + internal organ fibrosis**
- **American Rheumatism Association criteria (ARA criteria 1980) for systemic sclerosis**

Major criteria	• Scleroderma proximal to digits affecting limbs, face, neck, trunk
Minor criteria	• Sclerodactyly • Digital pitted scarring • Bilateral basal pulmonary fibrosis

  - 97% sensitivity; 98% specificity
  - One major + two or more minor

Ans: (b) Dermatomyositis

Ref: *Rook's Textbook of Dermatology, 8th edition, page 51-120*

7. Koebner's phenomenon is not seen in:

(a) Vitiligo (b) Psoriasis

(c) Dermatitis herpetiformis (d) Lichen planus

Explanation:

- The **Koebner phenomenon** is the development of **isomorphic** pathologic lesions in the **traumatized uninvolved skin** of patients who have cutaneous diseases.
- Koebner phenomenon signifies activity of the disease.

TYPES OF KOEBNER PHENOMENON:

A. True isomorphic phenomenon:

There appear to be three disease processes that display the true isomorphic response of Koebner:

- Psoriasis
- Lichen planus
- Vitiligo.

B. Pseudoisomorphic phenomenon:

The Koebner phenomenon also seen in infectious diseases

- Warts
- Molluscum contagiosum
- Behcet's disease
- Pyoderma gangrenosum.

C. Occasionally occurring isomorpic phenomenon:

In this category, diseases occasionally localize to sites of trauma, e.g.

- Cancer (gastric, testicular or mammary)
- Darier's disease
- Erythema multiforme
- Hailey-Hailey disease
- Kaposi's sarcoma
- Kyrle's disease
- Lichen sclerosus et atrophicus
- Pellagra
- Perforating folliculitis
- Reactive perforating collagenosis.

Koebner response in psoriasis:

- The reported incidence of Koebner response in psoriasis varies from 11-75%.
- The latent period between injury to uninvolved skin and appearance of disease is usually 10-14 days, but it may range from 3 days to several years.

The "reverse" Koebner response:

The reverse Koebner reaction is seen when an area of **psoriasis** clears following injury.

Ans: (c) Dermatitis herpetiformis

Ref: *Thappa DM, The Isomorphic Phenomenon of Koebner, Indian J Dermatol Venereol Leprol 2004, 70:187-89*

ANESTHESIOLOGY

1. Drugs not metabolized by plasma esterase:

(a) Mucaine (b) Esmolol

(c) Clevidipine (d) Atracurium

Explanation:

Esterases are a heterogenous group of enzymes which hydrolyse esters through the oxygen bridge to form alcohol and alkanoic acid → inactivates ester drugs

- Found in plasma, NMJ, RBC, hepatic sinusoids
- High capacity pathway with high clearance
- Non-organ dependent metabolic pathway (except in severe hepatic disease → ↓production plasma cholinesterases)
- Metabolites are usually inactive Except laudanosine (atracurium/cisatracurium) and salicylic acid → which can be active at high doses

A. Red Cell Esterases

Drugs metabolised: – Esmolol
– Remifentanil

B. Plasma Esterases

Drugs metabolised:

- Remifentanil → predic and context-independent
- Atracurium/Cisatracurium
- Etomidate → plasma and hepatic microenzymes

C. Pseudocholinesterase (plasma cholinesterase) Drugs metabolised:

- Suxamethonium
- Mivacurium
- Ester LA (egamethacaine)

Affected by: Altered physiology/comorbidities → acquired/inherited

- Pregnancy
- Liver disease
- Inherited disorder (pseudocholinesterase deficiency) → autosomal dominant with variable penetrance → atypical 1:3000 homozygotes, 1:500 heterozygote ↓ by drugs

Anti-cholinesterases:

- Neostigmine
- LAs → dibucaine
- Metaclopramide

Ans: (c) Clevidipine

Ref: *Stoelting's Pharmacology and Physiology in Anesthesia Practice, fourth edition*

2. First to recover after spinal shock post complete cord injury:

(a) Neck righting
(b) Tympanic or stapedial reflex
(c) Labyrynthine reflex
(d) Withdrawal reflex

Explanation:

Spinal shock

- **Definition:** Spinal shock is defined as a condition of transient physiologic, rather than anatomic, reflex depression of spinal cord function below the level of injury. Spinal shock is usually temporary.
- **Duration:** Usually lasts for days or weeks after spinal cord injury and the average duration is 4 to 12 weeks. (Spinal shock is terminated earlier and the pyramidal tract signs and defense reactions occur sooner in incomplete lesions than with complete transverse lesions.)
- **Effect:**
  - All the fundamental functions of the spinal cord below the level of injury, including the cord reflexes, are immediately depressed, which is referred to as spinal shock.
  - Complete loss of autonomic nervous function below the level of injury resulting in loss of bladder tone and paralytic ileus as well as flaccid, areflexic paralysis of skeletal and smooth muscles.
- **Complications:** As the vasomotor tone is lost, the dependent lower extremities become edematous and patient may be particularly vulnerable to deep vein thrombosis and pulmonary emboli.
- **Recovery:** Occurs over a period of days to months, and spinal shock slowly transitions to spasticity.
- It has been suggested that this transition consist of four phases:

Phase 1	**Areflexia or hyporeflexia (0–24 hours),** Characterized by: • No deep tendon reflex • The first pathological reflex during this period is the delayed plantar reflex followed by a series of cutaneous reflexes such as the bulbocavernosus, abdominal wall, and cremasteric reflex • Sympathetic dysfunction
Phase 2	**Initial reflex return (1–3 days)** • During this phase, polysynaptic cutaneous reflexes are more prominent, while deep tendon reflexes still do not exist • It is not unusual for elderly individuals and children to experience recovery of deep tendon reflexes during this time • The Babinski sign can also be evident in the elderly
Phase 3	**Early hyperreflexia (4 days–1 month)** • Deep tendon reflexes may be returned in the majority of patients and the Babinski sign may appear
Phase 4	**Spasticity or hyperreflexia (1–12 months)** • Vasovagal hypotension and bradycardia generally improve within 3 to 6 weeks, but orthostatic hypotension may take 10 to 12 weeks to disappear • Episodes of malignant hypertension or autonomic dysreflexia

Ans: (b) Tympanic or stapedial reflex

Ref: Millers Textbook of Anesthesia and Critical Care, eighth edition

3. Fastest acting inhalational anaesthetic agent:

(a) Isoflurane
(b) Sevoflurane
(c) Ether
(d) Halothane

Explanation:

Onset of the effect of inhalational agent depends upon blood gas partition coefficient.

Blood-gas partition coefficient:

- The ratio of anesthetic concentrations in the blood and alveolar space when partial pressures in the two compartments are equal → The higher the blood-gas partition coefficient of an inhalational anesthetic, the higher the solubility of that substance in the blood
- The **lower** the blood-gas partition coefficient of an inhalational anesthetic, the **faster** the substance takes effect (less induction time)

Agent	BG coefficient	MAC
Diethyl ether	12	1.92
Methoxyflurane	11	0.2
Trichloroethylene	9	0.23
Chloroform	8	0.77
Halothane	2.4	0.75
Enflurane	1.9	1.68
Isoflurane	1.6	1.15
Sevoflurane	0.6	2.5
Cyclopropane	0.55	9.2
Nitrous oxide	0.47	105
Desflurane	0.42	5.72
Xenon	0.14	71

Ans: (b) Sevoflurane

Ref: *Stoelting's Pharmacology and Physiology in Anesthesia Practice, fourth edition, page 42-44*

4. Most preferred first line anesthetic for ECT in a depressive patient:

(a) Midazolam (b) Thiopentone

(c) Ketamine (d) Halothane

Explanation:

Anesthetic consideration during Elective convulsive therapy

- **What is ECT?:** The electroconvulsive shock is applied to one or both cerebral hemispheres to produce a therapeutic generalised seizure 30–60 s in duration. Electrical stimuli are usually administered until a therapeutic seizure is induced
- **Physiological effect of ECT:** Seizure activity is associated with an initial parasympathetic discharge followed by a more sustained sympathetic discharge. The initial phase is characterized by bradycardia and increased secretions. Marked bradycardia (< 30 beats/min) and even transient asystole (up to 6 s) are occasionally seen. The hypertension and tachycardia that follow are typically sustained for several minutes
- **Why anaesthesia required?:**General anaesthesia is require to ensure amnesia and neuromuscular blockade to prevent injuries
- **Anaesthetic management:**
  - Pre-oxygenation–with 100% oxygen
  - Premedication–Injection glycopyrolate or Atropine
  - Amnesia–Barbiturate (Thiopenthol/methohexitol) or Propofol
  - Akinesia–Injection Succinylcholine
  - Bag and mask ventilation till spontaneous ventilation resume

Anesthetic Drugs

- Methohexitone or thiopental are the the most preferred agent for ECT because they have very short duration of action.
- Propofol may be used but higher doses reduce seizure duration.
- Benzodiazepines raise the seizure threshold and decrease duration.
- Ketamine increases seizure duration but is generally not used because it also increases the incidence of delayed awakening, nausea, and ataxia and is also associated with hallucinations during emergence.
- Use of etomidate also prolongs recovery.
- Short-acting opioids such as alfentanil are not given alone because they do not consistently produce amnesia. However, alfentanil (10–25 mg/kg) can be a useful adjunct when very small doses of methohexital (10–20 mg) are required in patients with a high seizure threshold.

Ans: (b) Thiopentone

Ref: *Morgan's Clinical Anesthesiology, fourth edition, chapter 14*

5. Which of the following is not a definite airway?

(a) LMA (b) Orotracheal
(c) Nasotracheal (d) Tracheostomy

Explanation:

- Establishing a **definitive airway**, **defined** as a tube placed in the trachea with cuff inflated, below the vocal cords.
- **Orotracheal, Nasotracheal and trachestomy** are definitive airways as per definition.

Laryngeal mask airway (LMA)

- The LMA is a minimally invasive device designed for airway management in the unconscious patient. An inflatable mask is fitted with a tube that exits the mouth to permit ventilation of the lungs.
- The mask fits against the peri-glottic tissues, occupying the hypo-pharyngeal space and forming a seal above the glottis instead of within the trachea.
- **Disadvantages of LMA**
  - Risk of aispiration
  - Risk of displacement
  - Can't keep for long time (more than 4-6 hours)
  - Can't use in non supine position
  - Can't give PPV (Positive Pressure Ventilation)

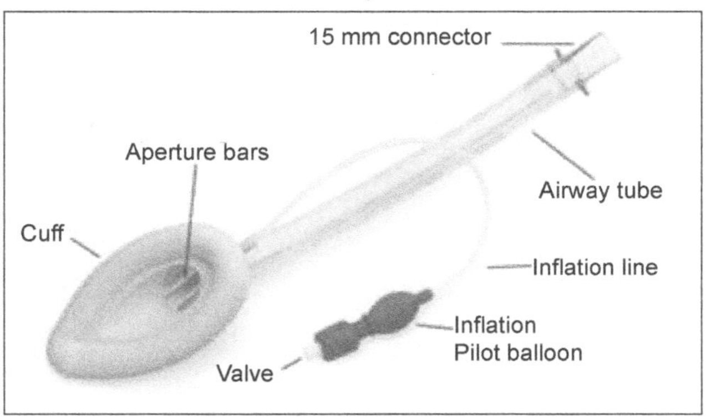

Figure: LMA

Ans: (a) LMA

Ref: *Benumof's Airways of Anaesthesiology, fourth edition*

6. Evidence based beneficial practice to prevent VAP are all *except*:

(a) Closed suction drainage of secretions

(b) Continuous/periodic subglottic suction of secretions

(c) Installing a filter for bacteria in expiratory tubes

(d) Head tilt of 10 to 30 degrees

Explanation:

Ventilator-associated pneumonia (VAP)

- Leading cause of death among hospital-acquired infections. Hospital mortality of ventilated patients who developed VAP is 46% compared to 32% for ventilated patients who do not develop VAP.
- **Five key components** for the VAP bundle:
  - Elevate the head of the bed to 45° when possible; otherwise, attempt to maintain the head of the bed at more than 30°
  - Evaluate readiness for extubation daily
  - Use endotracheal tubes with subglottic secretion drainage
  - Conduct oral care and decontamination with chlorhexidine
  - Initiate safe enteral nutrition within 24–48 hours of ICU admission

Pediatric VAP bundle:

- Elevate the head of the bed
- Properly position oral or nasal gastric tubes
- Perform oral care
- Eliminate the routine use of instil for suctioning

Additional evidence-based components of care:

- Hand hygiene
- Practices that promote patient mobility and autonomy
- Venous thromboembolism prophylaxis

Ans: (d) Head tilt of 10 to 30 degrees

Ref: *Poul Marino's the ICU book, third edition*

RADIOLOGY AND RADIOTHERAPY

1. Which is not true regarding technetium 99 MDP:

(a) More efficient in detecting osteolytic mets
(b) More efficient in detecting osteoblastic mets
(c) Can be used as bone scan to detect secondary's
(d) Can be used to diagnose osteomyelitis

Explanation:

Major drawbacks of ^{99m}technetium diphosphonates (^{99m}Tc-DP) bone scintigraphy (BS) influencing its diagnostic accuracy (i.e., low specificity, planar imaging, poor resolution images, impaired sensitivity in axial skeleton and lytic metastases)

Technetium 99m-methyl diphosphonate (99mTc MDP)

- Radiotracer used in nuclear medicine especially for bone scans. Any disease process which results in extracellular fluid expansion will lead to accumulation of this tracer.

Radionuclide profile

- Photon energy: 140 keV
- Physical half-life: 6 hours
- Critical organ: bladder

Uses

- To diagnose Osteomyelitis (three phase bone scan)
- Fractures, including stress and insufficiency fractures
- To diagnose **Malignancy**, e.g., **osteoid osteoma, bone metastases, soft tissue sarcomas**
- Painful scoliosis
- Post-traumatic haematomas, myositis ossificans, heterotopic ossification
- Tumoural calcinosis
- Metastatic pulmonary calcification
- Sickle cell disease

Ans: (a) More efficient in detecting osteolytic mets

Ref: *Radiopedia and Abdominal Trauma [HM DELANY], page 95*

2. Which is not used for thyroid scan?

(a) Iodine-131
(b) I-123
(c) I-125
(d) Tc 99

Explanation:

Iodine-125

- Half-life–60 days
- Commonly used in **brachytherapy** in the treatment of cancer especially in **prostate cancer**, enclosed in a implanted **titanium capsule**
- It is also widely used in **Radioimmunoassay** to show presence of **hormones** in **tiny quantities**

Iodine-123

- Half-life –13 hours
- Has **no beta activity only gamma activity**
- More suitable as nuclear imaging tracer to evaluate the anatomic and physiologic function of the **thyroid** (**thyroid scintigraphy/functional scan/radioactive iodine uptake/RAIU**)
- Abnormal results may be caused by disorders such as **Graves' disease** or **Hashimoto's thyroiditis.**
- **Tc99m pertechnetate** is also used for **functional imaging of thyroid** (used in India due to **nonavailability** of **I-123**)

Iodine-131

- Half-life–8 days
- Preferred for **Radioablation of thyroid gland** in **Graves' disease** and systemic **Radiotherapy**
- Widely used for localizing and treating **thyroid cancer** and **thyroid metastasis**
- Also used in **Imaging the thyroid**
- I-131 has **both beta and gamma decay**
- Destruction of thyroid tissue by Iodine-131 is due to emission of **Beta Rays**
- Iodine-131 is also used in **tissue targeting** radiopharmaceutical agents such as **MIBG**.
- The high energy **beta radiation** from I-131 causes it to be the **most carcinogenic** of the **iodine isotopes.**

Iodine-124

- Iodine-124 is a proton-rich isotope of iodine
- Half-life – 4.18 days.
- Its modes of decay are: 74.4% electron capture, 25.6% positron emission.
- Iodine-124 can be made by numerous nuclear reactions via a **cyclotron**.
- Iodine-124 as the **iodide salt** can be used to directly **image** the **thyroid** using **positron emission tomography (PET).**

	I-125	I-131	I-123	I-124
t1/2	60 days	8 days	13 hours	4.2 days
Emission	Gamma	Gamma	Gamma	Gamma
Energy	35 keV	364 keV	159 keV	606 keV
Use	RIA	Imaging/ablation	Imaging e.g., MIBG	PET imaging
Relatively long half-life and low energy photon emission are main criteria for preference towards I-125 for Radio Immuno Assay				

Also Note: Tc-99m pertechnetate thyroid scan is a functional nuclear medicine study used to assess the thyroid gland.

Ans: (c) I-125

Ref: *Basic Sciences of Nuclear Medicine, Magdy Khalil, page 34*

3. Which of the following differentiates a bone mets from a primary bone tumour?

(a) Epiphysis involvement
(b) Soap bubble appearance
(c) Periosteal reaction
(d) Vertebral pedicle involved

Explanation:

Skeletal Metastases

- Incite a mixture of **bone resorption and bone formation** and can thus take on one of three patterns, depending on the dominant process:
  - **Lytic metastases**
  - **Sclerotic metastases**
  - **Mixed lytic and sclerotic metastases**
- Additionally, metastases can have different morphological characteristics:
  - Diffuse
  - Focal
  - Expansile

Plain Radiograph

- As is the case with other bone lesions, skeletal metastases can be difficult to identify on plain films since extensive (30-50%) bone mineral loss is required before the density loss is radiographically-visible.
- In many other cases the lesion is visible due to **destruction of cortex**, or the presence of **visible sclerosis**.
- It is important to note that unlike primary bone tumours, in general metastases **incite no or only limited periosteal reaction**. The occasional exception to this general rule includes **prostate cancer**, some **gastrointestinal malignancies, retinoblastoma** and **neuroblastoma**.

Sensitivity and specificity of imaging modalities in bone metastasis

	Sensitivity	Specificity
18NaF PET/CT	100	97
MRI	95	90
SPECT	87	91
18 FDG PET	98	56
CT	74	56
Bone scintigraphy	78	48

Ans: (c) Periosteal reaction

Ref: *Radiopedia Internet Article Skeletal Metastasis*

4. Which of the following is not used in PET scan:

(a) 18 F (b) 11C
(c) Galium (d) Thalium

Explanation:

"Radionuclides used in PET scanning are typically isotopes with short half-lives such as **carbon-11** (~20 min), **nitrogen-13** (~10 min), **oxygen-15** (~2 min), **fluorine-18** (~110 min), **gallium-68** (~67 min), zirconium-89 (~78.41 hours), [37] or **rubidium-82** (~1.27 min)" *Ref: Radiology by Wolfgang*

*"**Fluorine-18 Fluorodeoxyglucose (FDG)** is the most common positron-labeled radiotracer in positron emission tomography (**PET**). In most tissues, including cancer, there is little phosphatase activity. The intracellular metabolite, FDG-6-phosphate cannot undergo further conversions and is therefore trapped inside the cell. FDG is useful in staging and metastasis of Renal cell cancer by PET" (Ref: Wolfgang)*

Positron Emission Tomography (PET)

- It is a nuclear medicine imaging technique that produces a three-dimensional image or picture of functional processes in the body.

- The system detects **pairs of gamma rays** emitted indirectly by a **positron-emitting radionuclide (tracer)**, which is introduced into the body on a biologically active molecule. Three-dimensional images of tracer concentration within the body are then constructed by computer analysis. In modern scanners, three dimensional imaging is often accomplished with the aid of a CT X-ray scan performed on the patient during the same session, in the same machine
- If the biologically active molecule chosen for PET is **FDG**, an analogue of **glucose**, the concentrations of tracer imaged then give tissue metabolic activity, in terms of regional glucose uptake.
- The electron-positron **decays** result in **two 511 keV gamma photons** being emitted at almost **180 degrees** to each other; hence, it is possible to localize their source along a **straight line of coincidence (**also called the **line of response**, or **LOR**).
- A **collimator** is a device that narrows a beam of particles or waves. Lead collimators are used in X-rays and linear accelerators

Ans: (d) Thalium

Ref: *Radiopedia and Radiology by Wolfgang Dahnert, 5th edition, page 1113*

5. Which of the following is not a commonly used window in CT Scan of Chest?

(a) Bone window
(b) Lung window
(c) Soft tissue window
(d) Blood vessel window

Explanation:

Typical window width and level values

Although this varies somewhat from institution to institution and vendor to vendor, window width and centres are generally fairly similar. The values below are written as width and level (W: x L: y) in Hounsfield units (HU).

- **Head and Neck**
  - Brain W: 80 L: 40
  - Subdural W: 130-300 L: 50-100
  - Stroke W: 8 L: 32 or W:40 L: 40
  - Temporal bones W: 2800 L: 600
  - Soft tissues: W: 350–400 L: 20–60
- **Chest**
  - Lungs W: 1500 L:-600
  - Mediastinum or soft tissue W: 350 L: 50
  - Bone windows
- **Abdomen**
  - Soft tissues W: 400 L: 50
  - Liver W: 150 L: 30
- **Spine**
  - Soft tissues W: 250 L: 50
  - Bone W: 1800 L: 400

Ans: (d) Blood vessel window

Ref: *Radiopedia*

6. Radio sensitizer for head and neck cancer is:

(a) Gefitinib (b) Cisplatin
(c) Oxaliplatin (d) Docetaxel

Explanation:

"**Cisplatin** is a potent radiosensitizer and the drug traditionally used for chemotherapy in head and neck cancers". **Ref:** *Indian J Otolaryngol Head Neck Surg 2011 Jul; 63(3): 229-236.*

RADIOSENSITIZERS

- Radiosensitizers are drugs that make cancer cells more susceptible to damage by radiation therapy. These drugs act by increasing the normally low level of oxygen in the cancer cells.
- Cancers with low levels of oxygen are less sensitive to radiation than cancers with normal or high levels.

Examples:

- Hyperbaric ***oxygen***
- Carbogen
- ***Nicotinamide***
- ***Metronidazole*** and its analogs (misonidzole, etanidazole, nimorazole)
- Hypoxic cell cytotoxic agents (***Mitomycin-C, Tirapazamine***)
- Membrane active agents (Procaine, lidocaine, chlorpromazine)
- **Radiosensitizing nucleosides** (5-Fluorouracil, Fluorodeoxyuridine, bromodeoxyuridine, Iododeoxyuridine, Hydroxyurea, Gemcitabine, Fludarabine)
- Texaphyrins (motexafin gadolinium)
- Supressors of sulfhydryl groups (N-Ethylmalemide, Diamide and Diethylmaleate)
- ***Hyperthermia***
- Novel radiosensitizers (***paclitaxel, docetaxel, irinotecan***)
- Cisplatin

Radiosensitizers used in head and neck cancers

- *Cisplatin*
- *Paclitaxel*
- *RSR 13*
- *Nimorazole*
- *Cetuximab*

Ans: (b) Cisplatin

Ref: *Indian J Otolaryngol Head Neck Surg 2011 Jul; 63(3): in recurrent cases, page 229-236*

7. Long term effect of craniospinal irradiation for medulloblastoma is:

(a) Secondary malignancy (b) Neuroendocrine abnormalities
(c) Neurocognitive effects (d) Hearing loss

Explanation:

SIDE EFFECTS OF CRANIOSPINAL IRRADIATION

(A) Early (during treatment and the first month after radiation)

- Anorexia, nausea and vomiting.
- Headache due to transiently increased intracranial pressure
- Mucositis (Posterior pharyngeal wall)
- Skin erythema within the treatment field and dry desquamation
- Alopecia
- Bone marrow suppression with low counts

(B) Early Delayed (up to 6 months after therapy)

Scattered astrocytic and microglial reactions, perivascular collections of mononuclear cells and demyelination seen.

- "***Somnolence syndrome***" and ***Lhermitte's sign***. Both are due to transient demyelination and start 6 - 8 weeks after the end of RT.
- The somnolence syndrome lasts for about 2 weeks (there are no consistent CT changes and diffuse slow wave activity on the EEG

(C) Late (90 days – Many years after therapy)

General

- Permanent alopecia in the scalp immediately adjacent to the high dose RT volume.
- Reduced bone marrow reserve
- Cataracts (lens usually gets less than 15% of the cranial dose).

Bone Damage

- After craniospinal RT patients will have a ***short sitting height*** (***reduced vertical growth of vertebral bodies***) and an increased risk of ***scoliosis***.
- Radiation to the whole brain can result in a disproportionately small cranium.
- ***Scoliosis and kyphosis*** are in part due to uneven growth of the paravertebral muscles after RT.
- Damage to bone is most likely due to direct ***damage to proliferating chondroblasts***, leading to ***arrest*** and ***destruction***.
- ***Intermitotic chondroblasts*** are the ***most sensitive*** cells in the skeleton, while osteoblasts are much less sensitive.
- There is also vascular injury leading to impaired bone and cartilage reabsorption.

Endocrine:

- ***Thyroid damage***
  - **Primary hypothyroidism** is **most common** (threshold at 2500-3000 cGy).
  - These patients must have their thyroid function tests checked at least on an annual basis in the long term.
  - There is a significantly increased risk of development of **benign thyroid nodules** and **papillary carcinoma of the thyroid** many years later.
- ***Pituitary/Hypothalamus damage***
  - Threshold at 24-29 Gy and ***growth hormone*** is impaired first.
  - Usually these children require ***growth hormone replacement therapy*** in the long term.
- ***Gonads***
  - ***Infertility*** is a risk after craniospinal radiotherapy (10 - 20% cases)

- **Male** gets less than **10%** of Total dose.
- Female gets **5 - 80%** of the total dose depending on the position of the ovaries.

CNS COMPLICATIONS:

Pituitary/Hypothalamus damage:

The pituitary gland is included in the treatment volume when the entire brain is irradiated.

The degree of pituitary hormonal deficiency is related to the RT dose.

- Growth hormone production is the most sensitive to treatment.
- Threshold at 24-29 Gy.
- Lower doses may produce isolated growth hormone deficiency and higher doses panhypopituitarism.
- Effect of RT on the pituitary axis is not immediate. Between 2 and 5 years after 30 Gy to the hypothalamic-pituitary axis 100% of children have biochemical growth hormone deficiency (this affects about 50% of children who receive 25 Gy cranial RT for ALL).

Hearing impairment

- Radiation to the posterior fossa significantly increases the risk of ***hearing deficits*** (***direct damage to the cochlea)***
- Related also to **cisplatin** chemotherapy (causes a sensorineural deafness) in combination with damage to the cochlea from RT.

Cerebrovascular Events

- Injury to endothelial lining and subsequent proliferation of small blood vessels
- There is a significant increased incidence of ***cerebrovascular events*** (strokes – both hemorrhagic and thrombotic) many years after RT.
- Cerebral vessel angiography shows arterial wall irregularities and focal stenotic lesions.
- ***Arteritis*** can affect medium and large vessels.
- ***Accelerated atherosclerosis***.
- ***Intracerebral cavernous malformations*** associated with cranial radiotherapy – within RT field associated with intracranial bleed.
- ***Radiation induced intracranial aneurysm*** can occur.

Necrotizing leukoencephalopathy

- Involves diffuse reactive astrocytosis, demyelination and multiple necrotic foci (no inflammation) that contain mineralized cellular debris.
- Patients often later develop ***cerebral atrophy*** and ***ventricular enlargement***.
- Clinical features are lethargy, seizures, spasticity, paresis and ataxia.

Radiation necrosis

- Occurs usually within 6 months to 5 years after RT (most 1 - 2 years later).
- Presents with signs of raised intracranial pressure and may have focal deficits.
- Radionecrosis appears as a mass lesion with surrounding edema on CT.

Seizures

Long term survivors after RT for brain tumors are at significantly increased risk for a seizure disorder. Most likely due to:

- Small vessel disease
- Cerebral necrosis
- Leukoencephalopathy

Intellectual Deficits:

The brain develops rapidly ***up to 3 years*** of age and very little after the age of 5 to 6.

The growth is due to an increase in the number of neurons as well as increase in size.

RT significantly affects brain development early in life.

- The most significant factor which adversely affects quality of life in long term survivors after RT for pediatric brain tumors is the long-term neurocognitive disability induced by their treatment.
- IQ is decreased, there are learning and behavior difficulties leading to impaired school performance and social difficulties.

Second Neoplasm: Patients are at risk of developing

- Astrocytoma
- Meningioma

Ans: (b) Neuroendocrine abnormalities

Ref: *Med Pediatr Oncol 997 May; 28(5):348-54 and http://www.pedsoncologyeducation.com*

8. In a child with coarctation of aorta, all the following are seen in plain chest radiograph *except*:

(a) Rib notching (b) Three sign

(c) 'E' Sign or 'Reverse Three sign' (d) Prominent ascending aorta

Explanation:

'E' Sign or 'Reverse Three sign' is feature of coarctation, but seen in barium swallow, not in plain chest radiograph.

Features of Coarctation of aorta

- Left ventricular configuration
- Prominent ascending aorta due to hypertension and bucuspid aortic valve
- **'Three sign':** The upper convexity is due to pre-stenotic dilatation and the lower convexity is due to post-stenotic dilatation. The mid portion represents the coarcted segment
- **'E' Sign or 'Reverse Three sign':** Seen in barium swallow due above aortic shadows
- **Rib notching:** Bilateral rib notching is seen between the third and eighth posterior ribs along its lower border usually after the age of 9 years.
- **Unilateral rib notching**: A feature of coarctation, if it involves the origin of the left subclavian artery also.

Differential diagnosis for rib-notching

- Chronic superior vena cava obstruction
- Chronic inferior vena cava obstruction
- Aortoarteritis in rare occasion
- Intercostal neurofibromatosis
- Intercostal arteriovenous malformations
- Post Blalock-Taussig shunt

Ans: (c) 'E' Sign or 'Reverse Three sign'

Ref: *Cardiac X-rays by V. Chockalingam and A. Chockalingam, 1st edition, Elsevier, 2008, page 99*

PSYCHIATRY

1. A 38-year-old male, known alcoholic, IV drug user presents with memory loss in last 6 months, motor incoordination, irritability, movement problems and confusion. Brain imaging shows cortical atrophy. What is the most probable diagnosis?

(a) Lewy body dementia
(b) HIV related dementia
(c) Heroin related dementia
(d) Alzheimer's dementia

Explanation:

Dementia

- Dementia is a syndrome characterized by:
  - **Memory loss**
  - **Executive dysfunction**.
- Ancillary symptoms like **confusion, mood symptoms** (irritability, depression, labile affect)
- **Motor symptoms*** (retardation or agitation or incoordination) are seen in **subcortical involvement**
- Risk factors assessment for all dementia cases is a must, since multiple factors may be present in a patient. The risk factors should be stratified based on the significance of association. Here, we have two such options, **HIV and Heroin**.
- **Alzheimer's** and **Lewy body dementia** affect elderly and "IV drug abuse" is the key in the question.
- **Heroin** is an opioid, which can produce confusion and incoordination in acute intoxication and irritability during withdrawal; but rare to cause cognitive decline.
- **HIV infection** is very common in IV drug abusers and HIV can cause all the symptoms mentioned in the question. Acute stage during seroconversion is characterized by delirium-like picture, called ad HIV encephalopathy. Chronic stage is characterized by dementia (both cortical–memory loss and subcortical – mood/motor Surgery).

Ans: (b) HIV related dementia

Ref: *Lishman's Organic Psychiatry, 3rd Edition*

2. Which of the following is a First rank symptom?

(a) Autism
(b) Made affect
(c) Ambivalence
(d) Loosening of associations

Explanation:

This question mixes Bleuler and Schneider. Let's be clear. Bleuler presumed following four aspects were fundamental in schizophrenia, which are famously called as 4As.

They are:

- **Loosening of associations**–the normal thought process which is well knit is disturbed resulting in formal thought disorder like word salad.
- **Ambivalence**–holding opposite ideas or emotions at the same time, resulting in conflict like unable to decide for or against
- **Autism** [not to be confused with autism–a childhood disorder of communication; though both share the baseline idea] – less or no interaction with environment (esp.social withdrawal), resulting in fantasy life – causing reality distortion

- **Affective disturbance**–reduced (blunting) or even complete absence (flattening) of emotions or incongruent expression of emotions like inappropriate laughter.

In contrast, **Schneider** proposed a set of symptoms which are highly suggestive of schizophrenia (provided organic pathology ruled out).

- **Audible Thoughts/Though Echo** [The patient experiences hallucinatory voices that echo or speak his thoughts aloud]
- **Voices Discussing** about the patient [Third person auditory hallucinations]
- **Voices giving commentary**
- **Somatic Passivity** [The patient believes that his body is controlled by external agency and he is just a doll]
- **Thought Withdrawal** [Patient experiences his thoughts being withdrawn or taken out of his mind by an outside force]
- **Thought Broadcasting** [Patient experiences his thoughts being disseminated to the world around him]
- **Thought Insertion** [Patient experiences thoughts being placed in his mind by an outside force]
- "**Made" affect** [Patient has the experience that his feelings are not his own, they have been imposed upon him]
- **Made" Impulses** [Patient experiences and generally acts upon a compelling impulse which he believes is not his own]
- "**Made" Acts** [Patient experiences his action and his will to be under the control of an outside force]
- **Delusional Perception** [Primary delusion, due to ascription of an idiosyncratic value to a normal perception]

*The **first rank symptoms** were incorporated in ICD as the diagnostic criteria for schizophrenia.*

Schneider also observed some symptoms called as "Second-rank Symptoms".

They are:

- Other disorders of perception.
- Sudden delusional ideas
- Perplexity.
- Depressive and Euphoric Moods.
- Feeling of emotional impoverishment.

Positive and Negative Symptoms of schizophrenia

Positive: Hallucinations, Delusions, Bizarre behaviors, Formal Thought Disorder

Negative: Affective flattening, Alogia, Avolition, Apathy

Ans: (b) Made affect

Ref: *Sims' Symptoms in the Mind, 6th Edition*

3. Defenses mechanism in "OCD" are all *except*:

(a) Undoing (b) Isolation of affect

(c) Displacement (d) Reaction formation

Explanation:

Defense mechanisms were described by **Anna O Freud** and others.

In psychoanalytic model, a defense mechanism is an "unconscious psychological mechanism" that reduces anxiety [which may be due to unacceptable or potentially harmful stimuli from id/ego/superego–as per structural theory of Freud].

A defense mechanism may be healthy or unhealthy [later case, explains the psychological symptoms]

Vaillant classified defense mechanisms into four categories viz.

- Pathological (psychotic denial, delusional projection)
- Neurotic (intellectualization, reaction formation, dissociation, displacement, repression)
- Immature (fantasy, projection, passive aggression, acting out)
- Mature (humour, sublimation, suppression, altruism, anticipation)

In OCD, there are three such defense mechanisms operate. They are {IUR}

- Isolation [unconsciously isolate and disown undesirable thoughts and feelings]
- Undoing [unconsciously cancel out an unacceptable desire or act by performing another act]
- Reaction formation [equalizing an unacceptable desire by taking on a lifestyle that expresses the opposite desire]

Displacement is a defense mechanism that shifts sexual or aggressive impulses to a more acceptable or less threatening target. For example, painting, poetry with themes of love; participating in racing or wrestling for aggression against some people.

Ans: (c) Displacement

Ref: *Concise Oxford Textbook of Psychiatry, Oxford University Press, 1994 page 86*

4. Which of the following memory and cerebral cortex are matched correctly?

(a) Association memory–Prefrontal cortex
(b) Procedural memory–Medial temporal lobe
(c) Reflex memory–Hippocampus
(d) Conditioning–Orbito frontal cortex

Explanation:

- Memory is the ability to store and retrieve information.
- It is both general [means, many areas of brain involved for a given type of memory] as well as specific [some regions play key role in certain types of memory e.g. emotional memory–amygdala]
- Basically, three types of memory and many subtypes exist. They are:
  - **Sensory**
  - **Short term**
  - **Long term**
- **Sensory memory** is stored in receptors itself very briefly and decay soon.
- Three subtypes:
  - **Iconic memory**–visual information.
  - Echoic memory–auditory information
  - Haptic memory–for touch stimuli.
- **Short term memory** is stored in synapses in the corresponding brain regions.
  - **Phonological loop**–temporal lobe
  - **Visual spatial sketchpad**–occipital and parietal lobes
- **Long-term memory** is divided into two major headings:
  - **Explicit/declarative memory**–facts, concepts, and experiences of conscious nature
  - **Implicit/Non declarative memory**–skills which may be learnt unconsciously.

- **Declarative memory** in turn divided into–**episodic and semantic**.
  - **Episodic memory**–storage of events, mostly personal [Flashbulb memories are critical autobiographical memories about a major event]. Medial temporal lobe, including hippocampus and prefrontal cortex involved here.
    - **Associative memory** is a subtype of episodic memory, defined as the ability to learn and remember the relationship between unrelated items [face-name pairs]. Apart from structures mentioned above, striatum also involved here.
  - **Semantic memory** is about general knowledge and same structures of episodic memory plus parahippocampal cortices [entorhinal cortex and perirhinal cortex].

Implicit memory: Mainly six subtypes

1. **Procedural memory** [Habit learning] which aids the performance of particular types of tasks without conscious awareness of these previous experiences. Areas: striatum, basal ganglia, cerebellum and motor cortex
2. **Emotional memory**–storage of feelings associated with events. Amygdala is key region
3. **Priming**–exposure to one stimulus influences a response to a subsequent stimulus, without conscious guidance or intention. E.g., ability to say a half-completed alphabet. *Perceptual learning is a type of priming-ability to differentiate different aspects of sensations through experience of stimuli, like appreciating tastes of different biriyanis! Occipito temporal cortex.*
4. **Conditioning**–reflex memory. Cortex, hippocampus and cerebellum.

Ans: (a) Association memory–Prefrontal cortex

Ref: *Kaplan and Sadock, Comprehensive Textbook of Psyhciatry*

5. Dose for severe depression in adults. Which dose is correct for adults?

(a) Amitryptilline 75 – 300 mg
(b) Fluoxetine 10 – 20 mg
(c) Amitryptilline 10 – 50 mg
(d) Sertraline 10 – 20 mg

Explanation:

Dosing of Antidepressants		
Class	**Drug**	**Range (mg/day)**
SSRIs	Citalopram (Celexa)	20-40
	Escitalopram (Lexapro)	10-20
	Fluoxetine (Prozac)	20-60
	Paroxetine (Paxil)	20-60
	Sertraline (Zoloft)	50-200
TCAs	Amitriptyline (Elavil)	100-300
	Clomipramine (Anafranil)	100-250
	Desipramine (Norpramin)	100-300
	Doxepin (Sinequan)	100-300
	Imipramine (Tofranil)	100-300
	Nortriptyline (Pamelor)	50-150

Ans: (a) Amitryptilline 75 – 300 mg

Ref: *Stahl's Essential Psychopharmacology, 4th Edition*

6. Which of the following is appropriate nonpharmacologic treatment for someone with narcolepsy?

(a) Exercise (b) Stimulus avoidance

(c) Progressive relaxation (d) Scheduled naps during the day

Explanation:

- **Forced naps** in daytime is the tested and recommended non-pharmacological treatment option for **narcolepsy**.
- **Stimulus avoidance** is not only difficult but also useless, since patient falls asleep in any situation {sleep is independent of stimulus}.
- Progressive relaxation is the method used in anxiety disorders, not as a primary in narcolepsy.
- Exercises may help in good night time sleep but that won't prevent daytime sleepiness completely.

More about narcolepsy:

- It is disorder characterized by irresistible bouts of daytime sleepiness
- **Tetrad of narcolepsy:**
  - ***Cataplexy***
  - ***Automatism***
  - ***Sleep paralysis***
  - ***Hallucinations [hypnopompic/hypnogogic]***
- Loss of **orexin [hypocretin]** producing neurons in lateral hypothalamus is the core pathology
- **Modafinil** is the drug of choice.

Ans: (d) Scheduled naps during the day

Ref: *Principles and Practice of Sleep Medicine, 6th Edition, Edited by: Meir Kryger and Psychiatry Made Simple, By P Arul Varman*